FOR ALL AMERICANS

★ ★ ★

The Dramatic Story behind the Stupak Amendment
and the Historic Passage of Obamacare

★ ★ ★

MICHIGAN'S 1ST DISTRICT CONGRESSMAN

BART STUPAK

ISBN 978-1-64003-090-9 (Paperback)
ISBN 978-1-64003-104-3 (Hard Cover)
ISBN 978-1-64003-091-6 (Digital)

Cover photo courtesy of the Associated Press and Harry Hamburg

Covenant Books, Inc.
11661 Hwy 707
Murrells Inlet, SC 29576
www.covenantbooks.com

CONTENTS

— ★ ★ ★ —

ACKNOWLEDGEMENTS

★ ★ ★

Linda Irving Smith, who edited my manuscript into this book.

Mardi Link, who served as my Story Editor and convinced me that I had a story to tell and that boring legislation is better understood with texture.

DEDICATION

I dedicate this book to the love of my life, Laurie, and to our sons, Ken and B.J. Laurie served as the book's corroborator, editor, story-teller, encourager, critic, and co-author.

Neither Laurie nor I could have completed this book without the love and understanding of our son, Ken. We are very proud of Ken and the dedicated, compassionate, and loving husband and father he has become. The words on the following pages do not begin to describe the joy, pleasure, and love that Ken, Cristina, and Nathaniel bring to our lives.

My life experiences growing up in a large Catholic family in Michigan's beautiful Upper Peninsula instilled in me a strong sense of fairness and a firm belief in social justice.

My election to Congress provided me the opportunity to act on these beliefs to improve the quality of life for my constituents and, with the passage of health care, for all Americans.

The loss of our son, B.J., reaffirmed my commitment to the sanctity of life and reinforced my belief that all life is precious and every day on Earth is a gift from God.

The Affordable Care Act could not have become the law of the land nor could this book have been written without the unceasing love, understanding, encouragement, and sacrifice of Laurie and Ken. I humbly dedicate this book to them.

PROLOGUE

★ ★ ★

The events portrayed in this book are my most accurate recollection of the behind-the-scenes negotiations and wrangling of ideas that took place over the fifteen-month period leading up to final passage of the Affordable Care Act. The discussions, comments and quotes attributed to individuals in this book are an accurate reflection of their words and deeds. The conversations, scenes, and characterizations of individuals are authenticated from my notes, interviews, documents, hearing transcripts, and the Congressional Record.

Immediately following my retirement from Congress, I was fortunate to be granted the opportunity to serve as a Fellow at the Institute of Politics, John F. Kennedy School of Government at Harvard University. During my Fellowship at the IOP, I taught a course on Congressional Investigations, which included lectures on food safety and the Food Safety Modernization Act, the BP Gulf oil spill, the Toyota sudden acceleration investigation, health insurance industry practices and rescissions, and passage of the Affordable Care Act.

While my book outline was drafted during my five months at Harvard, my serious writing did not begin until 2015, five years following my retirement from Congress. I credit my wife, Laurie, the case writers at Harvard University, and the BBC interviewers who encouraged me along the way.

This book is not an autobiography. This book explains, in depth, the strategic, political, and moral issues surrounding final passage of the Affordable Care Act. Although the Affordable Care Act is commonly referred to as Obamacare, it is much more than one person, one president, one Member of Congress or the political and ideological groups that supported or opposed its passage.

My story accurately reflects how, in this great country, the leadership and dedication of a few individuals resulted in meaningful legislation for all Americans. In this book, I demonstrate how dedicated and committed public servants rose above bitterly divided political parties, powerful lobbyists, and fervent members of frenzied and extremely polarized activist groups.

If, at times, my words seem harsh, rest assured that I do not hold any ill feelings toward any one person, group or individual. My comments only serve as an accurate reflection of my feelings and recollections during the time the events occurred.

My life experiences and upbringing in rural northern Michigan helped shape the positions on the issues that I felt most passionate about in Congress. My belief in health care for all Americans began with my motorcycle accident in 1972. The duty-incurred injury leading to my disability retirement from the Michigan State Police and the battle over balance billing during my term in the Michigan Legislature helped shape and sharpen my belief that health care is a right of all Americans and not a benefit reserved for the privileged few. My very personal belief in the sanctity of life comes from my strong Catholic faith and my strict upbringing in a large Catholic family. This book is a story of my own health care hell, which resulted in the passage of the Affordable Care Act *for all Americans.*

INTRODUCTION

★ ★ ★

I run. I probably should not be running, but I run along the shore of Green Bay, where I can hear the waves gently lapping over the sandy beachfront or violently crashing against the rocks protecting the roadway circling the peninsula comprising Henes Park in my hometown of Menominee, Michigan.

As I run listening to my iPod and alongside my dear wife, Laurie, my head is pounding with a combination of rhythms and thoughts. Both help to propel my aching body along the roadway just like the wind off the bay drives the waves. Today, the waves along Green Bay are angrily crashing over the rocks and sand. The wind is coming from the northeast and it reminds me of the political winds that swirled so viciously during the health care debate. Winds that were constantly changing direction and velocity, sometimes bringing warm, soft breezes and other times biting rain and bitter cold. Laurie doesn't like the wind; I view it as a challenge.

During the winter months, there are no waves crashing along the shore. Green Bay between Menominee, Michigan and Door County, Wisconsin freezes solid. Running outside during the winter months poses a more difficult challenge. Then, I must be vigilant. Snow and ice cover the road and I must choose my steps carefully. Black ice sometimes appears out of nowhere, causing dangerous slippery patches invisible to the eye. During the winter when the bay is frozen, what was sparkling blue water now more closely resembles the surface of the moon. The park is closed to traffic during the winter months and only the heartiest of souls are out walking or jogging. As I look out over the snowy, white expanse, all I can see is the occasional ice shanty, snowmobile, or ATV. Living in the Upper Peninsula during the winter can be brutal. We always joke that living here builds character and that we "Yoopers" possess a certain degree of toughness, strength, and endurance that is truly unique. Running in the winter also brings back memories of the healthcare debate: cold, isolated, precarious and unpredictable.

I no longer run for elected office, just for my health when my knees and my back say it is okay. Today, I find myself not on a run but on a plane back to DC. And there too, I will run. In DC, I run the crushed gravel trail along National Harbor and make my way along the shores of the Potomac. I continue up the corkscrew overpass and across the cement walkway over the Wilson Bridge. I continue to run across the bridge to Virginia. Here I hear the noise of the speeding traffic alongside me, the brisk winds blowing over the Potomac and the planes descending overhead on final approach to National Airport. Here, like at home, the winds are always a factor; and like at home, occasionally I see a bald eagle soaring over the treetops. I continue along the usually peaceful Mount Vernon trail up along the Tidal Basin where the wind blows the water up and over the sides of the cement steps and barriers. The political winds blow harder here in our nation's capital than anywhere else on earth.

Many years ago, Laurie and I attended one of our first summer congressional picnics, which were held on the south lawn of the White House. As I was a Member of Congress, we were the guests of President William Jefferson Clinton and Hillary Rodham Clinton. It was a truly gorgeous evening and we were awed by the beauty and splendor of being at the White House, surrounded by Members of Congress and their guests. Tables were set up on the lawn and guests mingled in line at the bar and along the massive buffet table as we listened to the band and enjoyed a wonderful evening of food, drink, entertainment and camaraderie.

The political atmosphere was much more pleasant back then. Members of both parties spoke civilly to each other and deep friendships developed across party lines. Laurie and I had to pinch ourselves to make sure we were really there and it wasn't just a dream. For two Yoopers from Upper Michigan from modest means, it was truly a dream. We didn't want the evening to end. As darkness began to fall, the crowd began to disburse and workers rolled up the sides of the tent. Laurie and I sat on our lawn chairs and looked out over the perfectly manicured green grass toward the Washington Monument. A good friend of mine, Congressman Earl Pomeroy from North Dakota, sat alongside me. Earl and I had come in together in the 1992 election. We were two newly elected congressmen from conservative, rural swing districts, and we shared many of the same views. We commented on the fact that we had been provided a unique opportunity to influence the future of our great nation and assist the people of our districts back home. Neither one of us took anything for granted. We pledged to work hard, do the best we could, and enjoy our time in Congress. We were grateful to be given the opportunity.

As the full moon rose over the Washington Monument and the Jefferson Memorial, I asked Laurie, "Where would you rather watch the moon rising, over the Washington Monument or over the pine trees of Northern Michigan?" Without hesitation, Laurie chose the pine trees of Northern Michigan. Right then and there I knew I would never be a "Lifer" in Congress. I never dreamed that I would serve for eighteen years, longer than any other congressman from Michigan's First Congressional District. But I felt in my bones that when it came time to leave Congress, it would be a very long walk home.

Six years have passed since the enactment of the Affordable Care Act, (ACA). I no longer have the desire to run for elected office, but I still occasionally attend political events. Now, the jeers have been replaced with cheers, especially among the party faithful. However, I am still amazed at the shortsightedness of some of the members of the Democratic Party, the arrogance of the US Conference of Catholic Bishops, and the hypocrisy of many of the activists in both the Right-to-Life and Pro-Choice movements.

With the passage of the Stupak Amendment in the US House of Representatives on November 7, 2009, Joe Cao (R-LA) had cast the only bipartisan vote on the House version of the national health care plan. Following passage of my amendment and with the health-care legislation sent on to the Senate for consideration, I had hoped that my health care hell would be behind me. Unfortunately, it was just the beginning. The second round of events would prove to be even more intense and life threatening. I no longer found solace in my runs, for with each step I could sense the coming of a nor'easter and I was afraid that the violent winds would engulf me, my family, and the entire nation. I didn't quite realize at the time that I would be right in the eye of the storm.

I was elected to the US House of Representatives in 1992 on my promise to raise the minimum wage, get our nation's fiscal house in order, and provide health care for all Americans. In 1996, Democrats succeeded in raising the minimum wage. Under President Clinton's leadership, we got our fiscal house in order. National health care was finally realized under President Obama. I felt like I had accomplished my mission; I had fulfilled my promises to my constituents. The race was won and I was exhausted. It was time to go home to the bay and the pine trees of Northern Michigan.

In the fall of 2012, I was headlining a campaign event for Democratic candidates for the Michigan Legislature on the western end of Michigan's Upper Peninsula. As I traveled throughout the weekend, campaigning and catching up with many old friends and supporters, I was constantly urged to run again for everything from president, state Senate, for my old congressional seat, and even for Governor of Wisconsin against the incumbent Republican Governor Scott Walker.

Four counties in Michigan's Upper Peninsula border Wisconsin. The counties of Gogebic, Iron, Dickinson and Menominee are in the central time zone and are influenced by Wisconsin's economy, geography, politics, media market, the Green Bay Packers and the Wisconsin Badgers. Michigan's First Congressional District is unique in the respect that the area is so large, it contains two time zones!

The following pages comprise my story of how I ran the race, kept my word, stayed focused, and never gave up. This is my story of the strategy, backroom discussions, and political arm-twisting that occurred behind the scenes preceding the final passage of the Affordable Care Act, better known as "Obamacare." This is also the story of how I was able to reconcile my inner conflict between my belief in national health care and my belief in the Right to Life. I truly believe that many years from now, the violent protests, threats, accusations, and intimidation that occurred during passage of the ACA will be looked at as one of the most serious and politically polarizing issues in our nation's history, rivaling only the passage of Social Security, Medicare and the Vietnam War. My family and I suffered considerably through health care hell but we derive deep satisfaction that now all Americans have access to affordable, quality health care.

CHAPTER 1

★ ★ ★

Beginnings (1952-1970)

Growing up in the Upper Peninsula of Michigan, I was like any other kid- active, curious, loved the outdoors, the Great Lakes and baseball. "Up North" in the Upper Peninsula of Michigan, you loved God, Country, and the Green Bay Packers and not necessarily in that order.

Gladstone Public Schools and the City of Gladstone sponsored the Recreation Center or "rec center," which was my social center, but when the church bell rang at six o'clock I knew I had better run home for supper or I would not eat. So, when All Saints Catholic Church rang that bell every night, I left the baseball field, the rec center, or the bay and headed home. The Stupak family supper always started with the Roman Catholic *Prayer before Meal*, which my family still says today. Then it was eat fast because there were ten kids at the table, plus my parents, and when a dish was passed, it never came back to you for "seconds."

Yes, there were twelve people at the table and often a friend was over for dinner so you never knew who was going to be at our house or how much there would be to eat. The Stupak home on Minneapolis Avenue in Gladstone, Michigan was truly like Grand Central Station with friends, cousins, and whoever else happened to be invited that day all gathered around the dinner table.

Our dining room table was rather unique in the respect that it also served as the pool table. My mother placed a 4x8 piece of plywood on the top of the pool table and covered it with a tablecloth at mealtime. The kids would all grab whatever chair happened to be closest and that pool table was immediately transformed into a dining table for twelve. My father loved to initiate a discussion on politics or the day's events, and the conversations always outlasted the meal. At the end of the discussion, my father would leave us with a social justice lesson intertwined with the Catholic *Prayer after Dinner*. As we grew older, we still had to ask for permission to be excused from the table and though the *Prayer after Dinner* dropped from our dinner ritual, the politics and the lessons in social justice remained.

The 1970 Michigan Gubernatorial election was a mixture of religion and politics. In addition to the Governor's race, there was a statewide ballot initiative to allow taxpayer funds to be used to support parochial schools. Parochial aid became a passionate election year issue. Our Democratic candidate for governor switched his position on parochial aid as the election cycle drew to a close; the voters rejected both parochial aid and our Democratic nominee.

The defeat of parochial aid meant the immediate closing of Escanaba Holy Name Catholic School. The announcement of the closing of Holy Name was bitter fruit for the large Catholic population in our Escanaba-Gladstone area. It was my first lesson in politics and in dealing with the Catholic bishops. Due to the defeat of parochial aid, the Bishop of the Marquette Diocese abruptly decreed that all Catholic high schools in the Upper Peninsula would close at the end of the current school year. This pronouncement came with little or no input from the Body of Christ- us daily parishioners- who supported and sacrificed for our Catholic schools. I should have learned from this lesson. The Bishop chose to shut down all the Catholic schools because he did not get his way with parochial aid. My father warned us that the Bishops were not truly concerned about the lives and souls of their parishioners, only the largesse of their contributions to the Church and the power and control they asserted over their congregations. I guess my father was onto something. I didn't quite understand it at the tender age of eighteen, but I certainly do now after my "health care hell."

My father's insight to the bishops' motivation was based on the fact that he almost became a priest himself. My father was the oldest child in his family and therefore, as they were Eastern European Catholics (Slovaks), it meant he was to be given to God. He was to be the priest. As an eighth grader, my father dutifully left for the seminary in St. Paul, Minnesota. While in the seminary, his mother died unexpectedly. My father was extremely close to his mother and I don't believe that he truly ever recovered from her death. Three and a half years later, his father died. My father would say that my grandfather died of a broken heart after the death of his wife.

My father remained in the seminary and was within a few months of his ordination when he began to question whether the priesthood was truly his calling. During the last few months in the seminary, he struggled with his decision to become a priest. While home on break with a friend, he met my mother, after which his internal struggle to remain in the seminary intensified. Although he was uncertain of his commitment to the priesthood, the seminary allowed him to participate in classes as he struggled and prayed about his decision to continue his studies and receive the sacrament of Holy Orders.

I learned of my father's conflicted feelings about remaining in the seminary from Father Arnold Thompson of Mary Queen of Peace Catholic Church in Kingsford, Michigan, who had been his close friend and a fellow seminarian. Father Thompson confided in me about my father's struggle in the seminary when I knocked on his rectory door while canvasing for re-election to Congress in 1994, seven years after my father's death. For reasons that I will never know, my father very rarely spoke about his time in the seminary.

In February of 2015, Laurie and I spent a long weekend with my eldest brother, Frank A. Stupak, Jr. and his wife, Penny at their rental home in Florida. During our visit, I asked Frank if my father had ever talked with him about his time in the seminary. My had father confided in Frank that one of the saddest days in his life was the day he gave final notice to his superiors that he would not continue with his studies to become a priest. Even more painful for him was returning the leather-bound "priest prayer book" given to him by the Bishop. Returning his priest prayer book meant walking away from his ten-year journey to the priesthood. Returning his priest prayer book meant letting down his deceased parents, who had expected their eldest son to become a man of the cloth. Returning his priest prayer book meant saying goodbye to the seminarian family he had come to know and love over the past decade. Returning his priest prayer book symbolized the end of his faithful journey. The sadness of that day stayed with my father until he died of a heart attack at the young age of seventy-three in Florida, where he had lived in retirement with my mother.

In my father's eulogy, my brother Frank acknowledged my father's deep faith when he commented, "instead of saving souls, he decided to create them." So, with my mother and all ten children we laid my father to rest in March of 1987, one year prior to my first election as Michigan State Representative. It was my father's teachings and examples that instilled in me my strong Catholic faith, my passion for politics, my compassion for those in need, and my belief in social justice. I can still hear my father's words as he shook his finger at me from the opposite end of the dining room table, "Bart, be kind to the bum on the street, for tomorrow, he may be your boss." No truer words could have been spoken to an aspiring politician. My father's words have remained with me through all these years.

CHAPTER 2

★ ★ ★

Growing Up Stupak (1966-1972)

Unlike my wife Laurie, my formal Catholic school education ended as soon as it began. Catholic education became too great of a financial burden for my mother and father, with six children attending at any one time.

My father taught school at Nahma High School, twenty-six miles east of Gladstone. Nahma High School was made up of a large Native American population and was considered a poor school district. After many years in the classroom and due to the consolidation of several smaller school districts, my father advanced in his career as an educator and became superintendent of the Big Bay de Noc High School District.

To supplement his income and give back to his community, my father was active in local politics as a City commissioner, mayor of Gladstone, member of the Delta County Board of Commissioners and eventually served as chairman of the County Board.

Whether it was his attempt to unionize the veneer plant in Gladstone, providing city services of water and sewer to the outskirts of town, or saving Marble Arms and the jobs created there, my father was a populist with a social conscience, which he instilled in me.

I enjoyed being with my father as he attended meetings or entertained commissioners at our home and discussed the issues of the day over a brandy Manhattan or two. I distinctly remember candidates coming to our home seeking my father's endorsement in the Democratic primary and/or general elections.

Every two years, my father wrote a letter to his constituents outlining his position on issues and his vision for community progress. My brothers and I would load up our paper route bags and deliver his message to the voters. My father's letter to his constituents taught me an important lesson, which I followed throughout my political career: I learned to develop and organize my thoughts on issues and explain my positions in a clear and concise manner, communicate directly with the voters, and keep my word. Like my father, my word is my bond.

The BJ Fund, named after our deceased son, Bart, Jr., grants a $2,500 annual scholarship in honor of my father, Frank A. Stupak, Sr. This Memorial Scholarship is awarded to a Big Bay de Noc high school senior who excels in leadership and community service throughout his/her high school career.

I participated in many Democratic Party events and was an active and enthusiastic volunteer. Whether it was acting as a human billboard or peddling literature at the early age of six, if it involved politics, I was there helping candidates, meeting the voters, and learning the value of grassroots organizing.

I specifically remember walking home from All Saints Catholic School and praying for the election of John F. Kennedy. It was not until the day after the 1960 presidential election that Kennedy was declared the victor. Three years later, I was home for lunch from Gladstone Public School when President Kennedy was shot in Dallas. Later that afternoon on November 22, 1963, I delivered the sad news to the good folks along my paper route.

It certainly was a sad day for this young paperboy who followed the daily activities in the lives of our energetic, charismatic, charming young president and his growing family. It seemed like we had just grieved over the loss of his infant son and now the President himself had been assassinated. I walked a little slower with my head hung low as I delivered the paper with tears in my eyes. Along my route, my customers quietly accepted the paper and did not want to believe the headline, that President Kennedy was dead. What would come next? We simply had to turn to our faith and prayers for our country as we turned the page of the *Escanaba Daily Press* in disbelief about our stricken leader, our devastated country and our intense grief.

The only time I remember seeing my father cry was as he watched the television coverage of the assassination of President Kennedy. I could not watch. I went outside and played in the newly fallen snow. At least something was new, fresh and pure even though our world was not.

I was attending Mass when Jack Ruby shot and killed Lee Harvey Oswald. I was disappointed that I missed the coverage of the shooting on television. The next day, Monday, I delivered the headline that Oswald was dead, and that Ruby admitted to killing him. I thought Ruby was acting like he should receive a medal because he had done the country a favor by killing Oswald. Instead, Ruby gave the conspiracy theorists more ammunition that the CIA, the military, or "the mob" was behind the President's assassination. We were denied the opportunity to understand why Oswald killed Kennedy. Was Oswald a lone wolf as the Warren Commission claimed, or was there more to the death of our young president?

I tend to believe that Oswald acted alone because he wanted to be somebody and achieve his fifteen minutes of fame. Unfortunately, Oswald was nobody but a tragic figure who denied all Americans the leadership of our youngest and only Catholic president. While our prayers may have helped elect him, they could not save John F. Kennedy.

Three years later, during the 1966 campaign and as a member of the Democratic Party youth honor guard, I was granted the opportunity of welcoming Senator Robert F. Kennedy to Escanaba. As I listened to his speech, I learned a very important lesson about knowing your audience when Senator Kennedy remarked in reference to the high school mascot, "Now I know why they call you the Eskymos. It is really cold up here!" Senator Kennedy really knew how to relate to his audience and everyone cheered and applauded.

I followed Senator Kennedy's example when speaking to groups throughout my vast district. I learned about the school teams and mascots of every small town I campaigned in and had the honor of representing, and worked them into my remarks when it was appropriate. It is an effective, easy way to connect with the local population.

Twenty-eight years later, during my first re-election bid as congressman, I brought Congressman Joe Kennedy to Escanaba. While we were on different social levels, Joe and I talked about how we had so much in common. We both came from large, Catholic families. We learned our politics from our fathers, but neither of our fathers lived long enough to see either of us take an oath of office. Joe's trip to the Upper Peninsula was bittersweet for both of us and I still maintain strong ties with the Kennedy family.

It is difficult to summarize all that I learned as I tagged along with my father on the campaign trail or watched or listened to the election results broadcast on TV and radio. I would stay up as late as I could on election night until I couldn't keep my eyes open any longer and fell asleep on the couch.

In 1966, I worked very hard to help re-elect our Democratic state and federal legislators. But the 1966 election was brutal for the Democrats. The only bright spot was that my father won re-election to the County Board of Commissioners.

Einar Erlandsen, the State House Appropriations Chairman, was defeated by a young schoolteacher, Republican Charles Varnum. Our Democratic Congressman Ray Clevenger lost to Republican Phil Ruppe. I learned several very important political lessons that year: national issues truly can impact state and local politics and elections, and never give your constituents the impression that you take them for granted. A well-executed Get-Out-The-Vote (GOTV) is critical to any successful election. Clevenger served one term and was our last Democratic congressman until my election in 1992, when I defeated Phil Ruppe.

Following the 1968 assassinations of Robert F. Kennedy and Martin Luther King, Jr., and with the loss of so many brave young men and women during the Vietnam War, the United States slid into a tumultuous period of unrest. Here at home the civil rights movement was becoming more and more violent. The anti-war protests were becoming more and more frequent and the tragic shooting of unarmed Vietnam War protesters at Kent State University further divided our country. This was my generation. Innocent, safe, and secure lives were unraveling all around me. I went off to college in the fall of 1970 to become a police officer and to play sports. I had not given up on our country; I wanted to hold it together and stop the violence on our streets.

I enrolled in Northwestern Michigan College and earned my Associate's Degree in law enforcement. At Northwestern, I was elected college council president and was a member of the basketball and baseball teams. Politics, sports, and college- it was a great time for me.

I applied for and was accepted to Michigan State University in the fall of 1972. I returned home to find meaningful work and earn enough money to pay for my tuition at MSU. I applied for a patrolman position with the Escanaba Police Department. I scored very high on the exam and was hired as the youngest police officer in Escanaba City Police history. At age twenty, I was walking the beat in Escanaba, and anxiously waiting my twenty-first birthday so that I could apply for a Trooper position in the Michigan State Police. I held the utmost respect for the Michigan State Police and becoming a Trooper was my dream job.

I was enjoying my job as a police officer for the City of Escanaba and I was gaining valuable law enforcement experience. So, in the fall of 1972, instead of continuing my college education at MSU, I spent the weekends campaigning for my father's re-election to the County Board of Commissioners and the rest of the Democratic ticket.

CHAPTER 3

★ ★ ★

Vietnam Sorrow (1972)

One week before the 1972 General Election, Charlie Stewart, my childhood friend, was tragically killed when his helicopter was shot down over Vietnam. The Democratic nominee for president, George McGovern, seized on Charlie's death as a rallying cry against President Nixon's failed promise that the Vietnam War would be over by Election Day. As I listened on my transistor radio, Senator McGovern urged citizens to vote against the war by voting against Nixon. I listened to Senator McGovern invoking my childhood friend's senseless death in Vietnam, and campaigned with a heavy heart. Unfortunately, President Nixon was re-elected by a wide margin.

Charlie was seventeen months younger than I and we grew up together five houses apart on Minneapolis Avenue. I vividly remember the first time I saw Charlie. He was only ten years old and was desperately attempting to push the family rowboat through the weeds out into the open waters of Little Bay de Noc. My best friend, Steve DeRoeck, and I watched nervously as Charlie pushed as hard as he could while his father verbally and physically abused him. Charlie's father cursed and berated his eldest son as he tried to push the rowboat through the thick weeds. That day, like every other day that we were with Charlie, no matter how hard he tried, he could never please his father. If I was over at Charlie's and his father was home, I could not wait to leave. I constantly told Charlie that he was a better man than his father. But Charlie loved his father, his family and his country.

Charlie had been elected senior class president at Gladstone High School. He had agreed to accept the role of class president because no one else wanted the job and the responsibility of governing in this Vietnam era. Charlie did a great job as class president and after graduation, like his father, Charlie enlisted in the Army. Charlie was just nineteen when he died alongside twenty-one other US servicemen when their Chinook helicopter was shot down by a heat-seeking missile while on a courier run.

I stopped by the Anderson Funeral Home in Gladstone to pay my respects to the family and say good-bye to Charlie. In my eyes, he had died a hero. However, I was alone in the funeral home with the casket and a picture of Charlie in his uniform. Charlie's family was not there to receive visitors, and during the time I was there, no one else came to pay their respects. I said my prayers and looked at the guest register and found that very few people, and none of our classmates, had signed his book of condolences. I was crushed that no one had come to say good-bye and thank you to Charlie. I questioned not only the continuation of the war but also the sacrifices made by Charlie and his brothers and sisters in the military. I wanted to believe that his family had been there to receive visitors. Maybe I just missed them.

Sadly, Charlie's parents had sent him a care package just before he was killed. The care package still haunts me to this day. It was never received and was returned to Charlie's parents with a label on it simply stating "KIA 10/31/72."

Charlie's care package is one of only a very few perishable items left at the hallowed Vietnam Wall Memorial and is now part of the Vietnam Veterans Memorial Collection kept by the National Park Service. The Park Service believes that Charlie's brother left the care package at the Vietnam Wall in 1993 with a note stating, *"Mom and Dad want you to have these cookies and Kool Aid... They send all their love."*

As congressman, I would see Charlie's father, Charles L. Stewart, Sr. quite often during my many visits to Gladstone. He did not like the fact that I invoked Charlie's name and memory in many of my veteran's speeches. It was just too painful for him. However, it was healing for me and I will never forget my childhood friend.

Memories of Charlie and the Vietnam War remained with me throughout my congressional career. I was always very serious and selective concerning my responsibility of voting to authorize war. I supported the military actions in Bosnia, Kosovo and Afghanistan. I strenuously objected to the war in Iraq as an illegal, immoral, and unethical war. As congressman, I considered my votes on whether to declare war the most difficult of my career.

I learned a great deal during my days growing up in Gladstone, Michigan. As a middle child, I learned the art of compromise. As a paperboy, I learned to be responsible, polite and considerate. As an Eagle Scout, I learned to be dedicated, trustworthy and loyal. As a member of our family, I developed a strong work ethic, a sense of compassion, and a commitment to public service. All the lessons learned from my parents, siblings, friends and neighbors enabled me to become the longest-serving northern Michigan congressman in modern times, run up the largest popular vote percentage, and become the only Democratic congressman to serve consecutive terms.

As I reflect on my early life growing up in Gladstone, it is fair to say that some of it was magic and some of it was tragic. But it was a good life.

CHAPTER 4

★ ★ ★

Michigan State Police (1972-1984)

When I turned twenty-one, I applied for a position with the Michigan State Police and scored high on their tests. However, the State was not hiring or training any recruits to become Michigan State Police troopers at that time and I continued with my patrolman duties at the Escanaba Police Department. I was certain my dream of ever entering the state police recruit school was shattered when I flipped my motorcycle in June of 1973 and severely injured my shoulder.

While the specialists did their best to put my shoulder back together, it was doubtful if I would ever be able to completely rotate my shoulder enough to withstand the rigorous physical requirements of the Michigan State Police. I underwent reconstructive surgery on July 5th in Marquette and immediately began physical therapy and rehab to strengthen my shoulder and regain my range of motion.

I entered the Michigan State Police recruit school on November 5, 1973. Despite the weakness in my right shoulder, I learned to do pushups with one arm and hid the bleeding from my shoulder. Armed with my prior police experience at Escanaba and an unshakable determination, I graduated from the Michigan State Police training academy in February 1974 and was assigned to the Caro Post.

Caro, Michigan is located 356 miles from Escanaba and a long way from the people and culture of us Yoopers. Agriculture is the dominant industry of Tuscola County and the topography is extremely flat. The residents drove too fast and drank too much. Motorcycle gangs from Flint and Saginaw terrorized the local communities and state campgrounds along the shores of Lake Huron. The Michigan State Police had just opened a new State Police Post in Caro to combat the unlawful conduct of the motorcycle gangs and to reduce the carnage on the highways of Tuscola County.

The Michigan State Police Post in Caro, Michigan opened in February 1974 and I was the post "cub." In other words, I was the rookie. Every dirty job that no one else wanted to do fell to the cub. The cub was expected to do the worst jobs without pay and without complaint. It was bad enough being the rookie but I was also 356 miles from my family and my friends. I found that dealing with death, motorcycle gangs, and a very authoritative, semi-military organization was very difficult. However, I was very stubborn and I wasn't about to give up. Before I departed for Caro, I proposed to my girlfriend of less than eight months, Laurie Olsen, and she accepted. I was miserable without her; we were to be married in September but moved the date to June to enjoy the summer together. While we enjoyed the summer, Laurie and I missed our families and longed to be back home in the Upper Peninsula.

To keep herself occupied as I worked full time and performed my hours of "volunteer" overtime, Laurie enrolled in college. Laurie then talked me into taking a few classes toward my bachelor's degree. Unfortunately, Laurie and I saw each other less and less as my work shifts swung every seven days. My fellow troopers at the Caro Post were more than happy to trade me their midnight shifts in exchange for my afternoon 3-11 p.m. shift. To attend evening classes I had to work either the day shift, which ended by 4:00 p.m., or the midnight shift. Each weekday, I left Caro to drive the forty-five miles to Saginaw Valley State University for the start of my night classes. Laurie was working 8:00–5:00 p.m. and then she left for Delta College, forty miles from Caro. We never saw each other; we had been married for less than three months and our schedules of work and college drove us in different directions. By January, Laurie put the brakes on her studies but encouraged me to continue mine. I still joke with her that she talked me into going back to college and she quit after one semester.

With Laurie's help and support, within two years I had earned my bachelor's degree in Criminal Justice along with a minor in Political Science and graduated Magna Cum Laude. After requesting a transfer from Caro to the Michigan State Police Capitol Post in Lansing, I enrolled in the Thomas M. Cooley Law School and earned my law degree. Once again, I worked special assignments, led a team of six troopers and conducted special investigations, which allowed me to work the day shift and attend law school at night. My law school graduation present was the birth of our son, Kenneth Lee Francis, named after our fathers.

After graduation from law school, I sat for and passed the Michigan Bar. In 1981 and for several years, I was the only attorney in the Michigan State Police. I conducted special, sensitive investigations of legislators and state employees at the State Capitol. One of my investigations involved Republican State Representative Charles Varnum (R-Manistique) in one of his less-than-flattering acts. Varnum was accused of urinating on the desks of the leadership of the Department of Social Services. At the time, Varnum only had a few weeks left in office. He had already been defeated in the November election by Democrat Pat Gagliardi. Politics had changed Charles Varnum and not for the better; he was bitter in defeat and did not resemble the young schoolteacher who sixteen years earlier had defeated State House Appropriation's Chairman Einar Erlandsen.

Another more interesting and contentious investigation I led was of Democratic State Representative Daisy Elliott (D-Detroit), Chair of the Michigan House Labor Committee. Daisy Elliott had a stolen Cadillac in her possession. After a grueling investigation and jury trial, Elliot was convicted of receiving and stealing stolen property valued over one hundred dollars, a felony in Michigan.

The Charles Varnum and Daisy Elliot cases taught me that in politics, as in life, you never burn your bridges, and you never believe that you are above the law.

Although I was an attorney, my plan was to remain in the Michigan State Police until I secured a vested retirement after ten years of service. While on special assignment with the Elliott case, I was injured in the line of duty while in pursuit of a bicycle thief. After several operations on my left knee, I was medically retired from the Michigan State Police. I truly enjoyed police work and hated to leave my profession and dream job, but State Police policy was that an injured trooper had to be able to return to work one hundred percent physically fit and pass all fitness tests. I could not drag a human-sized dummy more than a few yards before my knee would collapse. Therefore, I was unfit for duty and medically retired from the Michigan State Police.

Looking back, I never worried about how my surgeries and therapies were paid for. Having blown out my knee while on duty, my medical expenses were paid for by my excellent health insurance coverage through the Michigan State Police health and pension plan. Any unpaid medical bills were picked up by the State of Michigan because my injury was covered under worker compensation laws. More than one insurance carrier was picking up my medical bills and workers compensation provided me with a steady paycheck for the seventeen months that I was off active duty as a result of my knee surgeries.

I was fortunate. Not only did my employer provide excellent family health insurance, my paycheck was also protected. Our youngest son, Bart Jr., (B.J.) was born just before my injury and he was constantly seeing a pediatrician. B.J. was eventually labeled chronically ill due to his many childhood illnesses. If Laurie was not at the hospital with me, she was there with B.J. We were grateful for good health insurance and never thought about how we were going to pay for all the medical bills generated by B.J. and me.

Today, employer-provided health insurance usually covers only the employee and not the employee's family. Worker compensation laws have also changed. It is difficult for injured workers to collect a full paycheck based on worker compensation and disability insurance. The cost to carry full family health insurance and disability insurance is now very expensive and every injury seems to be contested by the employer's insurance carrier.

I often think about many of my colleagues in the State Police who were injured or killed in the line of duty and how they and their families must have struggled to make ends meet or begin a new career. I was fortunate that I had my law degree; I was an attorney and a bright future still lay ahead of me at the age of thirty-two.

Laurie talked quite often about moving back to the U.P. to raise our children, Ken and Bart, Jr. (B.J.), and to be closer to our families. We promised each other that if we were ever given the opportunity, we would return to the Escanaba area. My retirement from the State Police had given us that opportunity exactly ten years from the day that I was the cub assigned to the Caro Post. Laurie and I sold our home in DeWitt, packed up our belongings, and with our two young sons moved 425 miles back up north to be closer to our families, practice law with my brother, and explore my political opportunities.

CHAPTER 5

★ ★ ★

Early Politics (1986–1990)

After going door to door campaigning for the 1986 Democratic state representative candidate and failing to defeat the Republican incumbent, I decided to run for the position myself in 1988. I believed the incumbent state representative was incompetent and had a conflict of interest on some of the votes he had taken. The campaign was bruising, but we gave it our all. We knocked on doors, walked in parades, attended meetings and candidate forums, distributed campaign literature, stuffed envelopes, and participated in all the grass roots campaigning activities humanly possible.

I still remember driving up to thank my supporters at Escanaba campaign headquarters on election night 1988. Laurie asked how I felt about my chances now that polls had closed. I explained that I was comfortable with whatever way the election went as I had done all that I could. I was proud of her and our family and I had no regrets. The voters were kind to me; I won the election by a 52-48 margin and was the only challenger to defeat an incumbent member of the State Legislature in 1988.

As a newly elected state representative, I signed up for the legislative health insurance. The Legislative Health Care Plan was considered a "Cadillac Plan" as there were no co-pay requirements. It was better than the health insurance I received based on my state police disability with all its new co-pays and restrictions. I did not have all these co-pays when I injured my knee.

During the campaign, I had pounded my legs walking and running in parades and climbing stairs during door-to-door canvassing. I had loose cartilage floating behind my kneecap and I needed another knee operation. I wanted my operation done as soon as possible so I could hit the ground running, so to speak, in my legislative career. However, the state legislative health insurance program denied my claim for the knee operation due to my pre-existing condition (six previous knee surgeries). Fortunately, I was able to transfer back to my State Police disability health insurance with its co-pays. Because my surgery was related to my previous injury, the state police health insurance covered most of the cost.

I learned a very valuable lesson regarding health care coverage: insurance companies will find any reason to deny a claim. Therefore, when I was elected to Congress in 1992, I chose not to take the Congressional Health Care Insurance even though I was repeatedly assured that the "Cadillac plan" offered to Members of Congress would cover any future knee operations and I would not be denied coverage because of a pre-existing injury or condition. Despite all the assurances and the calculations showing me how the Congressional Health Insurance Plan(s) would save me money over my current health insurance, I did not trust the insurance companies. I never enrolled in the Congressional Health Insurance Plan.

During several of my re-election campaigns and during the healthcare debates, when political and health care opponents claimed that I was not entitled to the lavish health care benefits (that they mistakenly claimed Members of Congress enjoyed), I stopped them dead in their tracks and told them that I was not receiving coverage under the Congressional Health Insurance Plan. I explained that Members of Congress did not have their own lavish health insurance but rather the same insurance options as any other Federal employee under the Federal Employee Health Benefit Plan(s). More on health insurance later but for now, it is sufficient to say that my family and I never participated in the Health Insurance Plans offered to Members of Congress. If I would have participated in the congressional plans, I am sure that my claims would have been denied as I had seven more knee operations, back surgery and neck surgery. Each surgery was a consequence of my degenerating knee, which will soon need to be replaced.

One more valuable health insurance lesson learned in the Michigan Legislature was that of balance billing for Medicare patients. During my first year as a state representative, legislation came on the House floor to end the practice of "balance billing" by health care providers. Balance billing occurs when the health care provider (physicians, hospitals, specialists, etc.) bill a patient for the difference between what the provider charges and what the health insurance will pay. In the Michigan Legislature, the Democratic proposal was to end balance billing by Medicare and Medicaid providers. The amount billed to the Medicare and Medicaid patients may not have been significant, but the policy was strongly opposed by all health care providers.

Most Medicare and Medicaid patients are on a fixed income. It is a financial burden on them to pay that portion of the physician bill not covered by health insurance. Medicare and Medicaid are government-sponsored programs but they do not regulate how much a health care provider may "balance bill" a patient. For example, for performing my knee operation, my orthopedic surgeon may charge $3,500 for his services and my insurance may only approve $2,500. Therefore, my orthopedic surgeon may balance bill me $1,000. This balance billing is also referred to as "out of pocket" expense. With my knee surgery example, I am just listing my orthopedic surgeon. This does not include the other health providers who may also balance bill me for services related to my knee surgery including the anesthesiologist, radiologist, MRI and lab tests, hospital room or outpatient clinic, and rehabilitation services, etc.

What the Michigan Democrats were focusing on in 1989 was to put a stop to balance billing on Medicare and Medicaid patients. I strongly favored ending the practice and worked hard to make sure all four Democrats in the Upper Peninsula delegation supported the legislation.

As we debated the bill, we were one vote short of passing the legislation. As we ran different Democratic amendments refining the legislation, I realized that State Representative Dominic J. Jacobetti, the longest-serving legislator in Michigan history and Chairman of the Appropriations Committee had not voted with us. Jake, as everyone called the Chairman, had silently voted against the Democratic amendments to end balance billing. I was shocked. As the final bill came to a vote I went over to implore my good friend, mentor and fellow Upper Peninsula colleague to vote with us to end balance billing. Jake stated that "he had to vote with his friends," meaning Blue Cross/Blue Shield of Michigan. Jake voted "nay" and the vote ended in a tie. We lost by one vote.

I couldn't understand why Jake refused to vote with us and instead chose to support the health care providers and insurance companies. It was as if Jake had turned his back on his colleagues and his constituents. Jake's friendship with the insurance companies, doctors and lobbyists was more important to him than the public policy issue. In my mind, the principles of social and economic justice were trumped by special interests. In my mind, Jake was wrong on this issue and I had a difficult time understanding his vote.

Despite my disappointment with this vote, Jake and I remained very close throughout our careers. He had the ability to form coalitions, such as the Upper Peninsula Representatives with the Detroit Representatives, across both geographic boundaries and political party lines to promote economic prosperity, protect the environment, and improve the quality of life for people throughout Michigan. His ability to form coalitions and get things done was more important to me than disagreeing with him on his balance-billing vote.

The last time I saw Jake was in 1994 at my major political rally with Vice President Al Gore. After the campaign speeches to a packed gymnasium at Northern Michigan University, the Vice President and I left the stage to work the rope line, where we were enthusiastically greeted by the crowd. Laurie drew my attention to the empty bleachers behind the stage. There was Jake sitting alone, leaning on a cane and looking more fragile than his seventy-four years of age. Laurie asked me to take Vice President Gore over to say a few words to Jake.

I pulled the Vice President away from the crowded rope line and we went over to say a few words to Jake, who lit up as he spoke to Vice President Gore. Twenty days later, Jake died of a heart attack as he prepared to travel to the State Capitol for the start of his twenty-first term. I was headed to Washington, DC for my second term. I am happy that Laurie had drawn my attention to Jake at the rally; he was a friend and a mentor and a tireless public servant. He loved and dedicated his life to serving the people of the Upper Peninsula.

While I only served two years in the Michigan Legislature, I learned many valuable lessons that would serve me well later in Congress and reinforced my belief that all Americans are entitled to quality, affordable health care. I argued that health care is a right for all Americans and not a privilege for only those who could afford it. Despite my best efforts, balance billing is still occurring under Obamacare.

CHAPTER 6

★ ★ ★

Skull and Crossbones (1990)

My two-year term in the state legislature was flying by and I was considered a political hot shot. In the early summer of 1990, State Senator Joe Mack resigned his seat and a special election was called. It was not difficult for Governor Jim Blanchard to persuade me to run in a special election to fill a vacant State Senate seat in the heavily Democratic western end of Michigan's Upper Peninsula. The problem was that I had to give up my House seat to run for the State Senate seat in the August primary. I could only declare for one office and I decided to run for the open State Senate seat. At the time, former State Representative Don Koivisto was also contemplating a run in the special election. I had the Governor on my side and Don had the Democratic State House Leadership, the U.P. state representatives, including Dominic Jacobetti, and geography on his side.

I was convinced that nobody could out-hustle me. So, every day away from Lansing I would drive the 400-500 miles back to the Senate district and I would campaign like hell. I was a crazy man as I traversed the western end looking for votes. I left my campaign strategy to the "pros" as I focused on the strength of my grassroots politics. I handed over the media to the political consultants hand-picked by the labor unions. Unfortunately, the professional consultants killed me politically.

The "pros" produced and maximized the airtime for a television ad that claimed that my opponent wanted to make our pristine Upper Peninsula into a nuclear waste dump. Featuring a skull and crossbones image flashing across television sets throughout northern Michigan, the commercial was extremely hard-hitting and the visuals were over the top. The graphics were too harsh and I heard from every person I met that my campaign had crossed the line. I was being bombarded with negative feedback and the backlash was fast and furious. Don ran a response ad that labeled me a dirty campaigner and compared me to a boiling pot of chili. I dropped hard and fast in the polls and the skull and crossbones ad was destroying my credibility and good will with the voters. No matter how much or how good I was at grassroots campaigning, I could not overcome that ad. I was losing the Senate race and with it my political career. From phone booths throughout the Western Upper Peninsula, I called my media consultants and demanded that the ad be pulled. They refused. I called the union officials and they said I was too soft. They had seen the ad and said that it was fine, that I had overreacted. My family and volunteers who were busting their butts for me pleaded with me to pull the ad. I finally convinced the consultants to pull the commercial with a week to go in the campaign.

Because it was a special election, the campaign cycle was short. The skull and crossbones ad had killed me. I was now expected to lose by well over a thousand votes, but I never gave up. We ramped up the grassroots campaign to reverse my falling fortunes but time ran out. Don Koivisto won the seven counties that were part of his state house seat. I won the two counties that were in my house district by a 10-1 margin, plus the largest county, Marquette County. Unfortunately, Marquette had a historically low voter turnout for the special election and primary. Not only had the ad turned voters against me, it turned voters off and they did not come to the polls. Overall, of the ten counties that made up the State Senate district, Don Koivisto won the seven counties he had represented and I won the other three. I lost by approximately 350 votes. I had turned my campaign over to the professionals, against the wishes of my wife and closest advisors. Another very hard lesson learned: never relinquish control over your own political campaign.

The worst part about the State Senate race was that I was required to give up my State House seat to run in the special election. Whoever won the special election would serve out the remaining four months of the senate term and would appear on the November General Election ballot as the Democratic candidate for a full four-year State Senate term. It seemed that my political career had ended after a quick twenty months; I was now considered a "flash in the pan." My political epitaph was already written and it was way too short.

One of the saddest days in my life came on Friday, December 28, 1990: I had to pack up my files and political memorabilia from my state representative office in Lansing, Michigan. I had driven my Chevrolet Blazer the 425 miles down to Lansing and tightly packed away all my political hopes and dreams. I did not know how, but I promised myself that someday I would return to public service. It may have been the snowflakes falling on my cheeks as I loaded the last boxes, but drops of water somehow fell from my face. It was 5:00 p.m. on Friday and I couldn't delay my exit any longer. I was leaving yet another job that I truly enjoyed and it hurt badly. My stomach was in knots. I deserved to be miserable; it was my own fault. I got ahead of myself politically and had jumped at the first opportunity to advance. I did not listen to Laurie or my friends and relatives who thought that I was moving too quickly. I bucked the state Democratic Party establishment and my political career had ended before it ever really got started. As the snowflakes began to multiply, I drove north, never dreaming that my loss to Don Koivisto would be a blessing in disguise.

The day after losing the primary I reached out to Koivisto and publicly endorsed him. I worked especially hard to make sure that our Democratic candidate for my former State House seat was elected. I wanted people to know that I was a team player and that I was committed to politics and public service. While out of office in 1991, I accepted speaking engagements and attended political events throughout the Upper Peninsula. I wanted to remain active politically as I attempted to rehabilitate my image and regain the respect of the voters that I lost with the skull and crossbones ad.

While my political career seemed to come to a screeching halt, Laurie's political career was just beginning as she ran for Menominee City Council in November of 1991. I may have lost my State Senate race, but the Stupak family did not lose its enthusiasm for public service and door-to-door campaigning. The Stupak family, Ken (age 11), B.J. (age 9), Laurie, and I, canvassed the neighborhoods for Laurie and she received the largest vote total of all the candidates, becoming one of eight City Council Members.

CHAPTER 7

★ ★ ★

Run for Congress (1992)

By 1992, the Democratic presidential nomination process was well underway and I traveled and attended Democratic political events across northern Michigan. By February of 1992, the constituents who knew me best were encouraging me to run for Congress against the Republican incumbent Bob Davis. I wanted to run but did not know if I could marshal the necessary resources after coming up short in the Senate race. The unions were disappointed and upset with my defeat. Governor Blanchard was narrowly defeated in 1990 by John Engler, and the Democratic State Representatives were still angry with me for jumping ship and opposing Don Koivisto in the State Senate race. During the Senate campaign, it was highly rumored that I was only running for State Senate to broaden my base and position myself for an eventual congressional bid. I had promised the voters that, if elected, I would not run for Congress in 1992. I vowed to complete the full Senate term through 1994. Fortunately for me, Don Koivisto made the same promise to serve out his full term as State Senator.

Therefore, in 1992, since I had *lost* the State Senate race, I was no longer bound by my promise. I was free to pursue the congressional seat against the popular seven-term incumbent, Bob Davis. Believing that I could once again beat an incumbent, I traveled the congressional district sounding out my chances with the voters. As is so often the case in both politics and life in general, there is much to be said for being in the right place at the right time!

The US House banking scandal broke early in February of 1992 and our Congressman Robert W. Davis (R-MI) had the third-highest number of overdrawn checks with 878 bounced due to insufficient funds. The General Accounting Office audited the House Bank and provided Americans with details on the scope and breadth of the problem, but it never publicly disclosed the names of the check bouncers. The House banking scandal seriously undermined the public's confidence in their Member of Congress as speculation swirled back in the congressional districts as to whether their Member was bouncing checks. Congressman Davis never indicated that he was involved in the House banking scandal until March 15, 1992, when the Detroit News broke the story. Davis immediately flew back to the congressional district to meet with angry constituents. They did not accept his reasons for floating outstanding checks for over three years before he had sufficient funds to cover his personal expenditures. Public reaction was swift and furious as constituents and a Republican National Committeeman from Michigan demanded that Davis resign and/or not to seek re-election.

The House banking scandal was known as "check kiting," wherein Members of Congress were permitted to write checks and float them for months, even years, without enough money in their accounts to cover the overdrafts, without any penalties. For any other American, a bank cannot allow overdrawn accounts without civil and criminal penalties or felony charges for repeat offenders. With the House Bank, Members of Congress were not only overdrawing their accounts, these overdrawn accounts were permitted to remain open for up to thirty-nine months. The voters were outraged and viewed the House banking scandal as political corruption and malfeasance. Moreover, they now viewed their Members of Congress- who apparently could not even take care of their own bank account, let alone the nation's finances- as inept. Finally, twenty-two Members of Congress were cited by the House Ethics Committee for abusing their House banking privileges, including northern Michigan's Congressman Bob Davis with 878 overdrawn checks.

Now the voters in northern Michigan had 878 reasons to vote *against* their incumbent Representative Bob Davis. Within a month of being named one of the worst check-bouncers, Bob Davis announced that he would not seek re-election to Congress.

In politics, big breaks come when you least expect them. Any aspiring politician must be nimble to take advantage of unanticipated opportunities.

Laurie and I drove to Detroit to attend the annual Democratic Jefferson Jackson Day Dinner with guest speaker Governor Bill Clinton of Arkansas. As we drove to Jeff-Jack, former State Senator Mitch Irwin and I were encouraged to run for Congress and we each promised to support the other if either of us did decide to run. The jokes were coming fast and furious about how things can change in a New York minute and the formerly invincible Bob Davis (who beat Mitch in the 1988 congressional race, the year I was elected to the State House) had received his comeuppance. We knew either one of us would have a good chance of winning, but who could best take advantage of the Davis scandal and win in a strong Republican seat?

Here was my political opportunity. However, one of my closest friends was the Democratic Party favorite to run. Mitch was a hard worker and great campaigner. At the time of the House banking scandal, Mitch and Cindy were focusing on new careers and had just welcomed a second child into their family. After a lot of soul searching and many discussions with family, friends, and supporters, Mitch chose to pass and deferred to me for the congressional bid.

The Michigan Pro-Life community was pushing me to run even though they would not contribute to my campaign, as there was a Republican primary that they would be involved in. The fact that Michigan Right-to-Life had encouraged me to run was not a surprise to anyone in the Upper Peninsula of Michigan. When I served in the Michigan Legislature, the four Upper Peninsula representatives were Democrats and Right-to-Life. Even today, I believe only one former Democratic State Representative from the Upper Peninsula was Pro-Choice. The Upper Peninsula State Representatives were usually Catholic and Right-to-Life. In northern Michigan, Catholics are the dominant religion, support Catholic elementary schools, and the Catholic Church remains a vital social institution in our small, rural communities.

The Republicans were mildly concerned that either Mitch or I could potentially win the congressional seat against the current GOP prospects. Since 1992 was a presidential year there would be a greater voter turnout, especially critical in rural swing districts. To play it safe, the Republicans brought back former Congressman Phil Ruppe, who was revered by the voters in the U.P. and hailed from the Democratic-leaning western end of the Upper Peninsula. Congressman Ruppe's wife, Loret, was serving under President George H.W. Bush as US Ambassador to Norway and was former director of the Peace Corps. The Ruppes were personal friends of President Bush and it was rumored that President Bush had personally asked Phil to run for Congress to keep the seat in the Republican column and bolster GOP turnout in the presidential race.

No Democrat had ever served consecutive terms in this congressional district; the voters only elected a Democrat every forty years or so and then only for one term. The First Congressional District was considered a solid Republican stronghold and the pundits expected it to remain so.

At the closing of the filing deadline in mid-May of 1992, there were six candidates who filed for the open congressional seat in Michigan's First District. On the Republican ballot were former Congressman Phil Ruppe, State Representative Stephen Dresch from the Houghton area in the Upper Peninsula, and Bill Kurtz, a county commissioner from Traverse City in the Lower Peninsula. On the Democratic side were two candidates from below the bridge, Mike McElroy and Dan Herringa. I was the lone Democratic candidate from the Upper Peninsula. Fortunately for me, the bulk of the Democratic votes in the primary would come from the fifteen U.P. counties.

The Michigan Democratic Party was unofficially supporting Mike McElroy for the Democratic nomination. McElroy was Pro-Choice and had already raised well over $100,000, and the labor unions and party activists were eager to jump on his bandwagon. My chances of beating a Pro-Choice candidate in the Democratic primary were good. But then, my chances of defeating Congressman Phil Ruppe in the general election were not good, to say the least.

With very little money- approximately $40,000 compared to Mike McElroy's $180,000- I once again relied on an aggressive grass-roots campaign concentrated in twelve of the twenty-eight counties that comprised the First Congressional District. These twelve counties were in the central and western Upper Peninsula. Our campaign was so poor we invented the ten-second commercial. With a black and white photo of me standing by my State Police patrol car or standing with my family, the announcer could say my name three times in ten seconds without rushing it and added that I was a family man or a former state police trooper or an Eagle Scout. My family, friends, and core supporters busted their butts and never gave up on me or on our commitment to make our country a better place.

While my ten-second commercials could hardly compete with McElroy's thirty-second spots describing his brother's battle with cancer and the healthcare industry's role in bankrupting his family's health and finances, I campaigned harder. McElroy's fight for health care gave credibility to my speeches on health care. I campaigned on the fact that doctors should not be balance billing our seniors, the fight I lost in the State Legislature. I campaigned on the fact that I was medically disabled from the Michigan State Police and while I received a small pension, what about our fellow citizens who became disabled and did not have a health care plan to take care of their medical and financial needs. I made health care my personal fight and Mike discussed his brother's fight. Both versions of health care struck a nerve with the voters and health care became the defining issue of the Democratic primary.

The determining factor in the Democratic primary was: which campaign understood and could best predict the turnout of Democratic voters? I knew that of the twenty-eight counties in the First Congressional District, only twelve of the fifteen counties in the Upper Peninsula would determine the winner of the Democratic primary. I knew this and pounded those twelve counties. I knew how to count the votes in each county, in each precinct and in every contested Democratic race from township supervisor to county commissioner to judge. I knew where the Democratic votes would be cast. I did my homework and it paid off; I easily won the twelve most Democratic counties.

McElroy won sixteen counties but lost the primary with 43.11% of the Democratic vote. Dan Herringa took 8.77% of the vote, coming mostly from McElroy in the sixteen counties that had low Democratic turnouts. I snared 48.63% of the Democratic votes, winning the Democratic primary with less than 50% of the vote. As amazing as my victory was, it only earned me the right to run against the revered Congressman Phil Ruppe. No one gave me a chance to win in November.

CHAPTER 8

★ ★ ★

1992 General Election

The day after the primary, the Democratic Party held a unity breakfast in Marquette. State Senator Don Koivisto introduced me as the nominee and presented me with my first contribution for the general election. Don's contribution would not cover the cost of my now famous ten-second commercial, but it was the symbolic gesture that demonstrated that any lingering doubts about whether Don and I could work together or that there was any bad blood from the skull and crossbones nuke ad were put to rest. The contribution also signaled that the Democrats believed they had an opportunity to win this congressional seat for the first time since 1964. In that year, Democrat Ray Clevenger won the seat after President Kennedy's assassination and promptly lost it two years later to Phil Ruppe. Congressman Ruppe then held the seat for twelve years until 1978, when he left the seat to seek the Republican nomination for the United States Senate.

Congressman Phil Ruppe and President George H.W. Bush represented the old guard and Democratic presidential nominee Governor Bill Clinton and I were the young, new team in the 1992 General Election in Michigan's First Congressional District. A popular third-party candidate, billionaire Ross Perot of the American Independent Party, was the possible spoiler.

Once again, I relied heavily on grassroots campaigning and money was very difficult to raise. I called the Democratic Congressional Campaign Committee (DCCC), for assistance even though it had sent Washington, DC consultants to the district to pressure me to drop out of the primary because of my Pro-Life views. Still, I called DCCC after the primary and asked for help now that they were stuck with me and the 1992 presidential race was shaping up to be a three-way contest. If neither presidential candidate secured 270 electoral votes, the race would then be decided in the US House of Representatives and every congressional seat would be critical to elect Arkansas Governor Bill Clinton as president.

It made no difference: every consultant suggested to me by DCCC was polite but firmly told me that they would not take a job with my campaign because I was Pro-Life. Once again, it was my family, friends, core supporters and my "kitchen cabinet" that held the campaign together with little to no money. Even though most of the members of my campaign were Pro-Choice, they understood and accepted my Pro-Life views. I did not and still do not wear my Right-to-Life credentials on my sleeve. I am who I am and the importance of protecting the sanctity of life is my belief and position.

I have always believed that to be successful, a candidate is required to provide three solid reasons for the voters to support him or her and three reasons to vote against the opponent. Therefore, in my 1992 race for Congress, I made three promises: I would vote to raise the minimum wage, fight for national health care and restore fiscal integrity in Washington, DC.

Our effort slowly picked up momentum as we campaigned throughout the fall and Democratic political operatives started to take notice. The United Auto Workers (UAW) hired my close friend and local union president, Russ Bovin, to provide outreach to other unions throughout the First Congressional District.

Ann Beser, a close friend who worked for the Democratic Speaker of the Michigan Legislature when I was in the State House, took leave from her job and moved up to Escanaba to run my campaign. Ann reached out to the Democratic Party, Pro-Choice groups and the Progressive community, telling them that I was a hard-working, practical politician whose views fit perfectly with the district- and that I could win.

Highly respected Washington political reporter and insider Bob Novak traveled to the First Congressional District to report on President Bush's re-election chances in a solid Republican stronghold while he campaigned with his friend, Congressman Phil Ruppe, at the annual Labor Day Mackinac Bridge Walk. Before compiling his report, Novak attended a candidate forum in the small town of Cheboygan, Michigan. In addition to Phil Ruppe and me, the other candidates participating in the forum were state representatives and local candidates. Following the forum, Novak interviewed me and reported that I could actually upset Ruppe and President Bush appeared to be in trouble in the traditionally reliable Republican region of northern Lower Michigan.

After Novak's article, interest in our campaign increased substantially. David Broder of the *Washington Post*, who owned a summer home on Beaver Island in the rock-solid Republican Charlevoix County, reported that a congressional upset was brewing in northern Michigan. The money started to trickle in and DCCC-approved consultants were now willing to help. I wanted nothing to do with them. I could still feel the sting of the skull and crossbones ad and their previous rejection due to my Pro-Life views, so I asked Ann Beser and Laurie to handle the consultants.

The Clinton-Gore team loosened up some money for our combined grassroots effort and we suddenly had real bumper stickers and lapel patches instead of our homemade signs. We suddenly felt like maybe we could pull this off. Ann Beser asked her friend, pollster Bill Cromer, to conduct a quick tracking poll. Cromer's poll showed the race very close with Ruppe at 100% name recognition but supported by only 45% of most-likely voters. I had 65-70% name recognition and 42% said they would vote for me. Thirteen percent of the voters were still undecided. I was running above the Democratic base in the Republican counties and below base in most of the Democratic Counties. Running above or below base is critical to understanding your strengths and weaknesses.

As a Democrat, my base support in the First Congressional District was 45% as determined by the percentage of votes cast for Democratic candidates running for the State Board of Education (SBE). The vast majority of voters have no idea who the Democratic and Republican candidates are for the State Board of Education. Therefore, to establish a party's base of support, consultants review the percentage of votes cast for the Democratic candidates for the State Board of Education in a congressional district. Consultants can break down the party support based on the SBE votes in each precinct, county, and political district.

According to Bill Cromer's poll, I was running three points below the Democratic base. Ruppe was running seven to eight points below his Republican base. With Cromer's help, we determined which counties and which media markets I was running below and above the base. As expected, I was running below base in Marquette, Delta and Dickinson counties in the Upper Peninsula. Because the campaign started to raise more and more money each day in October, we decided to increase our television and radio buys in these counties. By mid-October, the campaign also had enough money to place television commercials in the Green Bay media market, which was the most expensive market in the district. As we raised money and placed more television ads, our support increased. In every one of my campaigns, I ran below the Democratic base in the Menominee, Delta and Dickinson counties until we aired television commercials to remind my neighbors of my commitment to them and to public service. There is an old saying in politics that comes from the Bible: a "prophet [politician] is never known in his own land."

We also needed to energize and expand our Democratic support in the Upper Peninsula. I asked former Governor Jim Blanchard and his former cabinet member and U.P. Director Tom Baldini to help me persuade either Bill Clinton or Al Gore to campaign for me in Marquette, the largest Democratic county in that congressional district. There were not a lot of local races in Marquette County to keep the voter's interest in the November general election. I certainly did not want to see another low voter turnout in the largest Democratic county in that congressional district as in my 1990 State Senate race.

During the last week before the election, Senator Al Gore came to Marquette and we held a rally at Northern Michigan University. It was a huge success as Senator Gore fired up the party faithful, the unions became energized, and the campaign momentum swung in favor of the Democrats. We suddenly had money to run thirty-second commercials touting the youth and vitality of the Clinton-Gore-Stupak team. We hit the Republicans hard for being against minimum wage, not providing national health care and we blamed them for creating the country's financial crisis. Our commercial struck a nerve with the National Republican Party and they filed a Federal Election Complaint against the Stupak for Congress Committee for an "in-kind" contribution to the Clinton-Gore campaign. It was a ridiculous accusation, as my campaign did not have money to spend on commercials supporting the Clinton-Gore presidential campaign when it struggled to pay for its own advertising. Moreover, the Clinton-Gore campaign had plenty of money, whereas I had very little. When this political attack on our campaign was filed and publicized by the National Republican Committee, I started to believe that maybe, just maybe, we were about to upset Phil Ruppe and send a Democrat to Congress. We had one more week to go. Could we keep our campaign momentum going? The Republicans continued to attack me while the Ruppe campaign filled the airwaves with very warm and fuzzy, positive Congressman Phil Ruppe commercials.

I spent the early morning hours of Election Day shaking hands at the Mead Paper Mill plant gate in Escanaba. The Mead Plant had the largest concentration of workers and voters in the First Congressional District. The workers parked their cars on one side of the Escanaba River and walked across a long narrow bridge to the plant entrance. As these workers stepped off the bridge at 5:00 a.m., I shook their hands and asked for their vote. My goal was to get the workers to slow down and shake my hand as they entered or left the plant. On this cold, windy day with snowflakes swirling around, the workers stepped out and shook my hand. There was no chatter about gun control, abortion, or taxes; the workers knew it was Election Day and they wanted to wish me luck. My early morning hours at the Mead Plant Gate were beginning to pay off. I felt confident of victory when I left Escanaba at 7:30 a.m. and drove down to Menominee to vote and campaign.

The Mead Plant gate became legendary with my campaigns. I would receive permission to stand outside the main plant gate and shake hands with the workers in off-election years, during the holidays, the early mornings of the Upper Peninsula State Fair, and any morning that brought me to Escanaba. If I had a scheduled meeting with the plant management, I made sure I shook hands with the workers before my meetings with their bosses. While Mead was a union paper mill, I never took the workers or their votes for granted. I believe that no matter how many times a candidate stands for election, it is always important to ask for and earn their trust. Nothing is a given, and no vote is ever taken for granted.

After Laurie and I voted with our boys in the booth with us, I headed up to Menominee Township to shake hands outside the polling place until the polls closed at 8:00 p.m. It was very dark as I left Menominee Township, but it had been a good day of campaigning. In each critical election, I would stand 150 feet away from the Menominee Township polling place, wave to voters and shake their hands as they came to vote at the Township Hall where three precincts voted. This Township Hall cast more raw votes than any other location in the district. I wanted the voters to see me one more time before they pulled the lever, knowing that I was still campaigning hard right up until the polls closed.

Laurie and I then drove back up to our Escanaba campaign headquarters. We always asked each other on the drive up north how we felt about the campaign. Had we given it our all? This campaign was an effort that we would feel proud of regardless of the outcome. We felt good, but we were nervous, exhausted, and anticipated a long night of election returns over the vast rural twenty-eight counties and two time zones that comprised the First Congressional District of Michigan.

Over the last days of the campaign, the Escanaba Stupak Headquarters became the nerve center of the get-out-the-vote effort for the entire Democratic team. By the time we arrived in Escanaba, every staff person, volunteer, friend and family member was mentally and physically spent. The back room of the office was being transformed into a little stage so I could thank my family, supporters and volunteers for all their work in this remarkable effort to win the congressional seat. The results were just starting to trickle in, and they were encouraging, but they were mostly from my strength areas in the Upper Peninsula. As the results continued, Ann Beser became anxious and took first me and then Laurie for "a walk around the block." Beser tried to explain what it meant to be a Member of Congress and what would be expected of me and of our family. She had analyzed the returns and could see that the trends looked like Bart Stupak might actually become a congressman. Laurie and I tried to assure her that we were ready for the challenge of Washington, DC, but it was a clear, cold, starlit night and we walked a little faster to get out of the Upper Peninsula November chill. I think the walk was more for Beser because she had just helped to elect a friend and his wife to Congress and clearly felt the Stupaks really had no idea what they were getting into.

After a very long night of waiting for returns from the twenty-eight counties, we defeated Phil Ruppe, 53.93% to 43.11%. We won and we won convincingly. Our campaign staff members and volunteers were so excited that they began answering the phones, "Congressman Stupak's Office." I had to admit, it sounded pretty good. I was headed to Washington DC as the first Democratic Congressman from Michigan's Upper Peninsula in thirty-eight years. Washington, DC- a place that I had visited only once when I accompanied Laurie to a conference there- would soon be my home away from home. Was I ready?

Congressman Ruppe called me early the next morning and congratulated me on winning the election. As always, Phil Ruppe was a gentleman. As I hung up the phone, reality started to sink in: I was going to Congress. I had achieved a goal that no one thought was possible two years ago when I lost to Don Koivisto in the Democratic primary for State Senate. I had to pinch myself to make sure it was real, for I never dreamed that I would go so far so fast in politics. I was only forty years old, had served one term in the Michigan House of Representatives and now I was going to the United States House of

Representatives. But how long would I remain in Congress? Would I be there long enough to keep my campaign promises?

As the campaign unfolded throughout the primary and the General Election in 1992, health care had become the number one issue. Could Congress truly pass legislation that would allow me to fulfill my campaign slogan: "Health care is a right and not just a privilege for those who can afford it"? Now I had to prove that it could be done. Would the democratically controlled Congress let Bart Stupak pass health care for all Americans, a feat that Congress had struggled and failed to achieve over the past eighty years? At forty years old, I did not have the answers, but I dared to dream of a better America in which Congress would increase the minimum wage and provide health care for all Americans while getting our nation's fiscal house in order. It had been a hell of a campaign, maybe the most perfect campaign I had ever run, but now came the hard part: I had to deliver on my promises.

I knew the reality of partisan politics was that I would be a top Republican target in the next election. After all, northern Michigan voters historically elected a Democrat once every forty years and then threw him out of office after one two-year term. I was determined that I would not be a one-termer. But what did I know? I was young, idealistic and passionate in my beliefs. As Laurie always tells me, I may not be the most intelligent person she has ever met, but I am definitely the most determined person she knows! I resolved to work like hell, to keep my word and to stand with our newly elected President Bill Clinton to achieve the dreams and promises of the Clinton-Gore-Stupak team.

As I packed my clothes before catching the flights to Washington, DC, I reflected on my own experience with health care. I had been able to pay my medical bills for my shattered shoulder twenty years earlier; I doubted if I could afford it now. The numerous surgeries that I had required for my knee were totally paid for by my employer-based coverage over the past eight years because I had good health insurance through the State of Michigan. In my campaign for Congress, I learned that my State of Michigan-sponsored health insurance was the exception and not the norm. I was determined to provide all Americans with quality, affordable health care. I packed my hopes, dreams and passion for health care right alongside the bitter truth that health care no longer addressed the needs of the American people and headed for Washington, DC.

CHAPTER 9

★ ★ ★

The Early Days of Congress (1992-2000)

When Laurie and I visited the US Capitol in the spring of 1991, we were shocked as we observed Members of the U.S. House of Representatives on the floor voting. It was utter chaos. Members of the House did not even have a desk to sit at to conduct business. The House floor was a noisy, chaotic scene with no one even paying attention during votes! How did Members of Congress even know what they were voting on when they could not hear the Speaker Pro Tempore or the Reading Clerk announcing the legislation or calling for the vote? In the fall of 1992, I was elected to take a seat in the chaos of the United States Congress.

Now that I had won, I was getting advice from everyone on which committees to seek, who to hire and to whom I must speak. Funny, none of these folks bothered to help me in my campaign until the very end, and now they were all taking credit for my victory. The unions wanted me on the Transportation Committee, Marquette County leaders wanted me on Armed Services and Lower Peninsula residents wanted me on Agriculture and Interior Committees. I wanted a seat on Energy and Commerce because that was the committee with the greatest jurisdiction and where health care legislation would be written. In many of my post-election interviews, I mentioned that passing health care was my number one priority.

My mind was made up; I was planning to seek a position on the Energy and Commerce Committee. The Chairman of the Energy and Commerce Committee was John Dingell from Michigan, whom I had never actually met. I truly was a Washington outsider, seeking to play ball with the ultimate insider, John Dingell. Chairman Dingell was one of the most senior members of the US House of Representatives. I was the newly elected congressman from northern Michigan and I wanted a position on one of the most sought-after committees in Congress. The Republicans made it very clear that I should not receive a plum committee assignment because, like my Democratic predecessors, I would be a "one-termer." I was apparently already labeled as the Republicans' number one target for defeat in 1994.

I was experiencing quite an introduction to hard-core Congress and politics at the federal level. When I was elected to the Michigan House of Representatives, all of us newly elected State Representatives met together and vowed to move our state forward. Here in DC, every speech, every amendment, every piece of proposed legislation contained an "I gotcha" amendment, one solely designed to provide political fodder for the next campaign. Being the number one target of the Republicans, I had to scrutinize, understand, and defend every vote, speech, and move I made.

I had only been on the job for one day when Congressman Norm Dicks approached me and introduced himself. Congressman Dicks asked me where my district was in Michigan. I explained the district and he said, "Well, the Base Realignment and Closure Commission [BRAC] is closing your base, K.I. Sawyer." I had no idea that K.I. Sawyer Air Force Base was on the Base Realignment and Closure Commission list. Norm was a senior Democrat on Armed Services and was very familiar with BRAC. I do not know if Norm was trying to be helpful by giving me a "heads up" but he seemed just a little too excited to tell me about the closing of the base. Sure enough, we checked and K.I. Sawyer Air Force Base, home of B-52 bombers and the largest employer in my district, was on the Pentagon's hit list to be closed by the non-partisan BRAC Commission.

A few weeks later, I was on the House floor when Congressman Henry Waxman (D-CA) approached me. I was just to the right of the Speaker's rostrum discussing committee assignments with a couple of other freshmen Members. I was disappointed that I was not assigned the Energy and Commerce Committee. Waxman approached me and said that as a Member of the Steering Policy Committee, he could not vote for me for a seat on the Energy and Commerce Committee because I was Pro-Life. He further explained that, because health care policy is within the jurisdiction of the Energy and Commerce Committee, he would not support a Pro-Life Member for the committee. I was caught off guard by his comments. I told him that health care was important to me and I wanted to pass health care reform in this Congress. Waxman said that he doubted if the Committee could even pass health care out of the committee but he could not support me for a position. I thanked him for his honesty and I said something to the effect that if I was re-elected I would again seek a position on the Energy and Commerce Committee. I believe that was the first and only time I spoke to Henry Waxman during my first two years in Congress.

We were told that freshmen Members of Congress were rarely assigned to the big three committees of Energy and Commerce, Appropriations, and Ways and Means. Our freshmen congressional class was one of the largest in US history and we wanted freshmen, Democrat or Republican, to be assigned to the big three committees. Of course, I was hopeful that I would be one of the few selected freshmen for one of the exclusive Big Three.

I was not selected to an exclusive committee and only one member of our freshmen class was. Instead, I was given a position on Armed Services, Merchant Marine and Fisheries and Government Reform Committees. With my Air Force base selected for closure under BRAC, Armed Services was a critical committee for me. Merchant Marine and Fisheries included a Great Lakes subcommittee, which was also very important with my district bordering on three of the five Great Lakes. Finally, Government Reform was an investigative committee with oversight of the Federal Government, which suited my law enforcement, legal and state legislature background. While I was disappointed in not being selected to the Energy and Commerce Committee, these three assignments would serve me well during my first term in Congress.

Congressman Mel Reynolds of Chicago was the only freshman Member placed on any of the exclusive Big Three committees. Mel was placed on the Ways and Means Committee through the efforts of his fellow Illini, Committee Chairman Dan Rostenkowski (D-IL). Reynolds touted an impressive resume: he was a Rhodes scholar and held an MBA from Harvard. As it turned out, a stellar resume is not always an accurate predictor of success *or* integrity: both Chairman Rostenkowski and Congressman Reynolds would be out of Congress within three years. "Rosty" was convicted of mail fraud for converting his official House postage stamps into cash and Reynolds was convicted of statutory rape. Congressman Reynolds was succeeded into office by Congressman Jesse Jackson, Jr., who was convicted of tax evasion in 2013.

I established myself as a serious legislator. I was a little tense, took my job very seriously and won re-elections by wide margins in a Republican district. I was comfortable interacting with Republicans as well as Democrats. It was important to me to get to know every Member of the House, Democrat or Republican. This personal goal served me well when I was in the Minority for twelve of the eighteen years I served. I was not a showboat or a partisan bomb-thrower; I quietly did my homework and did not give knee jerk reactions. There was sound reasoning behind my positions on the issues. I was not caught up in the Washington, DC political glamour scene and I traveled back to Michigan every possible weekend. I did not speak much on the floor or in Democratic Caucus meetings.

Throughout my career, I stayed on as a Member of the Democratic Whip Team, where I would study the issues and learn the arguments for and against legislation. The Whip Team also provided me with an opportunity to discuss legislation with all Members and proved beneficial to those who congregated in the Pennsylvania corner.

Members of Congress are creatures of habit and they tend to congregate in the same general area on the House floor. As a Whip, it was important to know where Members hung out so you could "whip" them by asking and recording how they would vote and, if necessary, persuade them to vote with the Democrats.

On the House floor, there are areas known as the Pennsylvania corner, Blue Dog row, the Railbirds, Black Caucus, Hispanic Caucus, the Smokers and the Leadership tables. If you name a Member of Congress with whom I served a couple of terms, I believe I can tell you where that Member congregated for legislative sessions. Of all the places where Members sit and stand during session, the Pennsylvania corner is the best-known location. The corner is occupied by Democratic Members of the Pennsylvania delegation and moderate Democrats from the Northeast and Midwest. As you view the House floor from the Speaker's rostrum, the extreme right hand corner or northeast corner of the House floor is the Pennsylvania corner. The end seat in the top row of the corner is reserved for the senior Democratic Member of the Pennsylvania delegation. Other "Pennsylvanians" and like-minded Members take seats to the right, in front of, or stand along the rail behind the Senior Member's seat. No one dares to sit in the senior Pennsylvania Member's seat even if he or she is not present. Throughout my career, the senior Pennsylvania Democratic Member was Jack Murtha. My best friend in Congress is Mike Doyle of Pittsburgh and I was a constant fixture in "the Corner."

Because I had a good grasp of the issues from my Whip position and an understanding of the chaos that ensued every day when 435 Members gathered for a vote, I was sought out by Members and asked, what was the legislation being considered? Which groups supported or were against the legislation? And, how was I going to vote and why? The congressional staffs of each Member would provide insight and recommendations on how they believed their Member should vote, but it is always good to check that recommendation with fellow Members of Congress.

My desire to learn the nuances of legislation made me a natural member of the Whip Team. It also allowed me to sharpen my skill in breaking down complex legislation and making it easy for Members and my constituents to understand both the legislation itself and my legislative votes. In a few short years, I had an excellent grasp of the legislative process; I was able to make sense of the apparent chaos on the House floor that Laurie and I had observed in 1991. My colleagues viewed me as a knowledgeable, pragmatic legislator and often sought my advice prior to casting their votes. I had grown as a politician and legislator and I absolutely loved the job.

CHAPTER 10

★ ★ ★

"Nothing Is Ever off the Record" (Spring 1993)

While I was not assigned to the Energy and Commerce Committee during my first term, I did manage to distinguish myself with President Clinton and my Democratic colleagues. It was nothing that I set out to do; it just sort of happened. It was probably naiveté on my part, but my statements in our closed-door meeting were more of a reflection of who I was as a person and politician. My comments to President Clinton and my freshmen colleagues at the White House were a true display of my strongly held beliefs in social and economic justice.

In the spring of 1993, the freshmen House Members were summoned to the White House by President Clinton as he pressed us to vote for his economic initiative, the 1993 Deficit Reduction Package. President Clinton was the charming individual he can be when he needs your vote. He was pulling out all the stops. He reminded us of the special bond between himself and the Democratic freshmen Members of Congress as we ran for office together in 1992, were elected together, and now had to stick together to pass his Deficit Reduction Package with all its cuts in programs, tax cuts, and tax increases. President Clinton was rearranging budget priorities in

Washington, DC, just as we were elected to do six months ago. It was Clinton at his best, persuading us, cajoling us, and doing his best to win us over. It was not working.

The significance of the meeting was not lost on me. Six months ago, I was a rookie Member from Michigan bewildered by the apparent chaos of Congress. Now I was in the White House, being asked by the President of the United States for my opinion on his signature legislation. Although awed by the honor in my quiet moments, I was comfortable offering my thoughts as a wonky legislator. I had done my homework and fully understood the President's proposal.

Each of us freshmen had our concerns and difficulties with the Administration's proposal, including the BTU Tax that was designed to reduce America's dependence on fossil fuels. It was a radical new way to tax the American people and it was not popular. The BTU tax was really Vice President Al Gore's creation, as he was putting forth his initiatives on combating climate change and was insistent on his gas tax.

I had serious angst with the Deficit Reduction Package, not only due to the BTU tax but also because of all the cuts to programs important to my constituents and the closing of the K. I. Sawyer Air Force base, the largest employer in my district. If that was not enough reason, the Clinton Administration had just announced that the new NOAA weather station would not be built in my district as previously reported, but would instead be built to the south in Republican Dave Camp's district. With the NOAA weather station came federal employees and jobs for the community in which the weather station would be located. I had no reason to vote for this package.

For about an hour I listened to all the arguments on why we should vote for the package, with each of my classmates stating why he or she was having trouble supporting the President's plan. The bottom line was that we were afraid we would be targeted in the next election for raising taxes. We would be labeled the tax-and-spend Democrats, even though the President was telling us that his plan would balance the budget in five years. Needless to say, we thought the President's economic forecasting of a balanced budget was a pipe dream.

Finally, I summoned the courage to stand and speak. I addressed the group and told them that I had many personal reasons to vote against the plan. In addition to the proposed BTU tax, the planned closing of the last military base remaining in my district, the elimination of the Coast Guard cutter *Mackinaw,* and the construction of a new National Oceanic and Atmospheric Administration (NOAA) weather station, not in my district as previously reported but elsewhere, all spelled "political suicide" for my young career. The fact that no Democrat from my district had ever served consecutive terms in Congress meant that I was most likely toast in the next election. Still, I firmly believed that as Members of Congress we had a moral and ethical responsibility to do what we believed to be in the best interest of the country and not what was politically expedient for us personally.

By now you could have heard a pin drop in the White House East Room. I had everyone's attention as I continued to speak. I went on to say that I had studied the package and despite my reservations I believed that it was in the best interest of the country to vote for the President's Deficit Reduction Package, and I promised to do so. If I lost my election over this vote, so be it. I had come to Congress to do what was in the best interest of the country and not what was politically popular.

I sat down to a standing ovation. The next day, a small article in the Washington Post recapping my comments proclaimed, *"Freshman Brings Down the House."* We passed the President's package by a one-vote margin and it led to a robust economic recovery. This vote did, however, cost some of my freshmen colleagues their elections.

Well before my comments at the White House, a couple of my freshmen colleagues quickly and publicly announced- before they had actually reviewed the plan- that they were against the Deficit Reduction Package. Later, after reading the proposal, and some heavy lobbying in support of the President's plan, these same Members of Congress "flip-flopped," ultimately voting in favor of the DRP to the outrage of voters in their home districts.

These well-intentioned members of the Democratic freshman class of 1992 were defeated in their re-election campaigns due, I believe, to a failure to communicate effectively with their constituents. They could not or would not explain the valid reasons behind the difficult votes they had cast: why their votes were in the best interest of the nation or how they ultimately benefited their congressional districts. I was always aware that I needed to address my constituents' concerns about how my votes affected them directly. I have always said that there are no bad votes in Washington- just badly explained votes.

I very quickly learned a couple of political lessons from the votes on the Deficit Reduction Package that stayed with me throughout my career: even with no reporters in the room, the press still manages to get the story. The President's plan *was* very unpopular. I quickly became the number one target for the Republicans in 1994. BTU no longer meant British Thermal Unit- it meant Bart Taxes You!

During the 1994 campaign, I boldly and sincerely told my constituents that yes, I did raise taxes on a handful of citizens in northern Michigan who earned more than $180,000 per year. They received a tax increase, but my vote *lowered* taxes for 35,000 families through the Earned Income Tax Credit.

Whether it was my refusal to vote in favor of the impeachment of President Clinton, my vote to close the gun show loophole, my vote against the war in Iraq, or my very controversial vote in favor of national health care, I have always voted for what I considered to be in the best interest of our country. I would then travel to the parts of my district that most likely disagreed with my vote and explain my controversial position with conviction and without hesitation. In their books, *My Life* by President Bill Clinton and Hillary Rodham Clinton's *Living History,* both cited my willingness to directly take on the tax implications of the 1994 Deficit Reduction Package as an example of how to campaign on tough, difficult votes and still win re-election. A couple of my House colleagues have also written about my speech at the White House and my willingness to cast the tough vote even though it may have cost me my congressional seat.

CHAPTER 11

★ ★ ★

1994 Election

It was another late night on October 1, 1994 as I stepped off the House Chamber floor with my friend, Earl Pomeroy of North Dakota. Earl was a freshman and like me came from a conservative district: the whole state of North Dakota. Earl said, "Well Stupak, now we have to go home and campaign. I will see you in November." As we walked down the east steps of the Capitol into the darkness, I said that I doubted if very many of our friends would be back. It was ugly out there. Earl just nodded and said he was having a tough time at home but thought that he would be okay. I told him that I was working my butt off but history was not on my side. He said, "You will be back Stupak," and we departed to our respective apartments for a few hours of sleep before the first flights out of DC in the morning.

The 1994 campaign was the most grueling campaign of my life. For the first time ever, I was running as an incumbent in an anti-incumbent election year. Suddenly, I was part of the problem. I struggled to defend my votes and explain to the voters in Michigan how I was different from the Democratic Majority. The first debate of the campaign season was in my opponent Gil Ziegler's hometown of Kalkaska and he had stacked the crowd against me. Laurie and my District Administrator Scott Schloegel pulled no punches when they critiqued my pitiful debate performance. They read me the riot act and questioned whether or not my heart was really into fighting for re-election. They insisted that I had to do what I do best: break down an issue and explain it in terms that my constituents would understand. I took their advice and began referring to my opponent as Millionaire Gil Ziegler. I quickly rattled off on one hand five ways in which I differed with President Clinton and the Democrats. My distinguishing no-votes became my crib notes, which I summarized as "B-A-N-G". I did not vote for the Brady Bill, B in BANG. I did not vote for taxpayer-funded abortion, A. I feverishly opposed NAFTA, N. Finally, I did not support gays in the military, G. Each one of these Democratic legislative initiatives was passionately opposed by the voters in my district.

Millionaire Gil Ziegler and I were complete opposites in how we conducted our campaigns. Gil had all the high-paid Republican consultants and I had my faithful "kitchen cabinet." Gil traveled the vast district in his private jet; I traveled in my Oldsmobile. Gil's jet allowed him to be home just about every night, while I was never home. I attended events and stayed until the very end; Gil attended events and left at the first opportunity. Throughout the campaign, I expounded on the differences between Millionaire Gil Ziegler and Bart Stupak, a true man of the people. The voters ultimately identified with me and my campaign, and even the Republican landslide could not take down their number one congressional target. On election night, Gil Ziegler said with tongue firmly in cheek that he was going down to the courthouse in the morning to change his name to Millionaire Gil Ziegler. I had miraculously survived the Republican tidal wave sweeping the country, yet when the election was over I honestly had to ask myself the same question the Washington Post posed in their headline when it profiled my campaign: "Why Would Anybody Want This Job?"

Unfortunately, the Republican landslide wiped out more than half of the freshmen Democrats, as I had gloomily predicted to Earl. The Republicans won control of the US House of Representatives for the first time in forty years. Even the Speaker of the House, Tom Foley of Washington State, was defeated. The election was a total repudiation of the Democrats and the Clinton Administration. We were considered the problem and the Republicans were the answer with their "Contract with America." Throughout the 1994 campaign, I referred to the Republican plan as the "Contract *on* America"- a political gimmick that would not solve any of the pressing problems facing our country.

The morning after the 1994 election, I called the Democratic Congressional Campaign Committee (DCCC) to ask about the outcomes of a few of my friends. I was shocked to hear that I myself had lost my election. According to the young staffer on the phone, Bart Stupak was the first name they had crossed off as having been defeated. I had to convince the young person that I was indeed Congressman Bart Stupak and that I had in fact won the election. Once the young staffer was convinced, he apologized and said that they just assumed I had lost since the tidal wave had wiped out so many of my freshmen colleagues. My freshmen friends, such as Jay Inslee (WA), Maria Cantwell (WA), David Price (NC) and Ted Strickland (OH) all lost that year but came back to the US Congress in later elections. A total of fifty-four Democrats lost in the 1994 election and the Republicans had the Majority in the US House of Representatives for the first time in forty years. Newt Gingrich became Speaker of the House. As a defeated and deflated Democratic Party caucused in Washington, DC to elect our party leadership, I was pleased to see that my friend Earl Pomeroy of North Dakota had also been re-elected. Earl remained in Congress until he was defeated for re-election in 2010, the year I chose to retire from the House of Representatives.

CHAPTER 12

———— ★ ★ ★ ————

Election to the Energy and
Commerce Committee (1994)

A day or two later, I started calling around to garner support
for selection to the Energy and Commerce Committee. The
Democrats were in disarray, but I spoke with Congressman
John Dingell, who assured me there would be four to six seats available. Congressman Dingell encouraged me to immediately submit
my nomination to the Steering and Policy Committee. Dingell also
informed me that Richard Gephardt (D-MO) would be the new
Democratic Leader and he suggested that I reach out to Dick as soon
as possible to be placed on his leadership slate for selection to the
Energy and Commerce Committee. I did everything suggested to
secure a seat.

Congressman John Dingell now saw me as more than a "one-
term wonder". I had survived the 1994 Republican tidal wave that
wiped out so many of my freshmen colleagues. Dingell was present
at the White House when I gave my speech to the freshmen urging
them to support President Clinton's Deficit Reduction package. I
had cast the tough votes and I did not complain. I was a workhorse,
not a show horse. John Dingell now wanted me on his committee
even if I was Pro-Life. In late November of 1994, I went back to

Michigan believing that I had secured a coveted seat on the powerful Energy and Commerce Committee.

The Energy and Commerce Committee is one of the most sought-after committee assignments in the House of Representatives because of its vast jurisdiction and its rich history. As the only committee referenced in the Constitution, the Energy and Commerce Committee is the oldest committee of the United States Congress and it is estimated that sixty to sixty-five percent of all the legislation considered by the House of Representatives passes through that group. Thus, Members of the Committee have the greatest opportunity to influence legislation considered by the US Congress.

After the election and subsequent Caucus Leadership votes, Laurie and I flew down to our favorite vacation destination in Jamaica. I planned to keep in close contact with my office, as I knew votes for committee assignments would occur within the next week or two.

Finally, after three years of non-stop campaigning to win my congressional seat and then to fight off the Republican tidal wave, I was going to be able to relax in the warm Jamaican sun. There I could bask in the knowledge that although I had been the Republicans' number one target in the 1994 election, I had not only survived but had proven my mettle and earned consideration for a seat on the coveted Energy and Commerce Committee. At that moment I felt that I could probably withstand any political attack. Even though I was Pro-Life, Henry Waxman would not be able to keep me off that committee. It was time to relax.

My phone began ringing the moment we landed in Jamaica. The nervous nellies back in DC were insisting that I come back and sit outside of the Steering and Policy Committee to do last-minute lobbying for my seat on the Energy and Commerce Committee. I told my staff that this was crazy and that I really wanted some down time in Jamaica with my wife. However, they kept insisting that I come back to DC. Finally, I called Congressman Dingell and asked for his advice. John echoed what my staff was telling me: that I should come back and try to catch the Members of the Steering and Policy Committee before the vote because nothing was certain.

I discussed the issue with Laurie and it was decided that I would fly to DC for the vote and if all went well, I would be back on the beach within forty-eight hours. I returned to the Capitol and sat outside the Steering Policy meeting in the hopes of persuading any undecided Members to vote for me for a seat on the Energy and Commerce Committee. I was elected on the first ballot.

Because there were six members elected to the Committee, we had to draw lots for seniority. My Chief of Staff, Ann Beser, drew on my behalf as I had caught the first possible plane back to Jamaica. She drew sixth. Although I was the first member elected in terms of Steering Committee votes, I would be last in seniority. In addition, as a Democrat in a Republican-controlled House, I knew that I would have to work hard on the issues before the committee. Who knew what might happen as the years and congressional terms went on?

CHAPTER 13

★ ★ ★

Bart, Jr. (B.J.) (May 2000)

From my first date with Laurie on June 21, 1973, our mutual love of music played an important part in our lives. During the early years of our courtship and marriage, musical selections ranging from the Moody Blues to Bob Dylan blasted from my too-large sound system in my extremely small apartment and our first, tiny, one-bedroom rental home along the shores of the Cass River after we were married. Our favorite albums and artists accompanied us through many long days and nights of work, college, law school and the birth of our two sons, Ken and B.J.

As teenagers, Ken and B.J. both developed their own tastes in music, which they enjoyed on their disc players. Quite often on Saturday mornings, much to their dislike, the boys would be awakened by the sounds of the stereo blaring "Wake up Sunshine" by Chicago or "Get over It" by the Eagles.

After reviewing the outline of this book, Laurie said to me, "You do not have a chapter on B.J." I told her that a chapter on B.J. would be too painful for me to write, but I knew that I would need to include him in this book for he played a very significant role in our lives and in my own health care hell.

B.J. was a joy. He was fun, full of energy, and loved sports and politics. He was an active member of the high school student leadership class and served as treasurer of the Executive Committee. He had just been elected president of the student body for his senior year and was applying to colleges. As chairman of the student activities committee, he was working hard to make sure that prom week was fun-filled and inclusive for the entire student body. He had also been chosen as a member of the Prom Court. B.J. was upbeat, positive, and always had a smile on his face. He demonstrated a strong commitment to public service and possessed a deep compassion for his fellow students. He was charismatic, well liked, and well known throughout our entire community. He had a promising future and much to look forward to.

In the early morning hours of Sunday, May 14, 2000, Mother's Day, B.J. was found dead on our living room floor with a self-inflicted gunshot wound to his head. Lying alongside his body was my State Police-issued .38 snub-nosed handgun. In an instant, our lives were turned upside down. We couldn't believe what had happened, or why. We just knew that B.J. was gone. I don't know how we managed to get through the day. We were in shock, as was our entire community. I remember our parish priest, Father Patrick Wesneske, and Sister Ellen coming to our house to pray with us. The police came and cordoned off our home with yellow crime scene tape and asked us to gather some belongings and leave the premises so that they could conduct an investigation. Father Pat offered his camp as a place for us to stay until the investigation was complete. We made calls notifying our friends and relatives. Everything was a blur. Nothing made sense.

The first call I made to a Member of Congress was to my good friend, Mike Doyle. Mike notified my roommates at C Street and within a day or two they were all in Menominee. Congressmen Mike Doyle, Zach Wamp, Steve Largent, Tom Coburn, John Baldacci, and Marty Sherman came to help us and lend support.

President Clinton announced B.J.'s passing at the beginning of his speech at the National Law Enforcement Officers' gathering on the West Lawn of the Capitol. As a founding Member of the Congressional Law Enforcement Caucus, I had been scheduled to attend the event.

On Wednesday, May 17, it was time for our Upper Peninsula community, relatives, and friends to say a final goodbye to B.J. The visitation was held inside Holy Spirit Catholic Church, as none of Menominee's funeral homes were large enough to accommodate the expected crowds. I remember entering the church and seeing all the beautiful flowers and plants sent in honor of our son. We tried to stop to read some of the notes and cards but people were starting to come in to pay their respects. Laurie, Ken, and I stood alongside B.J.'s casket in front of the altar. Laurie's parents, along with my mother, and all my brothers and sisters, sat in the front rows. A sound system had been installed in the church basement and extra seating was set up to allow the people seated there to hear the Mass.

The line slowly wound its way through the church, past B.J.'s casket. We hugged, cried, or shook hands with everybody who came down the line. Many of the people were wet from standing outside in the rain before entering the church. We were told that the line extended all the way through the parking lot and down the block. B.J.'s baseball team wore their uniforms with black armbands and the student leadership class brought yellow carnations and laid them on his coffin. We were very touched and grateful for all the people who came to pay their respects. Laurie served as Menominee's Mayor and I had served as both their State Representative and Congressman over the past twelve years. We knew just about everyone and everyone knew us.

We had been informed that a congressional delegation would be joining us for the funeral Mass. It was a sacrifice for the Members and some of their spouses to make the trip from Washington, DC to Menominee. They flew from DC to Green Bay, WI and then chartered a bus to Menominee. Sixty-two Members of Congress including Speaker Dennis Hastert, Democratic Leader Dick Gephardt, and the wife of the Vice-President, Tipper Gore came to comfort us and show their support. Their support during our time of sorrow showed a spirit of bipartisanship, true compassion, and a human side of Congress rarely witnessed.

When it was time to begin our son's funeral Mass, we realized that this was the last time that B.J.'s physical presence would be with us. Priests from throughout the Marquette Diocese, including the previous Bishop, came to assist Father Pat with B.J.'s funeral Mass. The sight of dozens of priests walking down the aisle wearing their white garments was both moving and humbling. Somehow, we managed to get through the sad funeral Mass with Father Pat's emotional homily and my brother's touching eulogy. I kept my composure until we started walking up the main aisle behind B.J.'s coffin and the choir began to sing "Battle Hymn of the Republic." I couldn't hold my grief in any longer and the tears began to flow. I cried all the way down the aisle and out of church.

We are grateful to our parish priest, Father Patrick Wesneske, who was celebrating his golden jubilee but made time to support and guide us. In a later interview reflecting on his fifty years as a priest, Father Pat said that B.J.'s death was one of the saddest experiences he had ever dealt with. On behalf of our Holy Spirit family, I was given the honor of eulogizing Father Pat at his funeral Mass a few years later.

We appreciate all of our family and the many friends who helped get us through our darkest, saddest time. We continue to lean on our family, friends, and faith on the difficult days when B.J. weighs heavily on our hearts.

In the days and weeks following B.J.'s passing, we struggled to find an explanation for his drastic and deadly behavior. What was he thinking? What caused him to want to end his life? What were we missing? It didn't make any sense to our family, our friends, his classmates, or his teammates.

I remember returning home late one night from an out-of-town speaking engagement. Laurie was sitting upright in bed with a stack of papers alongside her. She looked up at me and said, "Here, look at this. I think Accutane may have played a role in B.J.'s suicide."

Laurie had spent the evening on the computer conducting research. What she found was that Accutane, a prescription drug used to treat severe cases of acne, had been linked to numerous cases of depression, suicide ideation, and suicide. B.J. had been prescribed Accutane and was just about to complete his course of treatment. At the time of his death, he had six pills left.

Ken, being two years older than B.J., was the first to be treated for acne. Ken is like me, serious and practical. When he was prescribed Accutane by a dermatologist in Green Bay, Wisconsin, we were given a brochure, which both Laurie and I read and discussed. I asked my housemate and fellow congressman, Tom Coburn, if he was familiar with the drug and if it was safe. Tom was also an accomplished physician and I trusted his judgment. Tom assured me that Accutane was safe in most cases as long as it was monitored properly.

During the time Ken was on Accutane, he seemed to tolerate the drug fairly well. His blood tests indicated that his cholesterol and triglyceride levels remained normal during his course of treatment. In the fall of 1999, following his graduation from high school, Ken began his college studies at Michigan State University. From an early age, Ken's goal had always been to attend and graduate from Michigan State. He was, and still is, a true Spartan.

As a freshman at MSU, Ken had the honor of being chosen as a student manager for the Spartan basketball team. Serving as a student manager meant long hours of practice with the team, breaking down film, and assisting the coaching staff with whatever needed to be done. I don't think any of us realized the amount of time that would be required of Ken as a student manager.

As Ken was completing his treatment on Accutane, MSU was making a serious run at the NCAA Championship. We were all excited about MSU basketball and were making plans to attend the Final Four in Indianapolis. At the time, Ken seemed a little down, but we attributed his lack of energy and enthusiasm to his long hours of breaking down film over the course of the tournament.

B.J., on the other hand, was over the moon with Spartan basketball. He watched every game and analyzed the players. He knew all the stats and coaching strategies. He was confident that the Michigan State Spartans would win the National Championship and he was planning on being there to celebrate with his big brother. Ken and B.J. spent a good deal of time together during our time in Indianapolis at the Final Four. Unfortunately, it would be one of their last times together. Five weeks later, B.J. would be dead.

The more information Laurie and I discovered regarding the serious side effects of Accutane, the more we became convinced that the drug had played a role in B.J.'s death. That fall, the *TODAY* show came to Menominee to interview us and ran a story on B.J.'s suicide and the possible link to Accutane. The response to the segment was overwhelming.

With the help of my colleagues on the Energy and Commerce Committee, I launched an investigation into Accutane and the serious and sometimes fatal side effects it can have on unsuspecting patients and families. I discovered that a "Med Watch" warning had been sent out by the FDA prior to B.J.'s death, specifically linking the drug to depression, suicide ideation and suicide. During my investigation, my efforts were constantly thwarted by both the FDA and Pharmaceutical and Research Manufacturers of America (PhRMA). In February 2008, the FDA documented in an internal memorandum stating that Accutane may have caused the deaths of numerous young people. A review of the FDA database revealed that young, perfectly healthy males like B.J., with an average age of seventeen, had, without explanation, spontaneously killed themselves with a firearm. After screening out all intervening factors, the FDA concluded that the only common denominator in the deaths of otherwise healthy, well-adjusted seventeen-year-old males was Accutane.

We consider our experience and the loss of B.J. the result of a perfect storm. We were not provided the proper warnings concerning the serious side effects of the drug. B.J.'s dermatologist never established a baseline to determine normal triglyceride and cholesterol levels. Had the doctor conducted the tests properly, they would have shown that B.J. was unable to tolerate the daily 40mg (maximum strength) dose of Accutane over the course of six months. The doctor failed to acknowledge the fact that B.J. was not tolerating the drug properly even though it was brought to his attention on several occasions when B.J. complained of severe headaches. The doctor also failed to conduct the appropriate follow-up tests. As a result of his autopsy, we found that B.J. only had one kidney. This fact came as a complete surprise to us, as he had always been healthy and athletic.

Having only one kidney would have caused a failure of his body to process Accutane properly and expel excess toxins from his blood stream.

To complete the perfect storm, B.J. had access to a handgun in our home. The unimaginable had occurred and we lost our son and brother.

As a result of our investigation, patients and families are now given a proper warning and have greater access to information concerning the serious side effects associated with Accutane. In fact, the FDA subsequently approved a black box warning, the most serious warning it can issue, concerning the use of Accutane.

To this day, we are still approached by strangers who tell us about their experiences with Accutane. Although we feel that many lives were saved because of our efforts, we know that similar tragedies still occur every day.

Following B.J.'s death, I could not turn on the stereo, the car radio, a CD or an old vinyl record album without Laurie asking me to turn it off. I found solace in my favorite songs; Laurie found sadness. It is only recently that I have been able to play Pandora, my albums, CDs, or Sirius radio with Laurie. Even the Boss, Bruce Springsteen, cannot soothe the pain or replace the emptiness. There is still a nagging pain and emptiness that time and faith will never heal.

Music is slowly creeping back into our lives, but something in the music is missing and somewhat hollow. I realize that nothing will ever be the same. I often think about Ken and how he offered to remain at home with Laurie in the fall after B.J.'s death. However, we insisted that he return to MSU and complete his studies. We both expressed concern about how Ken would handle the loss of his best friend and little brother. After graduating from MSU, Ken traveled to California to attend law school even though he knew no one there at the time. He graduated from Pepperdine Law School and is now married to a wonderful woman. They have a young son who quite often reminds us of B.J.

As much as we miss B.J., our family has stayed together and has become stronger. We are thankful for the joy B.J. brought to our lives as a son and brother. His spirit lives on through the B.J. Stupak Memorial Scholarship Fund administered through the M & M Area Community Foundation. The Fund awards scholarships to graduating seniors across the Upper Peninsula of Michigan who exhibit leadership skills and possess a passion for community service.

Recommitment to Life

When you lose a loved one, you would give anything to bring that life back. The words "sanctity of life" took on a deeper meaning for me; life became even more precious. After B.J.'s death, I was devastated and angry. I had too many irrational thoughts, wanting only my own selfish answers. I blamed God for taking our young son. I was angry with the random kid shuffling without purpose down the street. Why did B.J. die and that kid was still living? That kid would probably never amount to anything and B.J. had everything to live for. Lord, I would ask, why did you take my son?

I was being selfish and had an all-consuming need to turn back time and bring my son back. But it doesn't work that way. B.J.'s death increased my commitment to life; I saw all life as even more precious than I did before he died. I wanted every life to be fulfilled. That life may only be seventeen days, seventeen years or ninety-seven years but each life has a span that only God knows. I wish everyone could live life to its fullest. My passion to protect the unborn increased when B.J. died.

I also understood that there was a balance to life. As an individual and a legislator, I realized that I could not passionately protect all unborn life and not be equally passionate about those lives devastated by disease, illness and injury. The health care debate should not have been viewed as a competition between the unborn versus the sick and dying. Yet these two principles were on a collision course that I did not fully understand nor appreciate at the beginning of 2009. I believed in protecting the sanctity of life *and* in health care for all Americans. I did not view it as an either/or proposition as did so many organizations and some Members of Congress.

I also did not anticipate how often I would ask B.J.- each and every night of this turbulent period- whether I was doing the right thing. Was it appropriate to protect the sanctity of life at all costs and defeat the health care legislation? What was I failing to see? What mistakes did I make each day that would prevent health care from becoming a reality just because I continued to insist on a vote on my Right to Life ("RTL") amendment? What could I do better to protect the sanctity of life while providing access to quality, affordable health care for all Americans? Finally, I would ask B.J. and Jesus to turn off my brain and allow me to sleep during the turbulent days and nights of my own health care hell.

CHAPTER 14

★ ★ ★

Pelosi as Speaker (2007)

In November of 2006, Democrats picked up thirty-one seats in the US House of Representatives; we were back as the Majority Party. History was made with Nancy Pelosi becoming the first female Speaker of the House. Victory was ours and it was because President George W. Bush was so unpopular that in conservative- to moderate-leaning congressional districts, Democrats won and won big. After twelve years in the Minority, Democrats were reclaiming the Majority. As the song goes, "Happy Days Are Here Again!"

I was excited at the prospect of not only becoming Chairman of the Oversight and Investigations subcommittee of the powerful Energy and Commerce Committee but also that we picked up so many seats in rural areas that the ranks of our Pro-Life Democrats swelled. I suddenly found myself discussing Pro-Life issues with new Members of Congress from around the country. Not only were there many new Democratic Pro-Life Members, the newly elected Republican members were also Pro-Life. The Republican Pro-Life leadership, now as the minority party, were required to give greater deference to the Pro-Life Democrats.

The Congressional Pro-Life Caucus consisting of both Democrats and Republicans was a force to be reckoned with; we could influence any legislation if we stayed united. Staying united and voting as a block was especially important because Pro-Choice activists, including the Speaker, held the gavel of key legislative committees in the House. To make matters even more difficult, Congresswoman Louise Slaughter, the incoming Chair of the Rules Committee, was co-chair of the Women's Pro-Choice Caucus. While our Pro-Life numbers grew, our ability to influence legislation in the new democratically controlled House waned. Speaker Nancy Pelosi is Catholic, but she would not allow Pro-Life legislation to come to the floor unless the President was Pro-Life. For Pro-Life legislation and our traditional RTL riders on the appropriations bills to be permitted under a Pelosi speakership, there had to be a Pro-Life counterforce equal to or greater than the Speaker.

In 2007 through 2008 the Right-to-Life counterforce to Pro-Choice Speaker Nancy Pelosi was President George W. Bush. During the 110th Congress from January 2007 to January 2009, Speaker Pelosi, at the urging of Appropriations Chairman David Obey (D-WI), allowed the traditional Pro-Life Riders on the appropriation bills. However, Speaker Pelosi would not allow an expansion of the Hyde Amendment, which forbids the use of taxpayer dollars to be used to promote, encourage or pay for abortions.

The Hyde Amendment was the most important traditional Pro-Life rider that both the Pro-Choice and Pro-Life Members debated during the annual discussion of the appropriations bills. Other traditional Pro-Life riders stipulated no abortion coverage in Federal Employee Health Benefit Packages; no abortions on domestic or international military installations; no International Family Planning funds or Planned Parenthood funds could be used to pay for abortions; and the gag order preventing health care providers from recommending, encouraging or promoting abortions to their patients. Finally, there is the RTL conscience clause, which prevents retaliation, retribution or discrimination against a doctor, nurse or health care worker who refused to participate in an abortion.

From time to time, the RTL Members would push for or promote other anti-abortion amendments, but these amendments never reached acceptance as a traditional rider. Riders are nothing more than amendments that are attached to legislation and "ride" the bill through the legislative process. The RTL riders prevented federal tax dollars from being spent to promote, encourage or perform abortions. Thus, the RTL riders were attached to the appropriations bills, which allocate money for the program. The RTL riders are amendments offered each year for consideration on the underlying legislation, whether the House is controlled by Democratic or Republican Speakers.

In some legislative years, such as 2007 and 2008, the traditional RTL riders are written into the underlying bill or accepted in committee "markup" of the appropriations bill to avoid an emotional debate and legislative fight on the House floor.

In essence, there was a truce between Pro-Life and Pro-Choice forces, which had accepted the Hyde Amendment as status quo over the past thirty years. The Pro-Life forces were fearful of the 2008 presidential election, when a Pro-Choice Democratic candidate such as Senator and former First Lady Hillary Clinton, Senator Joe Biden, Senator John Edwards or Senator Barack Obama would be elected president. If a Pro-Choice Democrat was elected president and the Congress remained in Democratic hands as in the first two years of the Clinton presidency, taxpayer money would once again be used to promote, encourage and pay for abortions.

We could not worry about what might happen in the future as this was 2007 and Nancy Pelosi was about to become Speaker. The bipartisan Congressional Right-to-Life Caucus set out to work with Speaker Pelosi to ensure that our traditional Pro-Life appropriations riders stayed intact with Pro-Life President George W. Bush in the White House. The perfect counter to Speaker Pelosi and the Pro-Choice Democratic Chairs in the US House of Representatives was President George W. Bush.

With the Democrats in control of both the House and Senate in 2007, I became Co-Chair of the bi-partisan Congressional Right-to-Life Caucus. During my first fourteen years in Congress, Representative Chris Smith (R-NJ) was the Chair of the RTL Caucus. I had worked on many issues with Chris and had gained his trust. In 2007, Chris moved to elect co-chairs of the RTL Caucus, and although each party still caucused independently on RTL issues, more and more bi-partisan meetings were taking place with Chris and me serving as chairmen.

As Pro-Life Democrats, if we stayed united we controlled enough votes to block any legislation from coming to the floor under the House Rules. My role in the RTL movement was to work within our Party to convince leadership to allow Pro-Life amendments and to work out differences when a RTL issue threatened to derail legislation.

At the start of the 110th Congress, there was still mistrust between the two RTL Caucuses. I had to convince Republicans to vote for Democratic Pro-Life amendments and Pro-Life Democrats to vote for Republican Pro-Life amendments.

As the Democratic Pro-Life leader and co-chair of the US House of Representatives Pro-Life Caucus, I became a pivotal Democratic Pro-Life voter and spokesperson. The success of the Pro-Life movement depended on my personal, legal and legislative skills to protect the sanctity of life in a hostile environment and quite often at the peril of my own political career. It was with good reason that Pro-Life Democrats were very leery of Speaker Nancy Pelosi.

Nancy Pelosi said the right things and realized that the Democratic Party would never be in the Majority without us moderate and conservative Pro-Life Democrats. As Speaker, however, how would she treat us? It is often said that you cannot serve two masters in politics, so the main question was whether Pro-Choice Speaker Pelosi was going to allow Democratic Pro-Life amendments. Would she allow Republican Pro-Life amendments? Would she allow Republican Motions to Recommit, knowing that the language in the Motion would contain, in part, Pro-Life language? How could she keep a rambunctious Democratic Caucus together, let alone be viewed as protecting the legislative rights of the Minority Party? Would she challenge President George W. Bush on the Right-to-Life issues and appropriations riders?

In her speech to the Democratic Caucus the night before assuming the Speakership, Nancy Pelosi reflected on her Catholic faith, her faith in the caucus, her faith in each of us as individuals and her faith in our great country. She spoke from the heart.

Nancy (D'Alessandro) Pelosi was raised in the City of Baltimore, where her father and her brother had each served as Mayor. She vividly recalled people coming to their family home asking her father for help. He would try to help them with finding a job, assisting their son or daughter in gaining admission to college, or providing aid with food, clothing, or medical assistance. During her comments to the caucus, I remember Speaker Pelosi claiming, "My father knew who to call to help people out and many times it was the Catholic Church."

Nancy Pelosi reminded us that she hailed from the City of San Francisco, named after St. Francis. As she began to recite the prayer to St. Francis she told us that she felt that we Democrats had a spiritual calling to provide for the poor, the needy, and the sick. She then brought forth the current issues facing our country and that we, as Democrats, were elected to address the difficult issues like climate change, heath care, unemployment, and the wars in Iraq and Afghanistan. We, as Democrats, had a special opportunity given to us to govern, a moral imperative to make our mark in history, to address the challenges facing our great nation and to become a more compassionate, caring people for all Americans, including those who live among us illegally.

Speaker Pelosi went on to say that with our Democratic Majority we have an obligation to move boldly and swiftly for the sake of our nation, for the sake of the world, but most importantly for future generations, for our children and grandchildren. The Speaker then said that immediately after she was sworn in as Speaker, she was going to invite the children of Members of Congress, who were present on the House floor, to join her at the Speaker's rostrum. She then closed by reciting lines from the Prayer of St. Francis.

"Lord, make me an instrument of Your peace;
Where there is hatred, let me sow love;
Where there is injury, pardon;
Where there is doubt, faith;
Where there is darkness, light;
And where there is sadness, joy.

O Divine Master,
Grant that I may not so much seek
To be consoled as to console;
To be understood, as to understand;
To be loved, as to love;
For it is in giving that we receive;
It is in pardoning that we are pardoned;
And it is in dying that we are born to
Eternal Life. Amen.

Her speech was uplifting and spiritual in nature and she received roaring approval from the caucus members. As we left the Cannon Caucus room that January 3, 2007 our Democratic Caucus was united, determined and invincible.

Congressman Mike Doyle (D-PA) and I were both extremely impressed with her speech to the caucus. Mike claimed that if she gave the same speech the next day, she would hit it out of the park. I agreed and said that if she governed like she just spoke and was truly inclusive and seriously addressed our problems, she would be a great Speaker. Still, we both had our doubts and we would wait and see what tomorrow and the next two years would bring.

I was surprised when the Speaker's parliamentary staff asked me to take the Chair (Speaker's Chair) on the second day of Session in the new 110th Congress as we tackled our legislative business. Things were looking up and I thought that maybe I would be able to work out my philosophical differences on abortion with the Speaker and the Democratic Leadership as I had for the last fourteen years. I was hopeful.

CHAPTER 15

———— ★ ★ ★ ————

Motion to Recommit (2007–2010)

The 110th Congress started on January 6, 2007. The first order of business on the opening day of a session is to determine the House Rules, which govern the official actions of the Members and how legislation would be considered on the floor of the US House of Representatives. In recent years, Democrats were denied the right to offer a Motion to Recommit.

Motions to Recommit are used by the minority party to offer substitute legislation in the form of an amendment to the legislation being considered. In other words, if the democratically controlled House of Representatives were considering immigration legislation, the Republicans have the right to offer their version of immigration reform through a Motion to Recommit. If the Motion to Recommit is approved by a majority of Members voting, the whole issue is sent back to the committee of jurisdiction for reconsideration. The committee is authorized to make any changes the Members of the committee believe are appropriate. Seldom is a Motion to Recommit ever approved. On those rare instances where a Motion to Recommit is successful, the legislation is sent back to the committee, where it usually dies.

The minority party exploits the parliamentary procedure of Motions to Recommit for political messaging by inserting politically sensitive issue(s) into the Motion and making it difficult for Members of the majority in swing congressional districts to vote against it. Thus, the essence of a Motion to Recommit is to politically embarrass Members of the majority to vote for the Motion. If a member of the majority party does not vote for the Motion to Recommit, the minority party immediately sends out a press release stating that the Member voted, for example, against seniors, for gays, or against our military service men and women. The vote on the Motion to Recommit is a recorded vote, which would then be listed in television commercials claiming that the Member voted in favor of allowing taxpayer funds to pay for abortions on vote number such and such. These political ads are disingenuous and appeal to a select group of voters in a Member's congressional district- groups such as Right-to-Life voters, seniors, veterans, gun owners, or military service men and women. The Motion to Recommit is focused on emotional issues such as taxpayer funding for abortions, amnesty for illegal immigrants, or background checks for child predators. The fear of a Member of Congress is that if he or she would vote against the Motion to Recommit- for example, against senior citizens, for abortions, illegal immigrants, or child predators- a press release and radio and/or television commercials would immediately be aired in the Member's home district, upsetting a vocal constituency group which would work against the Member in the next re-election.

Regardless of the subject of the legislation, the Republican Motion to Recommit usually included provisions on abortion, criminals, guns, immigration and gays. The Motions to Recommit were designed to draw enough Democratic votes to send the legislation back to committee, where it would die. As Chair of the RTL Democrats, I would plead with them to vote against the Motion to Recommit, stick to the merits of the legislation, and reject the added provisions, which were meant to divide and embarrass Democrats in the next campaign. We usually stuck together and defeated the Republican Motions to Recommit.

I could only wonder what the Republicans' Motion to Recommit would entail if the Democrats ever brought national health care legislation to the House floor for a vote. I imagine it would be filled with emotional conjecture on immigration designed to peel off the conservative and moderate Democrats. I am sure taxes would be part of a Republican Motion to Recommit to portray Democrats as tax-and-spend liberals. Another favorite Motion would be language on homosexuality and the claim that Democrats allowed pedophiles to assault our children. These emotional pleas would have very little connection to health care, but it would sure make us Democrats think twice before voting for national health care legislation. Little did I realize in 2007-2008 that I was not too far off in my suspicions as to the substance of the Republican Motion to Recommit on Obamacare.

During the 110th Congress (2007-2008), Democratic legislation was moderate enough and included our RTL Riders only because the legislation still had to secure President George W. Bush's signature before it could become law. President Bush acted as a counterweight to Speaker Pelosi on the abortion issue and gave RTL Democrats cover with sufficient RTL language in the legislation to secure his signature. President George W. Bush protected the RTL Democrats against the politically charged Motions to Recommit during the last two years of his presidency.

Once President Obama was elected, Speaker Pelosi no longer granted us our RTL riders on the appropriations bills. The Democratic legislative initiatives became more progressive and partisan, which left me wondering: whatever happened to the passion and commitment to govern based on the ideals of St. Francis?

CHAPTER 16

★ ★ ★

Chair, RTL Caucus (2007-2010)

Although Congressman Jim Oberstar (D-MN) had turned over the Right-to-Life Democratic Caucus and his leadership in the Bipartisan Congressional Right-to-Life Caucus to me in 2007, I continued to consult with him on Right-to-Life issues. Jim and many RTL Democrats felt uncomfortable standing next to the Republicans who were displaying graphic photos depicting aborted fetuses and listening to their inflammatory rhetoric. Jim viewed the Bipartisan Right-to-Life Caucus led by Congressman Chris Smith of New Jersey as "seeing abortion" in every piece of legislation. Jim found that he could no longer participate with the RTL Republicans with their incendiary language and graphic, disgusting partial birth abortion photos. Although Congressman Oberstar remained committed to his RTL position, he could no longer stand side by side with the Republicans.

While the Democratic RTL leadership was formally passed on to me to continue working with the Republicans, circumstances changed with the general election in November 2006. After the November election, the Republicans were no longer the majority party in either the House or the Senate. No longer would the RTL amendments that Chris Smith attached to every conceivable piece of legislation be tolerated. It was Chris Smith who now had to work with the Democrats to secure support for his legislative proposals. If the Democratically controlled Rules Committee was going to look favorably upon his proposals and rule them in order, he needed Democratic support, for which Chris came to me. I enjoyed working with him even though I could not always support his positions.

Chris and I worked well together and I had no problem joining him at the Rules Committee requesting the traditional Pro-Life Riders on appropriations bills. Appropriations Chairman David Obey of Wisconsin, whose district was adjacent to mine and was also a close friend, made it clear that he did not want abortion fights over his appropriations bills. With President George W. Bush still in the White House, David supported our RTL riders and many times automatically included them in the twelve annual appropriations bills. Even Speaker Pelosi allowed the Pro-Life riders and amendments to come to the floor in 2007 and 2008, knowing full well that President George W. Bush would insist that the RTL riders historically attached to the appropriations bills be included before he would sign any legislation.

While Speaker Pelosi allowed the annual Pro-Life riders, she was not willing to allow other Right-to-Life initiatives to be considered by the House of Representatives. When it appeared that there may be a showdown between Right-to-Life and the Democrats, Chairman Dingell and the Appropriations subcommittee chairs would often come to me and implore me to find a way to work out the language to prevent divisive battles on the House floor.

Since most of the Right-to-Life policy issues came before the Energy and Commerce Committee, Chairman John Dingell would simply say, "Stupak, I do not care how you do it, just work it out so I can move the legislation." Dingell's statement meant that I had to work with Representatives Joe Pitts (R-PA) and Diana DeGette (D-CO) to broker a compromise. Depending on the issue, many times I would also include Congressman Chris Smith.

Once we worked out the matter in Energy and Commerce, I then worked very hard to keep Rep. Michelle Bachman (R-MN) and other Republican flame-throwers from disrupting the legislation during floor debate.

Democrats were still angry over the debates on partial birth abortion. During this heated and emotional debate, the Republicans would display photos of half-aborted children covered in blood. Chris Smith, Trent Franks (R-AZ), Michelle Bachmann, Todd Aiken (R-MO), Steve King (R-IA) and even Henry Hyde (R-IL) would get all wound up and their voices would rise as they pulled out bloody picture after bloody picture to drive home their point about the horrors of partial birth abortion. Pro-Life Democrats would come to me and complain that Chris Smith and Henry Hyde made excellent points during the debate, but then they became vitriolic with their graphic pictures and rebuked anyone who opposed their position. It was not that RTL Democrats disagreed with the underlying amendment. They were sick and tired of being berated and associated with the graphic displays.

I would argue with Chris Smith that it was not necessary for the Republicans to push the debate over the top with their inflammatory rhetoric and gruesome photos and suggested that they would capture more Democratic RTL votes if they would only tone it down and leave the pictures out of the debate. I could not convince Chris or any other Republican that they did more harm than good with photographic displays that turned off Democratic RTL votes.

I would constantly remind Chris Smith and my Republican colleagues that they could not pass any RTL legislation without Democratic support. Each RTL legislative proposal needed about thirty Democratic votes to pass. RTL Democrats would actually boycott the floor debate because they did not want to be identified with the gruesome photos and rhetoric being spewed by the Republicans on Right to Life issues. I kept reminding Chris that not only would Democrats not show up for the floor debate, they would not speak in support of RTL issues because the Republican rhetoric poisoned the water.

When Representatives Bachmann, Franks, Aiken and others would speak, the Democrats would just tune them out and not engage in any dialogue with them as they were viewed as extreme and delusional. I could not convince my Republican colleagues that when it came to Life issues you get much more with honey than you do with vinegar. They would just say that they were not going to sugarcoat the horrors of abortion; I would retort that there is a difference between speech and debate and incendiary rhetoric. I never won that argument with my Republican colleagues.

CHAPTER 17

★ ★ ★

GINA (2008)

A great example of how I had to walk a tightrope with both the Democrats and Republicans in the House and Senate and the Right-to-Life coalition and still pass legislation occurred in the 110th Congress with the GINA legislation. GINA is the Genetic Information Nondiscrimination Act and the prime sponsor of this legislation was Congresswoman Louise Slaughter (D-NY). GINA simply meant that employers and their insurance companies could not use the results of an amniocentesis test or access other genomic or heredity tests as a basis to refuse health or life insurance coverage or deny benefits and discriminate against the mother or the child based on anticipated health issues. While RTL applauded the idea behind GINA, they were concerned that Representative Slaughter did not adequately define an embryo as a child and that the GINA protections would not be extended to adopted children.

Rep. Slaughter was also the Chair of the Rules Committee and co-chair of the Pro-Choice Caucus. Over the course of twelve years, GINA passed the House but was never considered by the Senate. Early in 2008, the GINA bill once again came for consideration before the Energy and Commerce Committee. Diana DeGette asked me to work on the bill because Right-to-Life was blocking it in the Senate. Louise Slaughter was even more frustrated and asked me to meet with her on the GINA legislation. With a Democratic majority in both the House and the Senate, Slaughter believed could overcome RTL opposition and finally have GINA signed into law. Early on, Slaughter realized it was not that easy and that she needed my help and advice on how to deal with the Right-to-Life concerns. She also realized that if she was going to have her legislation signed into law, she would have to placate President George W. Bush as he would veto GINA if RTL still had concerns with the language.

My orders were made very clear by Chairman of the Energy and Commerce Committee John Dingell, who barked at me, "Stupak, I do not know what the hell is going on with RTL and GINA, but work it out!"

Once I heard everyone's concerns it was not difficult to draft appropriate language to resolve the issue after twelve years of stalemate. As intended, GINA legislation would prevent insurance companies and employers from using genetic information as a basis for discrimination in determining various insurance rates and policies offered to consumers. Right-to-Life insisted that unborn and adopted children should also be protected against genetic discrimination. I believe Right-to-Life's concerns were either never adequately communicated or fell on deaf ears. Once we all understood RTL's concerns it only took a couple of drafts of legislative language to reach an agreement. Representatives Joe Pitts, Chris Smith, Diana DeGette, Louise Slaughter and I developed acceptable language which addressed RTL's concerns that children, including fetuses, embryos and adopted children, must be covered by the non-discriminatory protections of GINA. Once this RTL concern was addressed, the legislation easily passed both the House and Senate.

During the floor debate on GINA, Congresswoman Slaughter asked me to speak specifically on the Life issues and how they were resolved so there would be no last-minute withholding of votes by Right-to-Life Democrats and Republicans. During the debate on GINA legislation I emphasized how changes made in the bill "… cleared up any confusion as to whether families can be discriminated against based on the genetic material of their unborn child or a child under consideration for adoption." Further, I stated to my colleagues,

"As genetic testing becomes increasingly common, these provisions [in GINA] will ensure that genetic material gathered through pre-implementation genetic diagnoses, amniocentesis, or future techniques are not used to limit families' access to health care." I encouraged my fellow Democrats and Republicans to support the legislation without any further changes. GINA passed overwhelmingly in the House and the Senate opposition melted away.

On May 21, 2008, President George W. Bush held a bill-signing ceremony for the GINA legislation at the Ronald Reagan Building with Louise Slaughter, Jim Oberstar, and me offset by a gaggle of Republicans.

Sadly, only one year later, I was constantly attacked by Louise Slaughter for my RTL position during the health care debate. In fact, in November of 2009, when I presented the Stupak Amendment before the Rules Committee chaired by Rep. Slaughter, she would not even sit in the committee room when I made my presentation. She and the other Democratic women on the Rules Committee walked out of the committee room in protest before I even testified. So much for a "thank you" for helping to pass her legislation, which had languished in the Senate for twelve years. Apparently, Louise Slaughter still couldn't understand or acknowledge the fact that Members of Congress with deeply held beliefs could still work together in a respectful manner.

CHAPTER 18

★ ★ ★

A Promise Made (November 4, 2008)

I never dreamed I would serve in Congress as long as I did but every time I resolved to leave I would be convinced to stay one more term. One more term turned into eighteen years.

I wanted to leave in 2004 because I was so angry with President George W. Bush for going to war with Iraq. However, I decided to stay in Congress with the intention of helping John Kerry defeat him in the presidential election of that year. I campaigned throughout my district, challenging President Bush to end his illegal, immoral and unethical war in Iraq. Despite my passionate crusade as I crisscrossed northern Michigan on behalf of Kerry for President, John Kerry lost when Ohio went for the incumbent, President George W. Bush. I was reelected by a comfortable margin.

In 2006, I had raised very little money for my reelection, as I had been ready to retire. I met with Rahm Emmanuel, who was Chair of the Democratic Congressional Campaign Committee to discuss my reelection. To Rahm's credit, he was meeting with all of the incumbent Democratic representatives to encourage them to prepare for a tough campaign. Rahm knew that if he could convince enough moderate and conservative Democrats in swing districts to run, we could take back the Majority after twelve years in the Minority.

I held a congressional district in which no Democrat had ever served consecutive terms. I was in my seventh term and was now contemplating retirement. When I made my intentions known to Rahm, he was pleasant at first and tried to convince me for the good of the Democratic Party to seek reelection. But once I reiterated my desire to leave, he unloaded a profanity-laced tirade at me for being so selfish and not caring about the Party. He told me that I was wrong to want a different life than that of being a Member of Congress. Rahm was wrong with his profanity but correct in his belief that I was the ideal candidate to hold the district. After being called "an ungrateful mother f_____," one too many times, however, I wanted to simply say, "Screw you, I am out of here."

Each time I thought about retiring, I found it difficult to do so because I had not fulfilled all three of my promises to my constituents. Congress still had not passed health care. In fact, we had never even come close and I was beginning to believe that health care was a promise that would go unfulfilled. I was not ready to throw in the towel, but it was getting harder to see a way forward for Congress to pass health care legislation. While health care and the cost of prescription drugs were issues that Americans were concerned about, Congress was still not willing to tackle the problem.

By now the war in Iraq was extremely unpopular and Democrats were on the verge of winning back the House. I had a real shot at becoming Chairman of the Oversight and Investigations subcommittee. I had defended the Democratic priorities on the O/I committee for the past twelve years and I was the de facto Ranking Member. So once again, I decided to stay.

The Democrats did in fact take back the Majority in the US House in 2006, and I became Chairman of the Oversight and Investigations subcommittee of the Energy and Commerce Committee. The Oversight and Investigations subcommittee was a natural fit for me due to my law enforcement and legal background. I loved being Chairman of Oversight and Investigations. I will write more about that role later, as many of my investigations pertained to the health care issues, which helped shape the Affordable Care Act.

The Energy and Commerce Committee was chaired by my close friend and mentor, John Dingell. The world and Congress were both better places for me than before.

Still, I wanted to leave at the end of 2008. But it was a presidential election year and regardless of whether the Democratic nominee was Hillary Clinton or Barack Obama, the Democrats were going to win. Both candidates promised to make health care a top priority in their presidency; I therefore felt that I had to stay for one more term. I would have one more opportunity to fulfill my last unmet campaign promise: to provide all Americans with access to affordable, quality health care.

On November 4, 2008, the Democrats continued to expand their majority in the House and Senate, and Barack Obama was elected the 44th President of the United States. As the President-elect addressed the nation from Grant Park in Chicago, I was with my small cadre of campaign staff and political supporters in Marquette, Michigan, and began to uncork the first bottle of champagne. I leaned over towards Laurie and said, "I have run my last race, we will pass health care and I will retire as Congressman." Laurie just smiled and said, "We will see."

I do not know if Laurie truly believed me at that moment, but I was tired of never being home. I could envision the accomplishment of my last legislative objective and feeling that I could finally retire from Congress. My district had become even larger geographically than when I first ran for Congress and now encompassed thirty-one and a half counties. The Republican gerrymandering had removed Traverse City from my district and it now stretched 600 miles from end to end. I was tired of traveling every weekend in a district that spanned 600 miles, two time zones, bordered a foreign country and was separated by three of the five Great Lakes. I was tired and I wanted to do something else with my life. I was ready to pass health care. I was ready to finish the race. I was ready to leave Congress.

On election night, I was happy, relieved, and could not wait to get started on health care reform. With my friend Congressman John Dingell chairing the Energy and Commerce Committee, we would pass bipartisan health care reform legislation. With Dingell as Chair,

I would be deeply involved in the process and the drafting of the historic legislation.

Let the good times roll. I had just crushed my opponent and President Obama had actually won the First Congressional District. I had pulled out all the stops for Obama and we had both won big. However, I knew that the real winners would be the American people when we passed national health care.

I did not know that sixteen days later the Democratic Caucus would vote to oust Congressman John Dingell as Chair of the Energy and Commerce Committee and replace him with Henry Waxman of California. John Dingell's removal and the way in which it was orchestrated only cemented my decision to leave Washington at the end of the 111th Congress. January of 2011 could not come fast enough for me after Chairman Dingell lost his election for Chairmanship.

CHAPTER 19

★ ★ ★

Waxman v Dingell (November 20, 2008)

The day following the November 4, 2008 general election, while I was basking in the glow of our ever-expanding Democratic Majority and reflecting on the historic significance and excitement surrounding the election of Barack Obama as the 44th President of the United States, I was anxiously awaiting the beginning of the legislative session of the 111th Congress.

Suddenly my home phone rang and jolted me from my thoughts. The caller was Congressman Henry Waxman. Henry was second in seniority on the Energy and Commerce Committee, had over thirty years in Congress, and was currently the Chairman of the Oversight and Government Reform Committee. He informed me that he would be challenging John Dingell for Chairman of the Energy and Commerce Committee. I asked him why he was challenging Dingell and he stated that he felt that we only had a limited amount of time to pass President Obama's agenda and that John Dingell would not move the legislation quickly enough.

While I questioned Henry, he stayed on his message that Dingell would not get the job done quickly enough and that now was the time to move on health care, climate change, and an energy package. Waxman's argument was that it would take John Dingell far too long to pass legislation and that Congress, with a large Democratic majority, needed to act quickly and decisively during the newly elected President's honeymoon period.

I countered Waxman's argument and stated that I believed that the American people wanted Congress to work together in a bipartisan manner and that they were tired of gridlock and infighting. The results of the election had just proven that fact with the election of Barack Obama, who had promised to change Washington and had stated, "There are no red states nor blue states, just Americans." Henry was not interested in bipartisan legislation; he was only interested in moving the Democratic agenda. I also told Henry that challenging Mr. Dingell after he just had his knee replaced a week earlier was a cheap shot, knowing that it would be difficult for John to personally meet with Democratic Members before the Caucus vote. I was convinced that nothing I said would have made any difference to Henry; I was not going to change his mind. Knowing how close I was to John Dingell and the fact that we were both from Michigan, Henry's call to me was probably the last of thirty-four courtesy calls to the Democratic Members currently serving on the Energy and Commerce Committee.

Although I vehemently disagreed with Waxman, I understood that he had given generously to members of the incoming freshman class who would be voting for the next Chairman of the Energy and Commerce Committee. These incoming freshmen Democratic Members had received thousands of dollars for their elections from Waxman's Campaign Committee; Henry would now call in a favor and ask for their support as he had supported them. I had a sick feeling in the pit of my stomach as I hung up the phone.

I quickly called Dingell's office and relayed my phone conversation with Waxman to Dennis Fitzgibbons. Dennis was Dingell's Committee Staff Director and he assured me that the staff members were taking the challenge to the Chairman very seriously and were confident that he would defeat Waxman. The Dingell staff accused Speaker Nancy Pelosi of encouraging Waxman to oppose him in the race for Chair so she would have greater control over the committee. Nancy Pelosi could control Waxman, but she could not control John Dingell. I advised the Dingell staff to start counting votes and stop pointing fingers.

Dennis said that Dingell had had his knee replaced and was at home recuperating but would be back in time for the Caucus vote for Chair. Chairman Dingell might be back in time for the vote, but what about campaigning for the Chairmanship? I felt that Dennis was not taking the Waxman challenge seriously and that the Dingell Chairmanship was in greater jeopardy than he realized. A few hours later, I received a call from John asking me to join his Whip Team. There was no question about it: I would work my butt off for Mr. Dingell. He provided me with a list of current Members as well as incoming freshmen with whom I should speak to garner support for retaining John D. Dingell as Chairman of the Energy and Commerce Committee. I also wrote a couple of checks from my campaign account to incoming Democratic Freshmen who had campaign debt. As I handed checks to these freshmen Members, I reminded them what a legislative giant Chairman Dingell had been and that we needed his wise leadership to promote the President's agenda.

Prior to the Democratic Caucus convening to vote for our Party leadership and Committee Chairs, the Democratic Steering and Policy Committee meets with all the candidates and makes recommendations to the Caucus. Even though Speaker Pelosi appoints most of the Members to the Steering and Policy Committee, it was believed by Dingell supporters that John had an excellent chance of winning the committee's endorsement. Both candidates viewed the Steering and Policy Committee recommendation to the Caucus as crucial to their chances of winning or retaining the Chairmanship of the Energy and Commerce Committee. Dingell's Whip Team counted the votes and we were confident that John Dingell would garner twenty-six votes to Waxman's twenty-five. Even if it ended in a tied vote, neither candidate could claim that they had the endorsement of the Steering and Policy Committee. If it was a tied vote the Dingell supporters were ready to argue that since there was no endorsement by the Steering and Policy Committee, there was no need to switch horses in the middle of the stream.

Pelosi was also counting votes and she did not "...allow three of Mr. Dingell's supporters on the steering committee to vote because their committee chairmanships had not yet been ratified, and a fourth was absent." (Waxman Advances in Struggle to Wrest Committee from Dingell, *New York Times*, November 19, 2008). Nancy Pelosi not only used her considerable influence as Speaker to deny Chairman Dingell the Steering and Policy Committee endorsement, she had employed parliamentary tactics as well.

On November 20, 2008, the Democratic Caucus convened in the Cannon Caucus room to approve the recommendations of the Steering and Policy Committee. Losing the Steering and Policy Committee endorsement created an additional hurdle for us to overcome as the endorsement carried an especially strong influence with the in-coming freshmen.

The Pelosi-Dingell feud dates back to 2002, when Nancy Pelosi wrote a $5,000 check to John Dingell's primary opponent, Congresswoman Lynn Rivers. Reapportionment pitted the two veteran Democratic Members against each other when their districts were combined following the 2000 census. While Dingell easily disposed of Lynn Rivers in the primary, he would often joke that he had 5,000 reasons not to trust Nancy Pelosi. John Dingell often complained that when he was Chair, Speaker Pelosi would tell him that she wanted major pieces of legislation completed and reported out of his committee by such and such a date. Dingell would curtly reply that good legislation takes time and it is not determined by a date on the calendar. Chairman John D. Dingell did not appreciate the Speaker meddling in his committee affairs.

As the Democrats gathered in the Cannon Caucus Room, the Dingell whip team was confident but we knew that it was going to be a close race. Would Members who claimed they were supporting John Dingell actually vote for him, or were we doomed to experience the painful difference between a caucus and a cactus?

Quite often during my time in Congress the cactus/caucus quip attributed to Mo Udall came to mind. It is a classic retort from the quick-witted Udall. During his race for Majority Leader in the US House of Representatives, Mo fell a couple votes short. As he stepped out of the Democratic caucus room after narrowly losing his race for Majority Leader, Congressman Udall approached reporters and said that he now understood, "...the difference between a caucus and a cactus. With a cactus, the pricks are on the outside."

Right up until the time of the caucus vote, the Dingell Whip Team reviewed the lists detailing who was for us and who was against. I again reminded my colleagues of the difference between a cactus and a caucus. As many times as we went over the list, we knew deep down that some Members who were listed as John Dingell supporters might ultimately vote against him.

The night before the vote, Mike Doyle and I went over the Whip list one last time. We thought we had just enough votes for John Dingell to retain his chairmanship. However, we were unsure of the incoming freshmen Members of our Democratic Caucus. We knew that Waxman had supported many of the new freshmen Members financially; now he was calling in their votes. Did we have enough votes to offset those Members who claimed they were supporting Dingell but would actually vote for Waxman in the secret ballot?

As Congressman Dingell was still in a wheelchair following his surgery, it was decided that I would accompany him into the caucus room and Mike Doyle and several other Members would speak in support of Dingell's bid for Chairman. All the Members spoke eloquently and from the heart in their support of Mr. Dingell. We all knew it would be a close vote.

When the Waxman supporters began to speak, they complimented John Dingell on a brilliant career. They made it sound as if Dingell was retiring from Congress. They all were very gracious and put forth their best arguments as to why Henry Waxman should be elected chairman.

However, I was surprised and disappointed by the harshness of Congressman Bruce Braley's (D-Iowa) remarks. Braley attacked Dingell for not doing enough in the last session of Congress and for being too cozy with the Republicans. According to Braley, it would take John Dingell years, not months, to pass health care and climate change. He claimed that Dingell's better days had passed him by. Braley's comments were aligned with Waxman's, but Braley was blunt, rude, and insulting.

Braley had only been a Member of the Energy and Commerce Committee for two years and had little knowledge of John Dingell's legislative accomplishments during his fifty-year congressional career. Braley was the only speaker supporting Henry Waxman who attacked John Dingell personally during the speeches. Because of Braley's attacks on Mr. Dingell, I refused to support him in his 2014 US Senate run.

The two weeks of intense campaigning by both camps were over. Henry Waxman and John Dingell addressed the caucus and it was time to vote. I found myself wishing we did not have to vote at that moment because John had difficulty addressing the caucus. His voice was weak, he did not always speak directly into the microphone, and many of his words were lost. John Dingell suddenly looked all of his eighty-two years. Considering his health situation, Dingell did very well but he physically could not stand erect and his weak voice portrayed a feeble leader. He was not the John Dingell many of us had come to know, respect, and sometimes even fear. This was not the impression one would wish to showcase to newly elected Members of Congress who never heard or knew of John Dingell before their election to the US House of Representatives.

Each Member of the caucus cast his or her vote on paper ballots and placed them in large wooden ballot boxes. Each camp had three tally keepers who would count the votes outside of the Cannon Caucus room. As the tally keepers returned to the Cannon Caucus room to announce the results, we all strained to determine the vote count from the faces of the tally keepers. Our man Bob Brady (D-PA) was on the tally team. Mike and I locked eyes on Brady as he entered the caucus room and we instantly knew that Mr. Dingell had lost.

When the vote was announced, Henry Waxman had received 137 votes to Mr. Dingell's 122. Henry Waxman was now the Chairman of the Energy and Commerce Committee. I wheeled Mr. Dingell to the back of the Cannon Caucus Room and into an anteroom where Mike and the rest of our Whip Team had gathered. It was the first time that I had witnessed Members of Congress shedding tears over a caucus election. Mr. Dingell held his head high and was very gracious. He reminded us that we had important work to do with a new president-elect and majorities in both the House and Senate. John Dingell reminded us that it was still up to us, as Dingell Democrats, to influence and pass legislation. It was up to us to move health care, climate change, and the President's economic package. Mr. Dingell held back his disappointment but we could not. The pain on Mr. Dingell's face as he spoke bravely of our need to move beyond the vote and support our new president spoke volumes about the character of John Dingell.

I was totally disgusted with the Democratic Caucus. As Mike and I discussed many times later when reflecting on the vote, it was obvious that John Dingell won the vote of the incumbent members of the caucus but lost the vote of the newly elected freshmen, who only knew him in his wheelchair appearing frail and weak. They could not envision the intellectual youth and vitality of this legislative giant.

Our suspicion that the newly elected Members of the Democratic Caucus elected Henry Waxman to the Chairmanship was reaffirmed when it was brought to our attention that Waxman had not paid his Democratic Congressional Campaign Committee (DCCC) dues but instead had funneled his money to Democratic challengers in the November election. These newly elected freshmen who had been the recipients of Henry's financial support had been reminded that they owed him their votes.

In the meantime, John Dingell had raised over three million dollars for the DCCC. Although he gave some money to Democratic candidates, his contributions were not even close to the amounts that Henry Waxman had given. John Dingell fulfilled his commitment to the caucus, for the good of the caucus, and not for his personal gain. John Dingell did what was best for the Democratic Party, not what was best for John Dingell. Once again, it was the newly elected members of the Democratic Caucus who defeated John Dingell, not the people who knew him, worked with him, and loved him.

I was so disappointed with the Dingell/Waxman vote that I was ready to leave Congress immediately. Dingell had given his whole life to the Congress and they had thrown him out like a dog. If there was no loyalty or respect for the longest-serving Member of the US House of Representatives, why should my family and I continue to bust our butts to hold my historically Republican district? I had been elected nine times. I was the longest-serving Member of Congress from Michigan's Upper Peninsula. I was an anomaly; I was out of step with my party on abortion, gun control, and budgetary issues, but I always tried to find compromise and build coalitions to pass legislation. I could work with both Republicans and Democrats and the people of my district knew me and trusted me.

I knew my leaving Congress would disappoint Mr. Dingell, so I quietly filed away my feelings of disgust and vowed to keep my vow to Laurie that I had run my last race. There was no going back on my promise now. I would gladly leave Congress at the end of my two-year commitment, but we needed to pass health care first.

I could envision accomplishing my third, most difficult and elusive goal of providing health care for all Americans. The goal was within my sights but it had just become more difficult with Henry Waxman as Chairman of the Energy and Commerce Committee. Henry would ram through the legislation, he would be ruthless when necessary and he would piss everybody off in the process.

Suddenly, health care for all Americans seemed even further out of reach without Mr. Dingell wielding the gavel. We had come so far and we were so close. I vowed that I would not allow the Dingell loss to become a deterrent in my legislative effort to pass health care. But for now, the immediate question was: with the Dingell loss, would I still hold my seat as Chairman of the Oversight and Investigations subcommittee?

My Chairmanship could be in jeopardy due to the fact that Mr. Dingell was now just another Member on the Committee. I was one of John Dingell's closest confidants on the committee and in the Congress; would I be allowed to retain my Chairmanship of the Oversight and Investigations subcommittee now that Henry Waxman was Chairman of Energy and Commerce? Waxman had made no bones about the fact that he did not support me for a position on the Energy and Commerce Committee because I was Pro-Life. Now, I was afraid that Waxman would dump me as Chairman of Oversight and Investigations because not only was I Pro-Life, I was a staunch Dingell supporter.

A few hours after the caucus vote I received a call from Henry Waxman stating that he would like me and all the other subcommittee chairs to stay on. Henry said he had an aggressive agenda to pass and he needed the committee leadership to work with him to pass Democratic priorities in the limited period of the President's "honeymoon." Henry also asked if I would work with Phil Barnett, his incoming committee staff director, to conduct a series of investigations into several issues surrounding the health insurance industry. I advised Henry that I would welcome an opportunity to do so; health care would be my priority and I looked forward to passing landmark national health care legislation in the not-too-distant future.

Henry and I were on the same page when it came to health care, but our styles were different when it came to working with Republicans. We were both very firm in our investigative approach and, when appropriate, wouldn't hesitate to go after witnesses with piercing questions. However, Henry had no patience with the Republicans and put forth limited effort in working with them.

I did not tell Henry, Dingell, or anyone else that this would be my last term in Congress. I confided in Mike Doyle that I was ready to leave after the Dingell vote, but Mike just thought that I was still angry over the loss. In truth, I had lost my desire to remain in the US House of Representatives.

CHAPTER 20

★ ★ ★

Crisis Management (2009)

Barack Obama was sworn in as the 44th President of the United States on January 20, 2009. The largest crowd ever to witness the inauguration of a President stretched across the National Mall and spilled into the side streets between Pennsylvania and Independence Avenues. It was estimated that well over one million people came to witness history: the swearing in of the first African American President of the United States. Barack Obama had been a state senator four years earlier and now held the most powerful office in the world. During the campaign, President Obama promised to change the way Washington conducted its business, to end the partisan bickering and address the nation's problems head-on. The Obama campaign led people to believe that anything and everything was possible with Barack Obama as President of the United States. President Obama told the admiring crowd during his inaugural address that the problems America faced were "…serious and they are many. They will not be met easily or in a short span of time. But know this, America---they will be met."

The President went on to state that:

"Starting today, we must pick ourselves up,

Dust ourselves off, and begin again the work of remaking America."

The 111th Congress had convened and the Democratic Party held a large Majority in the US House with 257 Democrats and 178 Republicans. In the Senate, with two Independent Senators caucusing with the Democrats, the Democrats had counted on a super sixty-vote majority to prevent filibusters by the forty Republicans. The super majority that the President and the Democrats counted on to move legislation through the Senate ebbed and flowed with vacancies and the deaths of Senator Ted Kennedy on August 25, 2009 and Senator Robert Byrd on June 28, 2010. Even filling the US Senate seat left vacant by President Obama's election was a fiasco: Governor Rod Blagojevich solicited bribes for the appointment and was eventually indicted for trying to cash in on his power to select Barack Obama's successor.

The Minnesota US Senate seat went through several recounts until Al Franken was determined the winner and sworn into the Senate on July 7, 2009. Finally, the Senate Democrats had a sixty-seat majority. It was, however, short lived; seven months later, Republican Scott Brown won the special Massachusetts election and was sworn into the Senate on February 4, 2010. The opportunity to enact significant legislation and to remake America never materialized in the Senate. Witnessing the maturations of the Senate only reinforced what we, as House Members, often said: "The Senate is a place were good legislation goes to die."

I agreed with the President's inaugural remarks about remaking America and that the problems our nation faced were serious, they were many and they would not be met in a short span of time. I don't know if the Democratic leadership forgot the President's warning or were drunk on their own power with the size of their majority in both chambers, but they ignored the concerns of rank-and-file House Democrats. It appeared that the Democratic leadership did not have a strategy to pass meaningful legislation; instead, they would just bludgeon Members into voting for their legislative agenda.

I do not know if it was a lack of leadership or fear of political backlash, but the Democratic Senate leadership announced before the House voted on climate change legislation that they would not take up the legislation. So why then did President Obama and Speaker

Pelosi require Democratic House Members to walk the plank and vote on climate change legislation? Why was climate change one of the first polarizing, politically charged issues in the 111th Congress and not health care?

President Obama's first initiative was the economic stimulus package, which was aimed at reversing the financial meltdown in the United States and cost more than one trillion dollars. Once again, I do not know if it was lack of experience or simple arrogance, but Members of Congress had no opportunity for input regarding funding for projects and much-needed infrastructure that could help stimulate jobs in their congressional districts. One-third of the stimulus package was devoted to tax cuts in the form of a slightly lower payroll tax. The extra dollars in the workers' paycheck were so inconsequential that no one believed they had even received a tax cut at all. We tried to advise the Administration to send everyone a $250 check like President George W. Bush did, but our counsel fell on deaf ears. Members went home and touted a tax cut that no one believed existed.

The stimulus package turned out to be an albatross around the neck of every Democratic Member of Congress. The electorate became angry with us for spending a trillion dollars with nothing to show for it. Because of the way the stimulus package was put together and rolled out, Members of Congress had no say in the legislation and did not embrace it as their own. Members could not point to any credible benefits for their constituents. The Stimulus projects were selected and announced by the Secretary of some Department who none of our constituents knew or cared about. Constituents wanted to know where their Member of Congress was, and they wanted their questions answered.

The first seven months of the Obama Administration was a period of tremendous legislative action that was poorly managed. Legislation was passed over the political sacrifices of individual Members of Congress. The legislative initiatives were not ours but those of the new Administration. The Administration and the Democratic leadership put forth a legislative agenda without meaningful input from Members of Congress. They were tone-deaf to the needs of the Members, and seemed to care only about securing the 218 votes necessary to pass legislation in the House. In the Senate, they needed and had the sixty-vote super majority necessary to cut off debate and pass their ambitious agenda. Excellent ideas on the stimulus package were completely ignored and all decisions on the package were made in the White House. Even though the stimulus package was a disaster politically, it did manage to stabilize the free-falling US economy.

During those first several months of the Obama Administration, I was entrenched in legislation and devoted my time to trying to save the US auto industry with the government loans to GM and Chrysler and implementation of the highly successful Cash for Clunkers program.

In the Energy and Commerce Committee, I was also intimately involved with climate change legislation, introduction of the safe drug disposal of unused pharmaceuticals, health care reform and continual hearings on food safety and the unethical practices of the health insurance industry. While I was involved in many issues, I was focused on health care and my promise to Chairman Waxman to hold hearings on some of the questionable practices of the health insurance industry.

As Chairman of the Oversight and Investigations, I held hearings on the health insurance industry practice of rescission of individual health insurance policies without cause when the insured became ill. Hearings were held on meaningless catastrophic health insurance policies that were supposed to cover major medical costs but in reality covered very little. The O/I committee held hearings on the high cost of health insurance for small businesses and Medicare Advantage Plans, which provided private insurance for people over sixty-five. Medicare Advantage costs the government more than traditional Medicare coverage and is a giveaway to the rich and the health insurance industry. I also held the first hearing on nursing home standards, which had not been reviewed since the enactment of federal standards in the early 1980s.

Each of these Oversight and Investigations hearings was used to highlight the problems everyday Americans confronted as they attempted to maintain health insurance coverage for their family. Our challenge was not only to identify the problems in the health insurance industry but also to develop solutions to the problems. The results and recommendations of the Oversight and Investigations committee hearings formed the basis for parts of the health care legislation that was drafted by the staff of the Energy and Commerce Committee. The Energy and Commerce Committee had the greatest jurisdiction over health care in the US House of Representatives.

CHAPTER 21

★ ★ ★

Waxman's Committee (2009-2010)

nergy and Commerce Chairman Henry Waxman wasted no time bringing up controversial bills. First out of the shoot was climate change. Congressman Ed Markey (D-MA) had been chairing a special select committee on the issue for the past two years and was eager to pass climate change legislation. Several of the Democratic members on the Energy and Commerce Committee, including me, believed it was a mistake to begin the legislative agenda with climate change legislation. Many of us believed that climate change would be the most contentious issue between the two parties as well as politically sensitive to the voters back home- especially during an economic recession.

Chairman Henry Waxman pushed committee members to pass climate change legislation without any Republican support. Even though several moderate Democratic Members of the committee repeatedly told Waxman that we would rather deal with health care as opposed to climate change first, Henry simply said the Energy and Commerce Committee was going to pass climate change and health care would be second. I don't know if Speaker Pelosi ordered Chairman Waxman to make climate change the first order of business for the Energy and Commerce Committee or whether Waxman promised the liberal Democratic Members on the Committee in exchange for their support for his Chairmanship, but it was definitely a mistake to begin with climate change.

I believe climate change is a serious issue, especially after witnessing the water level in the Great Lakes swing widely from record high to record low levels within just ten years. However, it was too divisive of an issue to start off the Committee's ambitious legislative year, especially as the Senate had announced that it would not consider climate change legislation.

The Energy and Commerce committee went to work holding hearings and floating legislative trial balloons on climate change, none of which had any appeal to me or to Midwestern or oil patch Democrats such as Gene Green of Texas. Waxman kept pushing legislative proposals and holding individual meetings with Democratic Committee members to gain their support for climate change legislation.

The climate change legislation was very contentious and there was some question as to whether we had enough votes to pass the bill out of committee. The Democratic Members of the Energy and Commerce Committee were invited to the White House to meet with President Obama on May 5, 2009, to discuss climate change legislation with the President and Department of Energy Secretary Steven Chu. This was the first time in the history of the Energy and Commerce Committee that all Democratic Members of the Committee were invited to the White House to confer with the president on legislation. It was extremely rare for a whole committee to be invited to the White House to discuss legislation.

To me, this invitation presented an unexpected opportunity to express my concern to President Obama that the Committee was not taking up health care. I asked him why we were taking up climate change legislation when the Senate had declared that it would not do so. I suggested to President Obama that the Energy and Commerce Committee should instead be discussing health care legislation. He responded that he had to first address the dire economic meltdown the country found itself in and, thanks to Democratic Members, we had passed the Economic Stimulus package. The President went on to say that the House Democratic leadership now wanted to move to climate change legislation.

Perhaps the concerns that Members had voiced during the White House meeting with President Obama about not addressing health care helped to spur some action on the issue because eight days later, on May 13, 2009, Chairman Waxman held a briefing to exchange ideas on potential national health care legislation.

The briefing was held late in the morning and most Democrats attended to discuss health care reform. As of May, very few Democrats had had input on the proposed draft legislation on health care. It was unusual for most of the Committee Democrats to attend a briefing, but this was health care legislation and Members were interested in what would be proposed. The Democratic Members of the Energy and Commerce Committee campaigned on national health care and had offered ideas on health care reform to the Energy and Commerce Committee staff.

As a senior member and subcommittee chairman, I took my usual seat on the upper row of the dais in the Energy and Commerce Committee Room. As Members filed in they took their usual seats as if we were holding a formal committee hearing. Chairman Waxman called the meeting to order and quickly turned it over to the Energy and Commerce health care staff. Chairman Waxman simply said that the staff had been working very hard to put together legislation and incorporate the concerns of Members into a legislative proposal, which was now taking shape. The Chairman and the staff wished to bring Members up to date about the proposed legislation, and indicated that health care would be the next major issue the committee would tackle. Chairman Waxman stated that the staff would brief Members and seek input before the final draft would be presented. The other Members and I sat back and listened while the committee's health care policy advisor Karen Nelson explained its version of health care and complained about all the considerations special interest groups had requested in the legislation.

I listened and took minimal notes on the proposed health care legislation outlined by the staff. It became clear to me that the Health Committee staff had already written the health care legislation. Members pressed Karen Nelson as to why this program or that program was being placed in the health care legislation. Karen just kept repeating that this would be the only opportunity to pass health care and everything related to health care would be included in the legislation.

Finally, I could not take any more and just blurted out, "This proposed legislation is already written, it is too complex and it will never fly." I told my colleagues that this legislation was way too complicated and reminded them of the KISS concept: Keep It Simple Stupid. Therefore, I advocated for health care legislation that would expand Medicaid, SCHIP, and Medicare for individuals fifty-five years of age and older. Then, for all the rest of the uninsured Americans: allow them to buy into the Federal Employees Health Benefits Package. I further explained that federal employees accessed health care under the Federal Employees Health Benefit Package in every part of nation from Menominee, Michigan to Monterrey, California and from Alaska to Alabama.

> "We should allow uninsured individuals to buy into the Federal Employees Health Benefit Package (FEHBP). The FEHBP can work for all Americans. There was no reason to reinvent the wheel in the health care legislation. All of these programs that the special interests insisted upon are wonderful programs but they cannot be included in this health care bill or you will kill the bill under its own weight."

> Finally, I said, "Let me be the skunk at the party. I want to be very clear, abortion MUST NOT BE part of health care. Abortion is the one issue that will destroy our caucus and derail health care reform. There should be no public funding for abortion. It is an issue that you cannot win. Do not include abortion in health care."

While I was emphatic in my statement, I could tell it fell on deaf ears.

I saw Mike Doyle a little later on the House floor and he said, "Well, I guess you were indeed the skunk at the party and you made your feelings very clear." I told Mike that abortion will kill health care, if all the bullshit they are putting in the bill doesn't kill it first. Mike laughed and said, "That is what I like about you, buddy- you don't sugarcoat anything!" I just smiled and shook my head. This health care bill was going to be a disaster.

From that briefing by Karen Nelson and the health subcommittee staff, I was convinced that I had better take my concerns about abortion being included in the health care legislation to Speaker Nancy Pelosi. I would need to convince my fellow Democratic RTL Members to sign a letter to the Speaker, even though they believed it would be a waste of time. The members of the Democratic leadership were all Pro-Choice and would simply ignore our warning.

If John Dingell had remained Chairman of the Energy and Commerce Committee, I believe he would have immediately begun holding hearings on health care and would have worked to formulate a bipartisan bill. No doubt it would have taken John Dingell longer to develop a consensus on health care between Democratic and Republican committee members, but the legislation would have been bipartisan and it would have undergone a smoother legislative process in Congress.

CHAPTER 22

* * *

Shot across the Bow (July 2009)

In a CBS interview on June 6, 2009, a few weeks after our White House meeting, President Obama declared, "I'm Pro-Choice, but I think we also have the tradition in this town, historically, of not financing abortions as part of government-funded health care. My main focus is making sure that people have options of high quality care at the lowest possible price." The President's comments gave the RTL Democrats a shot in the arm and fostered a new willingness to sign a letter to Speaker Pelosi expressing concerns about abortion coverage in the proposed health care legislation.

In the Congressional RTL Caucus, we discussed the possibility of elective abortion coverage being included in the health care legislation. It was decided that I would write a letter to Speaker Pelosi, signed only by Democratic RTL Members, stating that RTL Democratic Members would not support any health care legislation that included abortion coverage as a medical service or created a funding mechanism to pay for abortions. My fellow RTL Democrats and I worked on the correspondence. We went back and forth with drafts, attempting to craft the exact wording on abortion coverage without the benefit of seeing a draft of the health care legislation. We felt it was critical to make our feelings known on abortion coverage before a final draft of the legislation was presented to the Democratic

Caucus. It was hoped that by addressing the abortion issue early in the legislative process, we could write language that would avoid a lengthy debate and vote on abortion coverage in the health care legislation. As with the GINA legislation, I believed a reasonable solution to the issue could be reached to avoid a protracted, emotional battle that could ultimately derail health care.

Finally, on June 25, 2009, nineteen RTL Democrats speaking with one voice agreed on the wording in the letter to the Speaker. We made our intentions very clear that we would not support health care legislation if it contained funding for abortion or abortion service was a covered benefit. As we stated unequivocally, "… we cannot support any healthcare reform proposal unless it explicitly excludes abortion from the scope of any government-defined or subsidized health insurance plan. We believe that a government-defined or subsidized health insurance plan should not be used to fund abortion."

RTL Democrats had made their feelings known. It was now up to Speaker Pelosi to decide how far she wanted to push the abortion issue in health care reform. We made it clear that we would not vote for any legislation that contained public funding for abortions. The two Democratic Right-to-Life Members from West Virginia, Alan Mollohan and Nick Rahall, due to their Committee Chairmanships and because they were generally opposed to signing onto Leadership letters, independently made their feelings known to Speaker Pelosi that they agreed with the RTL correspondence and would not support health care legislation that included abortion coverage. Therefore, twenty-one Democratic Members made it clear to the Speaker that they would not support health care reform that included funding for abortions.

Speaker Nancy Pelosi never answered our correspondence. Maybe she believed that the abortion issue would just go away or she was too busy trying to placate other factions of the Democratic Party to support health care reform. Maybe the Speaker just did not seriously take our promise not to vote for health care if it contained public funding for abortion. Whatever her reason, Speaker Pelosi ignored us. It would come back to haunt her.

The June 25 Democratic RTL correspondence to the Speaker was picked up by some of the mainstream media such as the *New York Times, US News & World Report* and *Time* magazine. In its July 8 issue, *Time* magazine wrote an article about the warning letter to Speaker Pelosi. This edition of *Time* delved into the whole abortion issue, stating that it could sink health care reform. Still, the Speaker remained silent.

Even though Speaker Pelosi never answered our June 25 correspondence, the Congressional RTL Caucus continued to dutifully appear before the Rules Committee and asked for our traditional RTL riders to the appropriations bills that were beginning to make their way to the House floor for approval. RTL riders had always tagged along as amendments to the appropriations bills, preventing the federal government from promoting, encouraging or paying for abortions.

The yearly RTL riders, which the Speaker had allowed in the last Congress, were now being shut out of the appropriations process. For the last thirty-two years (1977-2009), the Right-to-Life Riders to the appropriations bills were either included in the base legislation or were made in order by the Rules Committee as a House floor amendment for debate and vote. But in 2009, the RTL riders were being excluded from the appropriation bills and our requests for amendments were silently denied by the Rules Committee. With each appropriations bill, I was joined by Congressman Chris Smith (R-NJ) as co-chair of the bi-partisan Congressional Right-to-Life Caucus. We personally appeared and requested that our traditional amendments, known as riders, be made in order. Congresswoman Louise Slaughter would simply smile, thank us for our testimony, and then behind closed doors deny our riders without explanation.

I complained to Speaker Pelosi, the Majority Leader Steny Hoyer (D-MD), and the Majority Whip James Clyburn (D-SC) about the RTL riders not being included or allowed on the appropriations bill. I was told that our RTL riders would be in the final appropriations bill, after the Conference Committee between the House and Senate, and that I had to be patient. I was not going to be patient; I believed the Democratic leadership was going to run the string out on our RTL amendments and on me personally. The Democratic leaders in the House and Senate were Pro-Choice and the President was the most Pro-Choice president ever elected. I harbored serious doubts that the RTL riders would ever be included in the appropriations bills.

The most critical appropriation bill for RTL riders was the Labor-HHS Appropriations Bill, which funded Medicaid and federal health grants and loans. If there was one critical appropriations bill that could reverse the last thirty years of *no* public funding for abortions, it was Labor-HHS. I became more and more concerned that the Hyde Amendment language would never be made part of Labor-HHS Appropriations. The last time public funding for abortion was allowed under Medicaid was through the Labor-HHS Appropriations Bill in 1993-1994. Back then, Bill Clinton was president and Democrats controlled both the House and Senate. When the RTL amendment to ban coverage for taxpayer-funded abortions was presented on the floor, we lost the vote.

Despite a united effort by the Congressional RTL Caucus, we lost the vote to prevent public funding on the House floor in 1993 and 1994 because there were simply more Pro-Choice than Pro-Life House Members during the 103rd Congress. Pro-Life Members at least had the right to vote their conscience on protecting the sanctity of life. As disappointed as I was with the vote in 1993-1994, I had learned a lesson and was not going to sit by and let Speaker Pelosi push through the appropriations bills without our critical RTL riders. So, I huddled with my fellow RTL Democrats.

It was decided that Chris Smith and I would appear as co-chairs of the bi-partisan RTL Congressional Caucus and ask for our crucial RTL rider on the DC appropriations bill. (The technical name for the DC Appropriations Bill is the Financial Services and General Government Appropriations Act of 2010). If the Rules Committee failed to make our amendment in order, we would attempt to defeat the Rule allowing debate on the DC Appropriation Bill.

The Rule accompanying an appropriations bill is almost always a party line vote. The Rule simply begins the legislative process and allows the legislation to come to the floor for consideration and debate. In the US House of Representatives, the Rule accompanying a proposed piece of legislation sets out the length of time for debate, which amendments are to be offered, length of time to debate each amendment, and whether the minority party will be granted a Motion to Recommit.

On July 16, 2009 the Democrats, as the majority party, offered the Rule to accompany the District of Columbia Appropriations Bill. As is customary, the Rule was debated for sixty minutes, with the time equally split between the Democrats and Republicans. Once again, our RTL rider to this appropriations bill was not made in order. After the Rule debate, the vote approving the Rule for consideration of the DC Appropriations was called and nearly all 435 Members of the House of Representatives proceeded to the House floor to vote. I had secured a commitment from the RTL Democrats to vote No on the Rule. As the time to vote counted down to zero, the Rule was being defeated because approximately thirty-five Democrats joined the Republicans in voting No.

I stood in the well of the House by the Speaker's rostrum and watched as Majority Leader Steny Hoyer frantically urged Members to switch their Rule vote from No to Yes to support the Democratic Rule. The RTL Democrats did not budge and kept their No votes. I was urged by Congressman David Obey, Chairman of the Appropriations Committee, to change my vote and told him that I would not unless I elicited a promise from Leadership that our traditional RTL riders would be made in order. Further, I explained to David that not one of our riders had been made in order during this Congress. I told him that if the Speaker was not going to give us our riders, then we had no choice but to bring down the Rule on the appropriations bills.

With all the Republicans and approximately thirty-five to thirty-seven Democrats voting No, the Rule was going to be defeated.

Finally, with time expiring on the Rule vote, I walked toward Steny Hoyer, who was headed to the Pennsylvania Corner to find me. I called out to him and he turned around and yelled back at me, "What the hell are you doing?" I told him that we were taking down the Rule until our RTL riders were accepted. Hoyer said that

Leadership would include the RTL rider in the final appropriations bills. I told Steny that I did not believe it and that there would be no more games with our RTL riders. I went on, "Our taking down this Rule is a shot across the bow. We will also block the Rule for the health care legislation if we do not receive our RTL riders." Steny again asked me to change my vote and I refused.

I saw Speaker Pelosi on the floor twisting Members' arms to change their votes. Speaker Pelosi went right after the Committee Chairmen who were voting No and asked them to change their votes to Yes. The Chairs did not move to switch their vote. Speaker Pelosi then went to Congressmen John Dingell and Gary Peters of Michigan and convinced them to switch their votes from No to Yes. Of the thirty-seven Democratic Members who voted with me, Pelosi managed to convince two Members to change their vote. Neither Dingell nor Peters were Pro-Life but they felt that it was unfair of the Democratic leadership not to allow a vote on the RTL riders. By the time these gentlemen switched their votes, RTL Members had achieved their goal of sending a message to the Democratic leadership that we could and would take down the Rule on appropriations bills and even health care if RTL was not allowed our traditional riders. Even though all time for the votes on the Rule had expired, Pelosi twisted arms and the Rule passed, 216-213. Five Republicans were absent for the vote. If all the Republicans had voted, we would have had enough to defeat the Rule on the DC Appropriations.

Unfortunately, Steny Hoyer and I had a testy exchange on the floor during the Rule vote. Hoyer kept insisting that I should come to Leadership on this issue. I repeatedly reassured him that I had been to Leadership and that if Leadership continued to deny our RTL amendments, we would bring down every Rule. I also told him that if the Leadership presented the health care legislation with abortion coverage in it, RTL Democrats and I would defeat the Rule for consideration of the health care legislation. I emphasized that this was a warning shot. I asked him why Speaker Pelosi never answered our June 25 letter. Hoyer said that he did not know but that I could ask the Speaker herself as she walked towards us.

I turned and advised the Speaker that this was a warning shot on health care and on the rest of the appropriations bills, including Labor-HHS. Our RTL Riders had to be in the appropriation bills and the health care bill or we would block the legislation from ever coming to the floor. Speaker Pelosi was angry and said very tersely, "We can discuss this later off the floor." I shot back, "Later, like your response to our June 25 letter on abortion coverage in the health care legislation? We have never received a response." The Speaker repeated her statement, "We will sit down and discuss this issue later. The draft of the health care legislation has not been finalized." She wheeled and left the floor. I went back to the Pennsylvania corner to be harassed and congratulated by friends.

Right after this Rule vote the Republicans questioned the Chair as to the length of time allowed for the five-minute vote on the Rule. The questioning is best summarized by Congressman Westmoreland's (R-GA) question to the Chair, "So what is the reason for leaving the vote open? Clearly the outcome was changed by the vote being held open and people subsequently changing their vote." The Chair would only answer, "The vote lasted for the required minimum period."

Later, in the DC Appropriations debate, Congressman Todd Tiahrt (R-KS) offered an amendment to strike funding for abortions with federal tax dollars from the appropriations bill and the Democratic Majority tabled the amendment. Republicans and some of the RTL Democrats voted to defeat the Motion to Table the Tiahrt Amendment. We lost the Motion to Table by a vote of 225-195 and Tiahrt was not allowed to offer his amendment.

My Co-Chair of the Congressional RTL Caucus Chris Smith (R-NJ) came over and with a laugh asked, "Now do you have the Speaker's attention?" I told Chris, "Clearly Leadership understands my position now. They twisted arms to change votes this time, but next time, we will block the Rule." I mentioned further that I had told Leadership that this was a shot across the bow. If they messed with us on abortion coverage in the health care legislation, we would block the legislation from coming to the floor. Chris and I discussed writing a letter to Speaker Pelosi signed by all the Members of the bi-partisan Congressional RTL Caucus stating that we would not vote for health care if it included abortion coverage. Chris and I both felt that we could obtain more than 218 signatures on a letter, which would demonstrate that if the RTL Caucus stuck together we would block the Rule accompanying the health care legislation. We decided to write that letter to Speaker Pelosi following the August recess.

I pressed Speaker Pelosi for an answer to our June 25 letter and our subsequent RTL correspondence, but she never provided a verbal or written answer and thereby continued to ignore the concerns of the bi-partisan RTL Caucus.

CHAPTER 23

★ ★ ★

Oversight and Investigations Hearings (2009-2010)

"I think I speak for every member of the [Energy and Commerce] Committee on both sides of the aisle...that if in fact there is a practice of going in after the fact and canceling policies on technicalities, we have got to do whatever is possible to prevent that...If a citizen acts in good faith, we should expect the insurance companies who take their money to act in good faith also." Congressman Joe Barton (R-TX), Ranking Member of Energy and Commerce Committee, June 16, 2009.

Within six months of being asked by Chairman Waxman, I held hearings regarding the health insurance industry's abusive practices, which left Americans paying more and more for their health insurance yet left them with less and less coverage. Tens of thousands of individual health insurance policies were terminated or rescinded only after the policyholder became ill and needed coverage. In addition to rescissions of individual policies, the O/I subcommittee investigated consumer complaints about long-term care insurance, the predatory practices of Medicare Advantage, the worthless "underinsured" policies, and the increased costs of health care on small businesses.

Our hearings won rave reviews from my Democratic and a few Republican colleagues and provided Members of Congress with concrete examples to rebut the arguments against the need for national health care reform. More importantly, many of the health insurance industry abuses we exposed led to corrective provisions being added to the US House of Representatives' Public Health Insurance Option plan.

America's Affordable Health Choices Act, or HR-3200, was the US House of Representatives Public Option health care plan formally introduced in July of 2009. The US Senate had not decided on a plan to present to the American people, so the House of Representatives proceeded with a Public Health Insurance Option. The Public Option was a government-sponsored, not for profit health care plan. Like Medicare and private insurance plans, it was designed to be funded solely by the premiums it collected from policyholders. The health insurance policies offered under the Public Option were required to follow the same regulations placed on private insurance companies, including remaining financially solvent. No American would be forced into the Public Option because, as the name implied, the plan was an option and it would only exist as long as Americans paid into the plan. Section 162 of HR-3200 ended the health insurance practice of rescinding or terminating health insurance policies without clear and convincing evidence of fraud on the part of the policyholder.

While the Democrats had inserted a Patient Bill of Rights in HR-3200, our hearings were uncovering additional abuses in the health insurance industry that needed to be addressed to make health care accessible and affordable for all Americans.

I must give a heartfelt thank you to every Member of the Energy and Commerce Committee and our professional and personal staffs who worked diligently and with great intellect and integrity to bring forth examples of abuses that had built up over many, many years in the health insurance industry. Our staffs were incredible. They spent hours upon hours examining over 116,000 pages documenting 20,000 individual policies that were retroactively canceled or terminated once the policyholders became ill.

Our investigations spurred internal congressional and committee staff debates and fact-checking sessions to assure ourselves that our portrayal of the heartless actions of the health insurance industry were accurate and our proposed solutions were realistic.

The insurance industry abuses not only jeopardized a family's health and financial security but also led to parents divorcing so one spouse could claim Medicaid to cover their medical expenses. I hope that every staff member, Member of the Energy and Commerce Committee and Democratic Member of Congress who voted for the final Affordable Care Act is filled with pride and satisfaction when one of our solutions to these health insurance abuses is mentioned in the media, at the coffee shop, or overheard in a conversation among strangers. We may never realize just how much we improved the lives of many Americans; some of the most popular provisions of the Affordable Care Act were developed, refined and enacted through the efforts of the Oversight and Investigations Subcommittee Members and staff.

We conducted a field hearing in Congressman Baron Hill's Indiana district, which was the home of a couple of major health insurance companies. At this hearing, we were approached by individuals who initially had no intention of speaking but ultimately shared their heartbreaking stories of financial ruin because they were unjustly terminated from their health insurance policy when they became seriously ill. While they had recovered from their illness, they had not recovered from the financial devastation.

Our hearings investigating the health insurance industry did not end with the passage of the Affordable Care Act in March of 2010. Our hearings ended when Democrats lost control of the US House of Representatives after the November 2010 general election. It was an honor and a privilege to conduct and direct these hearings; below are a few examples of the real American health insurance nightmares we uncovered during our investigation.

Our hearings on the health insurance industry were exhausting, emotional and time-consuming but very important. Former

Committee Chairman Joe Barton (R-TX) and I challenged the insurance industry practice of rescinding individual health insurance policies for no legitimate reason when the insured individual's medical treatment became expensive. I began this chapter with a quote from Congressman Barton following the Oversight and Investigations Committee testimony from his constituent, Robin Beaton, on June 16, 2009.

Robin Beaton carried an individual health insurance policy with Blue Cross/Blue Shield of Texas when she was diagnosed with breast cancer. A week before Robin was scheduled to undergo a mastectomy, her health insurance policy was abruptly rescinded. Blue Cross/Blue Shield rescinded her policy after its "post-claims underwriting" was triggered by Robin's doctor visit for acne. Blue Cross/Blue Shield claimed that Robin falsified her application because she failed to disclose a rapid heartbeat that had been resolved years before she applied for health insurance with "the Blues." Robin was furious, put off her breast cancer treatment and sought to have her policy reinstated so she could afford her medical treatment.

It was claimed that Robin's review of her medical application and history was triggered when she visited her doctor for acne treatment. Acne has nothing to do with breast cancer, so why would it trigger a "post-claims underwriting" review?

Robin contacted her Congressman, Joe Barton, and he raised hell with Blue Cross/Blue Shield of Texas. Slowly and reluctantly, the Blues undertook a review of Robin's file and finally agreed to reinstate her policy. By then, Robin's cancerous tumor had grown to over five centimeters and she was forced to undergo a double mastectomy and removal of lymph nodes in one arm.

Following Robin's testimony before our subcommittee, we heard from other women who stated that they, too, had experienced cancellation of their insurance policies based on some flimsy excuse after being diagnosed with breast cancer.

Our investigation discovered that health insurance companies evaluated, rated and paid bonuses to their employees based on how much money the employee saved the company by canceling individual health insurance policies. WellPoint and its subsidiaries,

Anthem Blue Cross, entered into two separate settlements with states for improperly rescinding individual policies. In 2008, the insurance companies were forced to reverse 1,770 policies and pay a ten-million-dollar penalty. Then, in February of 2009, the company was required to pay an additional fifteen million dollars in penalties and reverse another 2,300 rescissions.

Instead of reviewing the health insurance application and the applicant's medical records immediately upon submission to ensure eligibility for coverage under their health insurance policy *prior* to enrollment, the insurance companies focused on immediately collecting the monthly premium. These insurance companies set up elaborate mechanisms designed to catch any possible expensive treatment that the insured required. Insurance companies automatically triggered a "post-claims underwriting" review when certain conditions, diagnoses, or prescriptions indicate a possible treatment for leukemia, ovarian cancer, brain cancer, breast cancer, or even a predisposition toward becoming pregnant with twins.

Insurance companies implemented computer programs which contain anywhere from 1,400 to more than 2,000 diagnostic codes, which trigger a review of an insured's application and medical records. The insurance companies will find any reason to rescind the individual's insurance policy, even when the insured faces the possibility of death if they do not receive the necessary life-saving medical treatment, as occurred with Mr. Otto Raddatz.

Otto Raddatz had purchased an individual health insurance policy with Assurant. The company launched an investigation into his health insurance application and medical records when he was diagnosed with lymphoma. Assurant rescinded his coverage days before he was scheduled to undergo a life-saving stem cell transplant. Assurant claimed that Mr. Raddatz failed to disclose that he had silent gallstones and an asymptomatic aortic aneurysm based on a CT scan five years earlier. Mr. Raddatz's doctor wrote to Assurant stating that he had never told Mr. Raddatz about either the gallstones or the aneurysm.

Assurant refused to reinstate Mr. Raddatz's health insurance to pay for his stem cell transplant. The Raddatz family contacted the Illinois Attorney General, who repeatedly pressed Assurant to reinstate his insurance coverage. Finally, Assurant relented and reinstated Mr. Raddatz's coverage, but by then it was too late. Otto's sister testified before our subcommittee because Otto died before he received the stem cell transplant that would have saved his life.

Health insurance companies rescind individual policies for pre-existing conditions, unintentional discrepancies on the insurance application, unknown medical conditions, omissions, and for unrelated incongruities. The current health insurance regulatory framework is a haphazard collection of inconsistent state and federal laws. Each state has its own regulatory system and in most states, insurance companies can deny coverage based on pre-existing injury, as I myself had experienced.

The CEOs from three insurance companies, Assurant, Golden Rule, and WellPoint, appeared at our June 16, 2009 hearing on rescissions. After receiving testimony from families devastated by their insurance companies' illegal, immoral, and unethical rescissions, I asked each CEO, "Would you commit today that your company will never rescind another policy unless there was intentionally fraudulent misrepresentation in the application?"

> Don Hamm (CEO, Assurant Health): "I would not commit to that…"

> Richard Collins (CEO, Golden Rule): "No, sir. We follow the State laws and regulations and we would not stipulate to that…"

> John Sassi (CEO, Consumer Business, WellPoint): "No, I cannot commit to that."

I was not going to allow these insurance executives off the hook and relied on my state police and attorney experience as I pressed them. I was finally able to wrangle a concession out of each of the insurance executives when I asserted to them that the passage of comprehensive health care reform would eliminate the abusive practices of health insurance denial without a finding of intentional fraudulent misrepresentation on the application.

Most Americans receive health insurance through an employer-sponsored group health insurance covering employees and sometimes their families. As the cost of health insurance has skyrocketed, more and more employers are covering just their employees and not the employees' dependents. The downturn in the economy in 2008 and 2009 left employers unable to afford health insurance for their employees. More and more individuals and families find themselves in the individual health insurance market without any negotiating leverage. Without leverage and knowledge of health insurance industry practices, individuals rely on insurance brokers to provide them with affordable, quality health insurance. Unfortunately, affordable and quality are not synonymous in the individual health care market.

Families rely on an insurance broker to provide them with a health insurance policy that will cover them for catastrophic illness or as David Null called it, "For the big 'Oh no!' moment- not for head colds." David Null and his wife had two young children and were the owners of a small air conditioning and repair service. Nulls' seven-year-old daughter, Tatum, became ill while the family was on vacation. Tatum spent seven days in a children's hospital as her kidneys began to fail. David felt secure in knowing that he had health insurance coverage through United American Health Insurance Company for this "Oh no!" moment. David was unaware that his "affordable" policy had a $30,000 cap per medical event.

Tatum blew through the cap after her first two days in the hospital. Tatum's hospital bill approached $100,000 for her seven days and she needed a kidney transplant, which would cost an additional $560,000. The hospital required a $200,000 deposit before Tatum could receive the transplant. The administrative director obtained a waiver from the hospital's key executives because David no longer had insurance that would pay any more towards Tatum's illness and upcoming treatment. The Nulls owed the hospital at least $70,000 and needed another $560,000 for the kidney transplant; Tatum's anti-rejection medication for the first three weeks after the surgery would cost an additional $86,000.

The Nulls faced financial ruin and bankruptcy to save their daughter's life, incurring $830,000 in medical expenses over a thirty-day period. The health insurance policy capped its financial exposure at $30,000, leaving the Nulls with an $800,000 debt. No matter how many insurance companies David contacted, none of them would cover Tatum or the Null family.

The Nulls worked with hospital officials, who directed the Nulls to immediately reduce their monthly income to $1,641 per month to qualify for Medicaid. Medicaid retroactively covered Tatum's hospital stay, transplant and medicine. The Nulls were forced to intentionally lower their income to remain on the government-sponsored Medicaid so Tatum could continue to receive her expensive medical treatment and anti-rejection medication, paid for by taxpayers.

Throughout our investigation, we learned of other families with individual health insurance policies who suffered a catastrophic illness or injury and found themselves "underinsured," with caps that never came close to meeting their medical and financial needs. These families confided that they had either filed for bankruptcy or, if they could not lower their monthly income, they had divorced. The custodial parent then went on Medicaid, which paid the current and future medical expenses.

The average family health insurance policy costs $13,375 per year and in Michigan's First Congressional District the median household income was $38,771. Therefore, thirty-four percent of a family's income would go toward paying for health insurance. It is no wonder many families went bare and did not purchase family health insurance or seek medical help when they became ill. In 2009, a great many individuals and families could no longer afford health insurance. The American Journal of Medicine reported that sixty-two percent of all bankruptcies in 2007 were linked to medical expenses. Incredibly, seventy-eight percent of those people filing for bankruptcy had health insurance. These bankrupt individuals were "underinsured:" they had paid for insurance that did not cover the very expenses for which health insurance is designed.

CHAPTER 24

★ ★ ★

Energy and Commerce Committee Markup of Health Care (July–Sept 2009)

After my little speech in the health care briefing conducted by Karen Nelson wherein I warned the staff and Members to leave abortion out of the health care legislation, some of my fellow Democrats approached me on the House floor and asked if I would consider one concept or another regarding abortion in health care. I would ask each Member to place their language and concerns in writing and I would be happy to work with them, but I was not going to respond or agree verbally to vague concepts. Plus, I wanted to learn what part of the proposed health care legislation their language would amend as I attempted to determine if abortion was a covered service or funded in the base health care bill.

Congresswoman Diana DeGette (D-CO) was especially adept at playing this game of "What do you think?" Then she would make a cavalier statement to Members of Congress or the media such as, "Bart and I will work this out" or "We will just have to sit down and work this out."

In the spirit of "working things out," Diana approached me numerous times with concepts on how we would resolve our differences. I politely listened and asked her to put her concepts in writing. She never did.

While Diana and I had conversations that were never committed to writing, I kept reading in the press that Speaker Pelosi had charged Congresswoman Rosa DeLauro (D-CT) to work out the Stupak Amendment with me. Rosa and I never had a meaningful discussion on my Amendment.

It was obvious that as we moved toward the annual congressional August recess and a possible markup of the health care legislation in the Energy and Commerce Committee, Diana DeGette's game was to keep me focused on her concepts and ideas, and then spring the language on me in committee. Diana DeGette and I never sat down or had a serious discussion to resolve the looming collision course on abortion before heading into the committee markup.

Committee markup is a term used to describe the Committee meeting when the proposed legislation is ready for consideration and amendment by all the Members of the Committee. During the markup and after all the amendments have been disposed of, Members then vote on sending the legislation to the full House of Representatives for consideration with a recommendation for passage. The Committee of jurisdiction also produces a Majority and Minority Report to accompany the legislation for consideration by the House. The respective accompanying reports address the pros and cons of the legislation and are available to all Members of the US House of Representatives prior to voting.

Throughout the month of July, my staff and I prepared for the markup of the health care legislation. Neither the Energy and Commerce Committee staff nor members of the committee would inform me if the Pro-Choice Members were going to offer an amendment in committee or roll the dice with an amendment on the House floor. I spoke to Rosa DeLauro, Diana DeGette, and Anna Eshoo and no one would admit to having any knowledge of an amendment to be offered in the Energy and Commerce Committee on HR-3200.

Without any indication that an amendment concerning abortion would be offered, RTL Democrats prepared to offer the Hyde Amendment in the Ways and Means and the Education and Labor committees. Both committees had limited subject matter jurisdiction over the proposed health care legislation but it provided RTL Members an opportunity, if necessary, to insert the Hyde language.

In mid-July, both committees held their markups of HR-3200, America's Affordable Health Choices Act of 2009. By the narrowest of margins, the committees rejected the Hyde Amendment.

It was now the Energy and Commerce Committee's turn to tackle HR-3200. The markup started with the introduction of HR-3200 on July 14 and would continue through July 31. In fact, the Energy and Commerce Committee would not truly finish its markup until September 23, 2009. The introduction, markup and legislative procedure to bring America's Affordable Health Choices Act of 2009 to the floor was a disjointed effort that skirted parliamentary rules and was highly partisan.

The proposed legislation was formally introduced on July 14 in the Energy and Commerce Committee, Ways and Means, and Education and Labor Committee. Previous drafts of the legislation had been provided to both Democrats and Republicans to secure their input, negotiate changes and prepare amendments to the proposed legislation. The goal of the Democratic leadership was to favorably report the legislation from the three committees with jurisdiction prior to the August recess and have it on the President's desk by the end of the year.

The goal of the Republicans was to delay the health care legislation until after the August break. They believed that the Tea Party protesters would make life so miserable for Democrats during the August recess that Democratic Members would not vote for health care in the fall. Senator Jim DeMint summed up the Republican strategy when he addressed the Tea Party Convention on July 17, 2009, "If we're able to stop Obama on this [health care], it will be his Waterloo, it will break him..." The Republican goal was not to simply defeat health care but to break the President's spirit and ability to govern.

America's Affordable Health Choices Act of 2009 was introduced with only the Democratic leadership of the three committees as the original legislative sponsors. There were only six original sponsors of Affordable Health Choices Act: lead sponsor John Dingell (D-MI) followed by Henry Waxman (D-CA) and Frank Pallone (D-NJ) (Energy and Commerce); George Miller (D-CA) (Education and Labor); and, finally, Pete Stark (D-CA) and Rob Andrews (D-NJ) (Ways and Means Committee). Democratic Members of the committees with jurisdiction and rank-and-file Democrats were not given an opportunity to be original sponsors of the legislation. Even if offered, I would not have co-sponsored or wished to be an original sponsor of HR-3200, America's Affordable Health Choices Act of 2009. I believed in the Public Option concept. I had studied and believed that HR-3200 as written perpetuated America's broken health care system. HR-3200 did not control rising health care costs, rewarded a health care system based on quantity, not quality of procedures, and did not encourage true competition in health care commerce.

In a committee markup, the committee clerk reads each title of the proposed legislation and Members offer their amendments relevant to the title and section number. In this case, the Republicans wished to slow down consideration of HR-3200 and demanded that the entire 1,000-plus page document be read verbatim before any amendment could be offered. Very rarely did either side require the committee clerk to read the entire legislation at the start of a markup. But it was late July and we were now beginning the markup of a very controversial piece of legislation; the Republicans hoped to delay the consideration of the legislation until after the August recess. If the Republicans were successful in doing so, Members of the committee would want to simply abandon the markup and go home. Anticipating that this delay tactic might occur, Chairman Waxman hired a speed-reader to read all 1,000 pages of the legislation to the committee Members.

It was amusing when the speed-reader began to read the legislation verbatim. He did a fantastic job! If you listened very closely, you could actually pick up a word or two as the reader swiftly enunciated through the pages before him. After speeding through the first one hundred pages or so, the Republican Members surrendered and waived the formal reading of HR-3200. The markup began in earnest.

The Republicans had done their homework and they filed hundreds of amendments to HR-3200. Democrats also filed numerous amendments. There were a number of bi-partisan amendments, which Chairman Waxman did not necessarily agree with unless he personally approved of them. For instance, one of the earliest amendments offered in our markup was by former Republican Chairman of the committee, Joe Barton of Texas. Joe offered an amendment on transparency regarding the cost of medical procedures. If we expected the consumer to help rein in the high cost of health care, then he or she should be empowered to learn the cost of a medical procedure and what type of care each medical provider performs. HR-3200 only required hospitals to post their fees for medical procedures and all included services online. If surgery was required, patients should be able to see whether the cost included the surgeon, anesthesiologist, lab tests, rehabilitation services, a private or semi-private room, etc. With this information, the consumer could shop and compare, keeping the cost of their medical procedures low through competition.

Gene Green (D-TX) and I had worked with Joe Barton on his amendment. We believed that all health care providers should be required to disclose their fees so consumers could truly comparison shop if they wished to make informed financial decisions about their treatment.

The doctors' lobbyists were adamantly opposed to disclosing physician prices for medical procedures. Under the legislation, hospitals would be pressured into keeping their costs low for medical procedures while the doctors could charge whatever they wanted. I thought that if hospitals were required to disclose their costs, the doctors should as well. Gene Green and I spoke in favor of the Barton Amendment and we were pleased to be part of a group calling for full disclosure and transparency of medical costs. After a long debate, Chairman Waxman called for the vote on the Barton Amendment, one of the first amendments to be considered and voted on in the national health care debate. If Congress could pass it, national health care would be the most important social policy enacted in our nation in the past forty-four years- maybe in the last century. Every amendment and every vote on every amendment was crucial.

As is the tradition with recorded roll call votes in committee, the voting began with the majority party and then moved to the minority side. Therefore, the voting on the Barton Amendment began on the Democratic side. Chairman Waxman voted No. Mr. Markey voted No. Mr. Pallone voted No. And so on down the line to Mr. Stupak of Michigan, the eighth in seniority of the thirty-six Democrats who voted on the Barton Amendment. Of course, I voted Aye.

The heads of the Democratic Members and their staffs virtually whipped off their shoulders. I had the guts to buck Chairman Waxman and my party on one of the first amendments offered by a Republican to America's Health Choices Act of 2009. I had the audacity to vote for what I believed to be in the best interest of health care for all Americans. I voted for full disclosure of what consumers would be charged by the principal players in the health care industry. This Amendment would enable the consumer to make informed decisions regarding the cost of their health care.

I will never forget the look on the Energy and Commerce Committee Staff Director Phil Barnett's face as he glared at me with total disgust. Phil was seated on the dais right behind Chairman Waxman. Then I saw Waxman lean over and say something to Phil. I knew right then and there that an ass chewing was coming. After the vote was completed and with the help of a couple of Democratic "Aye" votes, the Barton Amendment became, for now, part of HR-3200. As soon as the vote was announced, Phil Barnett shot out of his seat, walked over to me and said, "I need to talk to you," in the most disgusted tone. Anticipating this request, I jumped right out of my seat and went to the committee anteroom. Staff cleared the room and it was just Phil and me. Phil read me the riot act. "What are you doing voting with the Republicans? You are a 'senior' member of the committee and you are expected to vote with the Chairman!" In no uncertain terms, I told Phil that I came to Congress to pass health care and I would not give away my vote on health care over party considerations. I would vote for amendments that made sense and I would not be partisan.

After a few minutes of chewing on each other, Phil asked if I would tell him how I was going to vote on important issues and indicated that I was expected to oppose all Republican amendments. I once again explained that I would vote for amendments that made sense to me. I also told Phil that I did not realize that this amendment was a contentious one, as it was a bi-partisan effort that I had worked on. If the amendment was so important to Chairman Waxman, he should have informed the Democratic Members and should not have just assumed that we were going to vote with him. Phil said fair enough and I told him that I had no problem advising him how I would vote on any amendment in the future. For instance, I said with a smile, I would not be voting for and would vigorously oppose any abortion amendments. Phil failed to see the humor and said that my opposition was a given. Phil Barnett is an honorable individual and very loyal to Chairman Waxman. Phil and Chairman Waxman always treated me fairly but we had different styles of leadership and did not agree on a number of issues.

I then went back and took my seat as a senior Democratic Member of the majority party on the Energy and Commerce Committee more determined than ever to vote my conscience on every amendment to HR-3200. It was going to be a long, contentious markup and not just with the Republicans but also within my own Democratic Party.

I remained fully engaged in the markup with assistance from my senior legislative assistant and health care expert, Erika Smith, my Legislative Director, Nick Choate and my Chief of Staff, Scott Schloegel. I argued for and against Democratic and Republican amendments and we slowly slogged through each amendment offered in each title of HR-3200.

CHAPTER 25

★ ★ ★

Capps Pro-Choice Amendment (July 30, 2009)

Based on the President's public comments, the Democratic Pro-Life Members' correspondence to the Speaker, and the temporary blocking of the Rule on the DC Appropriations, I had hoped against hope there would not be an abortion amendment to HR-3200. Amendments that are filed with the committee in advance of the markup are given priority and are automatically called up when the appropriate title and section are being considered. While an abortion amendment had not yet been filed, I had repeatedly warned against offering such an amendment as it would further split Democratic support for health care reform. I wanted health care reform to pass *and* I wanted to protect the sanctity of life. I was prepared to continue the uneasy truce that existed between Pro-Life and Pro-Choice Members to simply maintain the status quo by granting our yearly RTL riders. However, with a Pro-Choice president and the Pro-Choice Democrats controlling both the House and Senate, the truce between the two groups had been shredded over the past seven months.

An amendment to allow public funds to pay for or authorize abortion coverage as an essential medical benefit was offered and narrowly passed in both the Ways and Means and Education and Labor Committee markups on health care. I was not naïve enough to think or believe that a similar amendment would not be offered in the Energy and Commerce Committee. I just did not know who would offer the amendment. Instead of dwelling on who might offer it, I huddled with Republicans Joe Pitts and Chris Smith and prepared counter-amendments.

Besides being my staff expert on health care, Erika Smith was also my Pro-Life staffer and worked with my congressional and Democratic Right-to-Life Caucuses. Erika also worked very closely with Autumn Christensen, Congressman Chris Smith's dedicated RTL staffer. Erika and Autumn worked with Congressman Joe Pitts' RTL staffer to prepare, draft and advocate for our RTL concerns within and outside of the Energy and Commerce Committee and the health care legislation. It seemed like Autumn was always in my office or Erika was at Chris's office working on RTL issues. These staff professionals were truly dedicated to the RTL movement; Erika's dedication eventually became her downfall as the national health care legislation progressed through Congress.

In trying to anticipate which Pro-Choice amendment might be offered in Committee, I studied the amendments filed in the Ways and Means and Education and Labor Committee markups. Then, after each markup, I huddled with the Pro-Life Democratic Committee Members. We relived each amendment: what was said and by whom? How had each committee Member voted? Did any Member switch his or her vote? I made notes after each conversation; the committee process had just begun, as had our battle to maintain current law prohibiting the use of public funding for abortions. Yet, in the two committees with limited jurisdiction over health care, the RTL Democrats together with the Republican Committee Members still did not have enough votes to maintain the Hyde language in HR-3200. Now, the fight moved to the committee with the greatest jurisdiction over health care, the Energy and Commerce Committee.

Joe Pitts (R-PA) and I prepared to offer up to four amendments to counter any abortion amendment and to, once and for all, codify the Hyde language. If we were successful, we would no longer have to rely on the yearly RTL riders in the appropriations bills to protect the sanctity of life. We would no longer have to appear before the Rules Committee to beg for our riders. It was going to be a struggle, but maybe with a break from the Senate, the RTL movement could finally codify Hyde language and make it permanent law.

Personally, I felt confident that we could defeat any Pro-Choice amendment to HR-3200 and with a little luck pass our Pro-Life amendments. The citizens in Michigan's First Congressional District also felt strongly about not allowing their tax dollars to pay for abortions and believed that every conceived child had a right to be born. The death of my son gave me a greater appreciation and desire to protect all life. I did not realize how precious life was until it was ripped from my heart and soul. Even though HR-3200 was silent on abortion, I diligently prepared to protect the sanctity of life in the Public Option health insurance plan pending before me. I had to succeed, both personally and for all the Americans that I represented.

Finally, on July 30, 2009, in the fourth day of the Energy and Commerce Committee markup of HR-3200, Congresswoman Lois Capps (D-CA) filed an amendment to allow federal funds to be used to promote, encourage and pay for abortions. Despite all our pleas with the Democratic leadership not to inject abortion into national health care and President Obama's public statements indicating his intent to maintain existing policy and law, the Democratic leadership chose to ignore us. The Democratic leadership was prepared to use every legislative maneuver and public pressure to stymie Pro-Life efforts to preserve current law.

In all honesty, I did not expect Lois Capps (D-CA) to offer the amendment, as Diana DeGette was the Pro-Choice Energy and Commerce Committee Member whom I had always worked with to resolve the differences on Life issues. In fact, Diana and I had worked out acceptable RTL language in the GINA Bill. Now, in the fourth day of the markup, the funding of abortions was front and center and it was time to debate and vote. I was never given an opportunity to review the Capps Amendment or invited to work out a solution as I had on so many occasions during my previous sixteen years in

Congress. Once again, the Democratic leadership ignored the pleas and warnings of RTL Members and believed they could roll us. We were not going down without a fight.

I was surprised that Lois had introduced the amendment and even more surprised when my best friend and former solid RTL voter, Congressman Mike Doyle, seconded the Capps Amendment. With Mike seconding the Capps Amendment, his support signaled to the Energy and Commerce Committee Members that the Capps Amendment was reasonable and enjoyed his Pro-Life support. Every Committee Member, staff person, and lobbyist in the committee room knew that Mike and I were very close friends and had lived together for the past ten years. Mike's support of Capps was meant to embolden Democrats to support the Capps amendment.

My friendship with Mike was being tested and his vote was viewed by some as a personal repudiation of my leadership and advocacy to protect the sanctity of life. If Mike Doyle believed that I was off base with my advocacy, then it might seem to be okay for other pro-life Democrats to abandon me and vote for the Capps Amendment. I felt bad for Mike, not because he supported the amendment, but because like many other Members of the Democratic Caucus, he came to Congress as a pro-life Member and was now voting as a Pro-Choice Member. While it was true that Mike's district was much more liberal (Pittsburgh) than when he was first elected from the more conservative suburbs in 1994, he now was voting pro-choice. I imagined Mike felt that the Capps Amendment was a compromise and that he would argue that since the abortions were being paid from segregated funds it was not taxpayer dollars being used to pay for abortions. Still, I was also convinced that Mike had not entirely abandoned his RTL beliefs.

When discussing Life issues with Members of Congress, their responses depended on how the issue was framed. If the issue was whether federal taxpayer dollars should be used to pay for abortions, as prevented by the Hyde Amendment, the answer was no. If you asked whether under the Federal Employees Health Benefits package should federal employees be allowed to use their own money to pay for an abortion? Most Members of Congress would answer YES.

I am always skeptical of pollsters when they claim that the country is divided 50/50 on the abortion issue. Constituent views on abortion and funding for abortion-related services truly depend on how the question is presented to the voter. In my own campaigns over twenty years, I always asked the question exactly the same way in each poll. Should the federal government use taxpayer money to pay for abortions? Do you consider yourself pro-life or pro-choice? Would you vote for or against a pro-life /pro-choice candidate? In my congressional district, pro-life narrowly eked out pro-choice voters. Like the two camps, pro-life and pro-choice, the voters in my district knew I was pro-life but it was not my main campaign theme and I did not wear the issue on my sleeve.

What also surprised me was how little Members understood about the scope of the Hyde Amendment. Hyde clearly states that the federal government and its policies shall not "support, pay for or administer programs or insurance policies which promote or encourage abortions." Members of Congress were well aware that the Hyde language prevented federal taxpayer dollars from being used to pay for abortions. Members did not realize that the Hyde language also forbade the Federal Government from offering health insurance policies that included abortion coverage and administering programs that supported or encouraged abortions.

At the time of the markup, there were thirty-six Democrats and twenty-three Republicans on the Energy and Commerce Committee. I needed thirty votes to pass or defeat any amendment. As Congresswoman Lois Capps offered her amendment, she angered me with the first words out of her mouth when she accused RTL Democrats of offering a "poison pill" amendment to defeat health care legislation.

Lois Capps stated,

> "You know, I would have preferred, of course, not to bring the abortion debate into the health care reform debate, but from long years of expe-

rience in this body and in this committee, it is
too often that tactics are used to poison good
pieces of legislation." (Page 268, Transcript of EC
Committee Markup of HR-3200 July 30, 2009)

By now I was seeing red. How could Lois Capps make a claim
that I had injected abortion into the health care debate when I tried
for months to keep abortion out of it?

In the April briefing, I told the Democratic Committee
Members in the first meeting on health care *not* to interject abortion
into the health care debate.

On June 6, President Obama declared, "I'm pro-choice, but
I think we also have the tradition in this town, historically, of not
financing abortions as part of government-funded healthcare. My
main focus is making sure that people have options of high quality
care at the lowest possible price."

On June 25, nineteen RTL Democratic Members wrote to
Speaker Pelosi and stated that they would not support health care
legislation that violated the sanctity of life. Speaker Pelosi never
addressed or responded to our letter.

In July, RTL Democrats sent a "shot across the bow" as Speaker
Pelosi refused to grant any of the traditional RTL riders on the
appropriations bills, so RTL Democrats voted against and almost
took down the Rule on the DC Appropriations Bill.

Now, on the fourth day of the markup in Title A and B of
HR-3200, Congresswoman Lois Capps offered an amendment to
allow federal funding of abortion. Capps offered the amendment, not
a RTL Democrat or RTL Republican. It was the Capps Amendment
that interjected abortion into health care. Her amendment had been
filed three hours earlier on the fourth day of the markup; three hours
before we began marking up the critical title and section which
defined the essential health care benefits that all health plans must
provide under HR-3200. Lois Capps arranged the timing so she
could present her Pro-Choice amendment.

Incredibly, Capps accused RTL members of interjecting abortion into health care debate and legislation. Capps also claimed that

this was compromise language. A compromise with whom? Herself? She had never presented nor asked any of us RTL Democrats to review her proposed language. Congresswoman Capps introduced her amendment, which no RTL Member of Congress had yet seen, just hours before she offered it. Yet Capps claimed that RTL Democrats inserted a poison pill to kill health care reform. The poison was that RTL Democrats did not agree with Capps and we opposed her amendment.

The Democratic and Republican RTL Members on the Energy and Commerce Committee made it very clear with the filing of our amendments that we were prepared to fight any attempt to reverse the longstanding principles of Hyde. The Hyde language states that the federal government shall not pay for, promote or administer programs in which abortions may be performed. We filed our RTL amendments on HR-3200 in the morning of July 19, eleven days prior to the filing of the Capps Amendment. An amendment is not necessarily offered simply because it is filed with the committee. In markups, Members often submit amendments but never actually offer them, staking their claim to an issue that must be addressed before the legislation is presented on the House floor.

As I stated earlier, we filed our amendments, learning from the markups in the Ways and Means and Education and Labor Committees that Pro-Choice Members had offered amendments to have abortions paid for under HR-3200. Still, I had held out hope that Members of the Energy and Commerce Committee would not interject abortion into our markup of the health care legislation. With the mean-spirited language in which the Capps Amendment was presented, I was drained of all hope that the abortion issue could be amicably worked out in this markup. For over sixteen years, I had been the go-between for the Pro-Choice and the Pro-Life Members of Congress and we worked out our differences as we had on GINA. But today, the Pro-Choice Members presented an abortion amendment after I pleaded with committee members not to raise the issue. The Pro-Choice Members had not even provided me with an opportunity to review the amendment before it was presented. I was not happy.

To be effective in my counter-argument to the Capps Amendment, I had to calm down. As I usually did, I sat back and listened to the debate and carefully read the Amendment. I had never seen this language before so it was important to fully understand everything about it. I had to assure our RTL Committee Members that there would be an amendment offered to preserve Hyde. As the debate in the committee began, Joe Pitts (R-PA), Joe Barton (R-TX), Cliff Stearns (R-FL) and Lee Terry (R-NE) succinctly stated our opposition to the Capps Amendment. I was concerned when a couple of the RTL Committee Democrats failed to speak up in opposition to it. Did we lose their votes?

Ranking Member Joe Barton asked for debate time and yielded to me as we had arranged. I am sure that Chairman Waxman would have recognized me but I did not want to take the risk of not being recognized to speak against the amendment.

I went straight after Lois' assertion that I had interjected abortion into the health care debate. I stated, in part, on the Capps Amendment:

> "As this debate started off on this amendment, I was really disappointed that the author of the amendment said that somehow, we [RTL Members] use this [RTL] as a poison pill."

> "For seventeen years, even before the author ever came to Congress, I have worked on these amendments. I have never used it as a poison pill. We have always based our legislation, and when I have worked with both sides on this issue, on principles, on what our ethics and our morals may be. So, it is not a poison pill."

> "Secondly, early this year, in January [June], 180 Members, Democrats and Republicans, wrote to the Speaker, wrote to the head of Appropriations, wrote to the Rules Committee, and said we have always [had] Riders on the amendments,

excuse me, on the appropriation bills. We heard nothing."

"And Commerce, Justice, State Appropriation, we lost our rider. Financial Services Appropriations, we lost our rider. Yesterday or earlier this week, the Senate actually took out the Hyde Amendment on the Federal Employee Health Benefit package, where it has always been".

"So, we write a letter, 180 of us. We get no response, every time we go to the Rules Committee and say keep our riders in place to protect our beliefs and the debate that we want, we are shut down. We are shut down."

"In fact, on this debate in this bill in particular, before it got going, twenty Democrats said we want to see some Pro-Life language. Okay. So, here is what we have [Capps]. Look at it. There are two principles, and most of us just cannot and will not retreat from [them]. Principles that we held before we came to Congress, and principles that we will have after we leave Congress. Abortion must be explicitly excluded from the scope of any authority anywhere in this bill to [be] define[d] a mandatory benefits package."

"Secondly, we must preserve the longstanding principles that public funds do not pay for abortion procedures, and do not flow through any plan that includes abortion. That is the policy that has long been applied by Congress..." (Pages 280-281 Transcript of Energy and Commerce Committee Markup of HR-3200, July 30, 2009)

I went through other problems with the Capps Amendment and at the end of my allotted time, I yielded back to Mr. Barton. Chairman Waxman immediately called for a roll call vote on the Capps Amendment. Everyone in the committee surveyed the dais to determine which Members were present and more importantly, which Members were absent. Even though no other Democrat spoke in opposition to the Capps Amendment, I knew the vote would be close. The mainstay Right to Life Democrats such as Mike Ross, Jim Matheson, John Barrow and Charlie Melancon were absent but I was confident that they would appear to record their vote and that all six RTL Democrats would vote against it. We could defeat the Capps Amendment.

As the Clerk called the roll, everyone on the dais and in the committee room tallied the votes as each Member announced their vote. After the Clerk finished calling the Democratic Members, she turned and called on the Republican Committee Members to record their vote. While the Republican Members voted, the Democratic Committee staff left the room to find the missing Democratic Members, especially Bart Gordon and Zach Space, as Chairman Waxman needed their votes to pass the Capps Amendment.

After the Clerk recorded the votes of the Republican Members, she then scoured the premises to determine whether any of the absentee Committee Members had returned to the room to vote. The fact that Members were absent from the committee room when a roll call vote was called was not unusual. Members of the committee may be in another hearing at the time or listening to the committee debate from their personal offices and then would walk down to cast their roll call vote.

The Clerk recognized Mr. Gordon and he voted Aye on the Capps Amendment. Then Mr. Ross voted No. Mr. Markey voted Aye. Mr. Barrow voted No. Mr. Space entered the committee room and voted Aye.

Chairman Waxman then asked the Clerk to announce the vote and she stated that there were thirty Ayes and twenty-eight No votes. Waxman repeated the tally and announced that the Capps Amendment was agreed to.

Ranking Member Barton objected to the vote and asked the Clerk to recalculate her tally. The Clerk reviewed her tally and again stated the Capps Amendment had thirty Ayes and twenty-eight No votes.

I was very disappointed but I still held out hope that we could reverse the damage of the Capps Amendment by approving the Pitts/Stupak/Blunt Amendment. The Pitts/Stupak/Blunt Amendment was drafted to counter the abortion amendments that had been adopted in the other committees with jurisdiction. We were prepared to counterattack the Capps Amendment.

As is customary in a markup, the Chairman's recognition of Members to offer amendments alternated between a Democrat and then a Republican. Since Capps had started Title A and B with her amendment, the Republicans then had an opportunity to offer one of their own. Without hesitation Congressman Joe Pitts (R-PA) offered the Pitts/Stupak/Blunt Amendment. Our amendment embodied the traditional Hyde language, which stated that no public funds could be used to pay for, promote or encourage abortions and that the federal government could not administer programs covering abortions.

In her argument, Congresswoman Lois Capps claimed to strike a balance by mandating that health insurance companies had to offer at least one plan that did not pay for abortions. The Public Option health insurance plans that offered abortion coverage to be administered by the federal government were in violation of the longstanding Hyde Amendment. While the Capps Amendment violated Hyde, we were also concerned that if HR-3200 was silent on abortion, the creation of the Health Benefits Advisory Committee would determine that abortion coverage was a benefit like any other and must be included in all the Public Option health insurance plans. Joe Pitts said it best when he argued in support of our amendment:

> "HR-3200 will require virtually every individual
> to have healthcare coverage that meets the mini-
> mum benefits standards. The bill then establishes
> a new government health board called the Health
> Benefits Advisory Committee to determine what

qualifies as a minimum benefit standard. This committee chaired by the Surgeon General and then in concert with the Secretary of Health and Human Services, will have the power to issue binding decrees on what type of healthcare coverage individuals must have and employers must provide.

History has demonstrated that unless abortion is explicitly excluded, administrative agencies and the courts will mandate it. For example, the Federal Medicaid statute was silent on the issue of abortion but the administration and the courts deemed abortion on demand to be mandated coverage. In the case of <u>Planned Parenthood Affiliates of Michigan v Engler</u>, the Sixth Circuit Court of Appeals explained that 'abortion fits within many of the mandated categories including family planning, outpatient services, inpatient services and physician services'."

"Some of these same terms, such as outpatient services, inpatient services and physician services are mandated under this bill. If the courts used such terms to mandate coverage of abortion in the 1970s, they will surely do it again if the administration doesn't do so first, only this time the mandates will apply not only to publicly funded healthcare but also to private insurance coverage." (Pages 291-292 Transcript of Energy and Commerce Committee Markup of HR-3200, July 30, 2009)

Joe Pitts then yielded part of his five minutes to me as co-sponsor of the amendment. I echoed what Joe said about explicitly excluding abortion coverage and warned that the courts and the Health

Benefits Advisory Committee would add abortion as mandated minimum benefit standards in the essential benefits package.

> "So, history has shown us when you don't exclude it [abortion], it is included and that is why the statutory exclusion has been necessary in programs like the SCHIP program and in the Federal Employee Health Benefit package.
>
> So this bill [HR-3200] really does an end run, I think, on the current funding restrictions of the Hyde Amendment so I would ask that we support the Pitts amendment." (Page 293 Transcript of Energy and Commerce Committee Markup of HR-3200, July 30, 2009)

Congresswoman DeGette and Schakowsky insisted that Hyde was being followed in the Capps Amendment and that it only allowed private insurance companies to offer abortion coverage without restrictions from the federal government. Their arguments were false. They wanted the federal government to provide for and pay for abortion on demand.

Joe Pitts responded to the Congresswomen with this point:

> "...Capps Amendment has a loophole. If Hyde goes away, abortion coverage will be mandated in the public plan. Secondly, nothing in this [Pitts] amendment says anything about disallowing voluntarily offered abortion coverage. It simply says that the government cannot mandate abortion coverage. If private plans want to cover abortion, this amendment does not stop that. What it stops is the mandate to force abortion in every insurance plan in the country." (Page 299-300 Transcript of Energy and Commerce Committee Markup of HR-3200, July 30, 2009)

The debate on the Pitts/Stupak/Blunt Amendment became very intense and Members on both sides of the abortion debate passionately argued for or against the Amendment. Then it was time for the vote.

I was confident that we would win this vote and insert the traditional Hyde Amendment in HR-3200. The vote would be close, but we would prevail because the question was different than that in the just-passed Capps Amendment. I knew that most Members generally did not believe in abortion and felt strongly that taxpayers should not pay for abortion services.

As he was for the previous vote, Congressman Bart Gordon was absent when the vote was called and that had me worried because I believed Bart would vote for the Pitts Amendment. With Bart Gordon absent, I was the first Democrat to support the Pitts/Stupak/Blunt Amendment and then the other RTL Democrats voted for the Amendment. Mr. Matheson and Mr. Barrow voted AYE. Congressmen Hill and Melancon were missing initially but came into the room and voted AYE. Finally, Congressman Bart Gordon appeared and voted AYE. We had a solid thirty votes!

When everyone had voted, Chairman Waxman asked the clerk how he was recorded and my heart sank. The clerk stated that Chairman Waxman was recorded as No and then the Chairman informed the clerk of his "…wish to change his vote from No to Aye." Several of the younger Democratic Committee members who voted for the Pitts Amendment thought Henry Waxman was having an epiphany, but I assured them that this was a procedural move on the part of the Chairman to bring the vote up later after he had a chance to twist arms to move Members from "aye" to "no" on the Pitts/Stupak/Blunt Amendment. (Page 311 Transcript of Energy and Commerce Committee Markup of HR-3200, July 30, 2009)

Before Waxman had switched his vote, the tally on the Pitts/Stupak/Blunt Amendment was thirty Aye and twenty-seven No. We had won, but Waxman would get his votes against our Amendment before the night was over.

Under the Energy and Commerce Committee Rules, a Member voting for an amendment can ask that it be reconsidered later in the markup. By switching his vote, Waxman reserved an opportunity to have the vote reconsidered at a later time. My friend from California, Mr. Waxman, was not having an epiphany.

The next amendment was a bi-partisan effort between Mr. Markey (D-MA) and Congressman Dr. Michael Burges (R-TX) to create an "Independence at Home" pilot program, which sought to keep chronically ill Medicare patients at home and provide them with coordinated health care. The amendment was approved on a voice vote.

With the clock ticking towards midnight, Chairman Waxman moved to reconsider the vote in which the Pitts/Stupak/Blunt Amendment had passed earlier in the evening. The Republicans immediately objected and Congressman Ralph Hall (R-TX), who may have been on the committee longer than Chairman Waxman, questioned under what authority Chairman Waxman had the right to reconsider a previously passed amendment. In response, Chairman Waxman stated that he was relying on Clause 3 of Rule 29, which states a "…member who votes on the prevailing side on an amendment may offer a motion to reconsider the vote." The vote to reconsider ended up being a party line vote. Although I had voted No the rest of the RTL Democrats voted Yes as they viewed the Motion to Reconsider as a parliamentary vote. The Motion to Reconsider passed 35-24.

While it may have been a parliamentary vote, I knew that Chairman Waxman now had the votes to defeat Pitts/Stupak/Blunt Amendment and that at least one Democrat would have to switch their previous vote on the Amendment from Aye to No. Waxman was definitely voting against Pitts/Stupak/Blunt, but his vote alone would not change the outcome and Pitts/Stupak/Blunt would survive the reconsideration. So, which Democrat would switch his or her vote?

As the Committee Clerk called the vote, the outcome was going to be close and the presence of every Member would be required. Once again Mr. Gordon was not present for the vote and the RTL Democrats Stupak, Ross, Matheson, Melancon, Barrow, and Hill all voted for the Pitts/Stupak/Blunt Amendment. As the Clerk called the Republicans, I noted that none of the RTL Democrats had switched their vote and therefore Waxman could not win. Then I realized that Congressman Bart Gordon was going to switch his vote and we would lose by one. I knew the Republicans were unanimous in their support of the amendment and none of them would switch. We were up by one vote when Zach Space (D-OH), who did not vote earlier on the Amendment, was now present for this vote. Space voted No, creating a tie.

After calling the names of all the committee members, the Chairman asked if there were any other Members who wished to be recorded or if any Member wished to change his or her vote. The Clerk then recognized Bart Gordon as he entered the committee room. Gordon voted No and then immediately left. The tie was broken and the Pitts/Stupak/Blunt Amendment, which mirrored the Hyde Amendment, was defeated by one vote. Congressman Bart Gordon had switched his vote from Aye to No and Zach Space showed up to vote against the Pitts/Stupak/Blunt Amendment.

The Capps Amendment stood. In a matter of a few hours, thirty-plus years of a prohibition on public funding for abortion was upheld and then overturned by a seldom-used parliamentary tactic.

Ironically, the next amendment by Republican Dr. Mike Burgess on requiring the Secretary to negotiate 'fair' reimbursement rates for doctors under the House Public Option Plan ended in a 29-29 vote with one Member not voting. Therefore, the Burgess Amendment also failed to pass because it was a tied vote.

We completed one more amendment, which passed on a voice vote, and then Chairman Waxman called for a recess until 10:00 a.m. the next morning, Friday, July 31, 2009. Members were concerned about going home for the weekend, as the House was scheduled to finish its weekly business by 1:00 p.m. on Friday and then head home for the August recess. Energy and Commerce Committee Members were in their fourth intense day of the markup on HR-3200 and tempers were frayed after emotional debates on abortion and the essential benefit package.

When asked as to his intent for Friday's markup, Chairman Waxman retorted, "Well, we are going to stay as long as it takes, and

I want members to please arrange their schedules to recognize that we have a very important matter before us. However long it takes, we must complete this legislation."

Then the Chairman added, "I don't anticipate we will be here until midnight Friday night." Since it was now midnight on Thursday, Waxman recessed the committee markup until 10:00 a.m. the next morning.

As we finished voting on the markup for Thursday, I vowed that I would use every parliamentary procedure to secure a vote on the House floor for the Pitts/Stupak/Blunt amendment before HR-3200 became law. As Mike Doyle and I walked back to our rooms at C Street, I told Mike that the fight for Hyde was not over and that there would not be public funding for abortion in health care. Mike said. "I know you will not give up but you really do not have any other options." I quickly retorted, "Then there will never be a health care bill."

Mike and I were extremely close friends and I should have been angry with him for seconding the Capps Amendment. I saw it as a cheap shot at me. But we were friends and we had been through a lot together. Mike had read scripture at B.J.'s funeral Mass. I knew him as a friend and not as a cold, calculating legislator who would intentionally cause me any harm or embarrassment. We remained friends and we would get through this health care hell together. We just did not quite realize what we were walking into as we made our way back to our little C Street bedrooms after the fourth day of a contentious markup on national health care.

CHAPTER 26

★ ★ ★

Day 5 Markup (July 31, 2009)

On Friday, July 31, as the Energy and Commerce Committee tried to finish its markup, I had one more opportunity to attempt to insert the Hyde Amendment in HR-3200, America's Affordable Health Choices Act of 2009.

Halfway through the markup, I called up for consideration Pitts Amendment 2-001. Congressman Pitts and I agreed that it would be best for me to offer the Pitts Amendment 2-001, which was, word for word, the Hyde Amendment. We crossed out Congressman Pitts's name on the Amendment and inserted my name instead.

The Committee had reduced the amount of time that Members would be allowed to debate amendments to three minutes to hasten the markup on HR-3200. Therefore, I quickly summarized my arguments. I made it very clear that this was the Hyde Amendment and we wished to codify Hyde. I attested to the Committee Members:

> "As we all know, back in 1973 and 1976, Congressman Jim Oberstar and Henry Hyde put together the Hyde language. Since that time, since 1976, it has been part of our law. But we have to renew it every year in the appropriations bills.

So as we take a look at it – and in the Capps language last night, when we amended, we said abortion is [n]either required or prohibited. That means the legislation is silent on it [abortion]. Therefore, if the administrator isn't going to, then the courts can interpret it, as we see from the Sixth Circuit Court of Appeals.

So the Capps Amendment, as we have in this bill now, does not include any restriction on the use of Federal subsidies to pay for health insurance that covers abortion on demand. And because the bill authorizes and appropriates the funding for these subsidies, there is no need for Congress to pass future Riders like the Hyde Amendment.

The Capps Amendment that was approved last night is really an end run on the Hyde Amendment. We must get the Hyde Amendment language back into this bill right here and now or we will be looking at massive subsidies for abortion. And that is without even talking about the funding of abortions through Medicaid in the public plan." (Energy and Committee markup of July 31, 2009, page 199)

I then yielded my remaining two minutes to Congressman Joe Pitts,

"Now some of our colleagues have talked about the status quo. In these plans, the status quo is no federal funding for plans that include abortion. The Capps amendment last night repudiates this longstanding Federal policy and instead it established what I would call an accounting gimmick.

Instead, it created a bookkeeping measure to create the illusion of a prohibition of taxpayer support for abortion. This Amendment actually prohibits public funds from being used to subsidize plans that cover abortion. The amendment before us will correct the negative effects of the Capps Amendment." (Energy and Commerce Committee markup of July 31, 2009, page 200)

Both Rep. Capps and Rep. DeGette attacked the amendment, claiming that we were actually expanding Hyde by codifying and applying it to all health insurance plans. While the Congresswomen were correct on their first point- that we were attempting to codify Hyde- we could not prevent private health insurance plans from including abortion coverage. The only restriction we could place on a health insurance plan was that the plan would not receive any federal money. As was current law, if a Federal Employees Health Benefit Plan included a portion of the premium paid with tax dollars, then the plan could not offer abortion coverage. However, a beneficiary of the partially funded Federal Health Care insurance policy could purchase a rider with individual money. Under Hyde language, a Federal Employees Health Insurance Policy could not provide for, pay for or encourage abortion coverage.

The Hyde Amendment language could not and did not prevent states from using state money to provide abortion coverage under the state's portion of Medicaid coverage. At the time of the debate, seventeen states used state money to cover abortions for women on Medicaid. (Energy and Commerce Committee markup of July 31, 2009, page 205)

Finally, Congressman Lee Terry (R-NE) probably summarized our arguments best when he stated, "Our concern here is that we prevent the taxpayer dollars from going in there [public option/ exchange]. So, we can't stop what a State or an individual does, but we can stop the taxpayer dollars from subsidizing the exchange and the public plan."

The recorded vote was then called and the final tally was twenty-seven Aye and thirty-one No. The Stupak Amendment was defeated. At the very end of the roll call, Congressman John Shadegg (R-AZ) switched from "aye" to "nay" to preserve the Amendment for reconsideration. In reviewing the vote total, the only other Democrat who could have possibly voted with us was Congressman Bart Gordon, but he had switched his vote the night before to pass Capps so he was not going to help us now.

I was now out of options and there were no other sections of HR-3200, America's Health Choices Act of 2009, where I could insert the Hyde language. The fungible Capps language would allow individuals to use taxpayer money, in part, to pay for abortions. Plus, under Capps, the statutory language neither prohibited nor supported abortion. Therefore, the HHS Administrator and the courts, as they had in the past, could include abortion coverage as an essential health benefit. While the Capps Amendment tried to cleverly hide this fact, the Executive Branch would determine abortion coverage as an essential benefit of health care.

There was one more surprise awaiting us as we continued the markup. Chairman Waxman called a fifteen-minute recess with both parties caucusing on the continuation of the markup. There were between fifty-five and sixty amendments left to consider on this Friday night. Most Members of Congress had left Washington, DC to begin the August recess; Members of the Energy and Commerce Committee were anxious to complete the markup and return home to their districts.

Chairman Waxman and Ranking Member Joe Barton agreed on the following procedure: the Committee would report out HR-3200, America's Health Choices Act of 2009, to the full House with a favorable recommendation. The fifty-five to sixty remaining amendments would be handed over to staff to determine whether the amendment(s) could be placed "en bloc." A few significant amendments would be laid over for a vote on inclusion in HR-3200 in September when we returned from the August recess. Once back in session in September, the Energy and Commerce Committee would re-convene the markup and deal with the remaining amendments as agreed to by staff, Chairman Waxman, and Ranking Member Barton. The key to whether this process would be followed was the assumption that HR-3200 would be voted out of committee with a favorable recommendation to the US House of Representatives and then sent to the Rules Committee.

I was disappointed that the Committee leadership had taken this approach to deal with the remaining amendments. If this was such an historic piece of legislation, then we should stay and finish our work. The House of Representatives was about to become the first legislative body in our nation's history to debate health care. Yet, the House Committee with the greatest jurisdiction over health care had grown weary of the process and shirked its responsibility. The process was being abbreviated and the authors of the remaining proposals were being denied the benefit of presenting and debating their amendments.

Chairman Waxman explained to Committee Members that if we voted the bill out of committee, Members could also have their amendments considered for inclusion in HR-3200 by going to the Rules Committee. For our RTL amendments, the Rules Committee was a dead end as Chairwoman Slaughter had not allowed a single RTL amendment or our traditional RTL riders during 2009. Slaughter would not have a change of heart and allow our RTL amendments into the national health care legislation. Chairman Waxman's assurance that all amendments would be dealt with fairly by committee staff and/or the Rules Committee was not true.

Chairman Waxman called for a Roll Call vote and true to form I was the first Democrat to vote No on favorably reporting out America's Health Choices Act of 2009. My vote was then followed with "No" from Democratic Members Engel, Matheson, Melancon, and Barrow. All Republicans voted against reporting out the legislation but it passed by a vote of thirty-one Aye and twenty-eight No.

I packed up my files as I prepared to leave the Energy and Commerce Committee markup of HR-3200, America's Health Choices Act. I carried my big three-ring binder that staff had prepared for me with all the known and anticipated amendments that the Committee considered over the past few weeks. Knowing that

I was not going to let go of the Stupak-Pitts Amendment, I placed all of my RTL documents in a brown accordion file. My RTL file had grown to four inches thick with papers on studies, court cases, RTL talking points, letters from National Right-to-Life, the US Conference of Catholic Bishops and other groups supporting the Amendments offered by Joe Pitts and me and opposing the Capps Amendment. I felt that this accordion file would be with me for the remainder of the health care debate through to the final vote on national health care. My brown accordion file, health care, and I had many more roads to travel before any health care plan would pass through the US Congress.

For the first time in our nation's history, one chamber of Congress had positioned national health care legislation to be considered, debated and voted on by the House of Representatives. While I was pleased that national health care would finally receive a vote in Congress, I was bitterly disappointed in the process used to report out the legislation. I felt that with fifty-five to sixty more amendments still to be considered, members of the Energy and Commerce Committee had abdicated their legislative authority to unelected staff members who would determine which amendments would be considered when we returned from the August break.

I am convinced that if John Dingell had remained Chairman of the Energy and Commerce Committee, there would not have been hundreds of amendments, we would not have needed a speed-reader to read the legislation, and all amendments would have been considered or withdrawn. The Committee would have completed its work and not abdicated its responsibility to staff.

My concerns with HR-3200 were more than just how the legislation was reported out of the committee. I believed the legislation had become far too complex and did not drive down costs. I also believed that the legislation would only perpetuate a broken health care system without providing universal health care coverage.

Substantive changes to America's health care system were also lacking. In a November 2009 letter to my constituents, I wrote:

"Health care is a basic right that should be afforded all Americans, it is not a privilege. It is my belief that in reforming health care in our country, Congress needs to build on the existing framework by making it easier for employers to provide health insurance and providing access to government programs for individuals not covered by their employer.

Despite some improvements to our health care system provided in H.R. 3200, I remain concerned with the legislation. My concerns [are] that the legislation does not effectively control rising health care costs, does not do enough to encourage true competition in the health insurance market, and builds on a system that rewards ineffectiveness instead of quality and value were not addressed. Therefore, I voted against H.R. 3200 in the House Energy and Commerce Committee on July 31, 2009.

Over the next month, congressional leadership, the Obama Administration and those of us who work on health care policy, will work to merge the three proposals passed by House Committees into one bill for consideration on the House floor. Similarly, the Senate must merge its two bills into one for consideration in that chamber. Once the House and Senate pass their respective bills this fall, extensive negotiations will begin to craft one compromise bill that can pass both chambers. I fully expect a comprehensive health care reform bill will be signed into law this year. To gain my vote, I must be convinced the final product effectively reforms our health care system.

During my first campaign for Congress in 1992, I made a promise to my constituents that I would support health care reform and not accept the health insurance that is offered to members of Congress until all Americans had access to quality, affordable health care. I have kept that promise.

I hear every day the heartbreaking stories of my constituents – the insured, the uninsured and the under insured. I hear from those who the current health care system has left helpless, bankrupt and disillusioned.

Despite my concerns with H.R. 3200, I do believe Congress is making good progress toward health care reform. The issue is complex and deserves thoughtful consideration. A great deal of confusion exists regarding the House health care reform proposal. To help clear up some of the false claims being made against the legislation, I have prepared answers to some of the most commonly asked questions about the bill. I have enclosed a copy with this letter and the document can be viewed on m web site at *www.house.gov/stupak*.

Again, thank you for contacting me.

The purpose of the constituent letter was to advise them that I was still fighting for health care reform and that the fight was not over. I had not given up on my belief that health care was a right for all Americans and not just for the privileged few. Unfortunately, the objectives that I outlined in my Committee opening statement on HR-3200 were not met in the legislation that the Energy and Commerce Committee had just marked up and sent to the Rules Committee.

I needed to regroup to make sure that the sanctity of life was protected in health care reform and that meaningful health care reform could still pass the House and the Senate. I strongly believed that these two principles could coexist, but right now it appeared that neither would survive.

As we broke for the August recess, nerves were frayed. I became the face of the RTL opposition to abortion in the health care legislation. This was not a position I sought or intended to play. However, as the Democratic leadership ignored our warnings and prevented our RTL Riders from coming to the House floor for a vote, the media and Members of Congress looked to me for leadership on the issue. Over the years, I had served as the Democratic co-chair of the bipartisan RTL Congressional Caucus and Chairman of the RTL Democrats and senior Member of the Energy and Commerce Committee. I had quietly worked behind the scenes to find compromise RTL language to please both camps. Now, in August of 2009, both Pro-Life and Pro-Choice activists had dug in their heels and I was not so sure we could find common ground in the development of health care legislation.

I had no choice but to take up the cause of protecting the sanctity of life and providing health care for all Americans. These two noble principles that I deeply believed in were on a collision course, and I tried to walk a tight rope between them. The tight rope became longer and more precarious as we adjourned for the August recess. I did not then comprehend how long and arduous this journey would become, and I could not begin to foresee what lay ahead.

I was looking forward to heading home for August and helping prepare for our son, Ken's, marriage on Mackinac Island. I wished to turn my focus on the upcoming wedding and not spend August answering questions on health care, abortion and the President. Ken's fiancée and her family were coming in from California, Peru, and Japan. Laurie had assisted with the wedding plans and handled many of the logistics but still needed my help. We looked forward to the wedding and a very special family celebration; I vowed to leave the chaos of health care behind until after Labor Day.

CHAPTER 27

★ ★ ★

Tea Party Unrest (2009-2010)

The media picked up on the abortion fight and dubbed the Pitts Amendment 2-001 as the Stupak Amendment. My Amendment was word for word the Hyde language that had been part of the RTL riders for the past thirty years. Hyde was now the Stupak Amendment. It was interesting that the internal Capitol Hill reports on the Energy and Commerce Committee markup of HR-3200 only made a passing reference to the abortion fight and centered its reporting on other provisions in the health care bill.

On the morning of Saturday, August 1, I left Washington DC for my home in Menominee, Michigan. My usual flight home took me from Washington National Airport to Detroit Wayne County Airport, then from Detroit to Green Bay, Wisconsin. I would leave my car in long-term parking and then drive the fifty-four miles from Green Bay to Menominee. If everything went well, it was an eight-hour journey home. No matter how I tried to save time, the trip to and from Washington from my home in Menominee was a minimum of eight hours. I had all my time in for a full day of work just in travel. After a short night with the markup ending around 10:30 p.m., I was mentally and physically exhausted when I arrived home.

I could stay home for forty-eight hours and then I had to hit the road. Even though the media likes to portray Members of Congress as being on vacation during the August recess, nothing could be further from the truth. For me, it was anything but a vacation. The First Congressional District of Michigan spanned 600 miles from the Saginaw County line to Copper Harbor on the Keweenaw Peninsula. My congressional district encompassed two time zones and bordered three of the five Great Lakes and a foreign country, Canada. Traverse City is straight across Lake Michigan, ninety-two miles from my home in Menominee. Because there is no bridge over Lake Michigan you must drive around the lake- 322 miles- to Traverse City. The true boundaries of the First Congressional District of Michigan extend out into the Great Lakes, making it the largest congressional district in the nation other than those states that have only one Member of Congress such as Montana, Wyoming, Alaska, etc. The First Congressional District of Michigan contains more shoreline than any other congressional district except Alaska.

I left home early in the morning on Tuesday, August 4 to meet with constituents and honor meeting requests from around the district. I arrived back home on Friday evening to participate in Menominee's Annual Waterfront Festival activities and the parade on Sunday. The trip went well except for the Senior Center Visit in Petoskey, Michigan.

On August 5, 2010, I arrived at the Petoskey Senior Center about fifteen minutes later than I had planned. The Petoskey Senior Center was one of the largest senior centers in my district and always had a good crowd. I enjoyed going to senior centers, having lunch with the members and saying a few words about what was happening in our nation's capital.

As I pulled into the parking lot I could see non-senior citizens walking around with signs that I did not take time to read as I was late. When I checked in at the front desk to pay for my lunch, I was advised that the Senior Center had been receiving calls all morning asking if I would be there and if they, the caller, could join in the Senior Citizen luncheon. The Senior Center receptionist said the callers were told that since they had not signed up in advance for lunch, they would not be served but could stay for my comments afterward. As always, I paid for my lunch at the non-senior rate and offered to say a few words and take questions from the seniors before I had to leave for my next appointment in Traverse City.

I made my rounds, shaking hands with the seniors and answering their questions as their table numbers were called up to pick up their meals. I was one of the last to pick up my meal and I quickly ate and then rose to speak to the seniors. As I was standing in the middle of the room, the back divider was opened and about twenty or thirty people filed in and started shouting questions at me about the health care legislation, HR-3200.

I asked the group to please stop interrupting me as I was going to finish my comments and then take questions from the Senior Citizens, as it was their luncheon meeting. The group shouted back that they would ask the questions and I would answer. I turned my attention back to the seniors and told them how they were exempt from HR-3200 as they had Medicare. The group in the back immediately called me a liar. When asked if I voted for HR-3200, I said, "No." Again, they started yelling, "Liar!" I continued to ignore this rude group crashing the Senior Center meeting and their ignorant and crude personal comments directed at me. I thanked the seniors for their time and apologized for the unruly crowd but explained that I had to be moving onto Traverse City. One senior jumped up and said that I did not fully respond to his question and asked why I was ducking out fifteen minutes early. I explained that I was not ducking out early- I was a little late in arriving as I had driven down from Sault Ste. Marie in the Upper Peninsula and was running behind schedule. The senior would not accept my response and started to argue with me.

Then, the group crashing the meeting insisted that I stay and meet with them. I told the group that I could not meet with them as I was going to keep my schedule. The group blocked the front door so I could not leave the Senior Center. One of the workers caught my eye and motioned me to the back door. As I walked to my car, the unruly group that was inside the senior center had assembled outside and were waving their signs at me. I blocked one sign from actually hitting me in the face. I squared off with that individual and made it very clear that if he tried to hit me again, I would be the last person he would ever strike. The crowd stepped back and I was able to make my way to my car. The crowd then gathered around and started to beat on my car, so I picked up my phone and called the police. Both the Sheriff and City Police came to the Senior Center, cleared the group away from my car, and then cleared a path for me to leave the parking lot. As I was leaving the parking lot, a person with a sign jumped in front of my car and was grabbed by a police officer as I slammed on my brakes. This was the first of many encounters I would have with the Tea Party in August of 2009.

A few days later a letter to the editor appeared in the local paper claiming that I had been rude and refused to answer questions. The letter also stated that I was so intimidated by the Tea Party demonstrators that I fled the Senior Center early. Nothing could have been further from the truth. Fortunately for me, individuals who had actually been at the Senior Center weighed in on my behalf. After a number of letters to the editor were received from my supporters during the month of Tea Party activists, the complaints of my alleged unprofessional conduct soon died down.

Tea Party activists followed me throughout my district travels that August and attempted to disrupt town hall meetings, private meetings with constituents, and any public appearance that I made in Michigan. Many times, the Tea Party consisted of a lone protestor with a sign, shouting insults as I spoke. After a few weeks of shenanigans by the Tea Party, the local citizens who had invited me to their events began to step in. Local organizers made it clear to the Tea Party that they were not welcome and that the event was not open to the public. The citizens of the First Congressional District and I became frustrated with the activists because groups, organizations, their members and citizens were unable to ask questions or conduct meetings without being disrupted by the Tea Party. Eventually, the organizers publicly claimed that their meetings were closed and asked uniformed police officers to keep control of the Tea Party activists who continued to disrupt the events.

During the August break, the Tea Party activists also flooded the numerous daily and weekly newspapers in the district with letters demanding that I hold town hall meetings so they could question me.

In each little town, village and city in the First Congressional District, Tea Party supporters wrote letters demanding that I make personal appearances and conduct town hall meetings. I believe that within two weeks there were at least thirty demands that I hold town hall meetings in thirty different locations during the month of August. When I did not immediately respond to every request, I was accused of hiding and refusing to meet with my constituents. Even one or two of the daily newspaper editors joined in the fray and wrote articles accusing me of being afraid to hold town hall meetings due to citizen opposition.

Throughout my career I had held, on average, twenty-six to thirty town hall meetings per year. I was always accessible to my constituents. Now, because a radical fringe group was demanding that I hold town hall meetings in every community during the month of August, the less thoughtful editors piled on. It did not make any difference that I had more counties in my congressional district than there were days in the month. It did not make any difference that I had scheduled meetings with constituent groups throughout the district on issues other than health care. It did not make any difference that I had a family and that I wanted to at least spend one day a week with them. It did not make any difference to some of the newspaper editors and Tea Party activists that my son was getting married and that I wanted to take a few days off from traversing my massive district for a special family occasion.

No, the Tea Party activists and a few senseless editors insisted that I spend my August driving around the district attending Tea Party town hall meetings. Simply ludicrous, but that was the political atmosphere facing Democrats in August of 2009.

The Tea Party was not only a pain in the ass to me, but throughout the state of Michigan in Democratic congressional districts, Republicans and Tea Party activists were disrupting scheduled congressional meetings with constituent groups that had nothing to do with health care. The Tea Party just wanted to make life miserable for Democratic Members of Congress who had not yet voted on health care legislation.

I had consistently voted against the Wall Street Bailout in 2008. Therefore, I had good relations with the Tea Party activists. But this good will was quickly coming to an end. I had problems with some of the Tea Party members who would show up at town hall meetings with their recording devices and intimidate citizens trying to ask questions. If there was a sensitive issue that a constituent wished to raise, I would ask the Tea Party members to turn off their cameras and give the constituent the courtesy of discussing the issue in private. These sensitive moments where I requested that they turn off the recording devices involved grieving parents and relatives of brave servicemen who had died or a child killed in an accident.

Quite often, Tea Party activists would shout down my requests, claiming that it was a public meeting and that they had a right to record everything. The insensitivity of the Tea Party activists wore on my constituents. If I knew of parents of soldiers killed in war or of other sensitive matters that might arise when I was in a community, I agreed to meet with relatives in their homes to avoid those types of confrontations.

The Tea Party was against anything that the government proposed. The irony of their actions and comments was that most of the Tea Party activists were receiving government benefits, especially government-sponsored health insurance through Medicare and Medicaid. Based on their comments during town hall meetings, I also believed that they were against our president simply because he was Black.

CHAPTER 28

★ ★ ★

President's Call and the August Recess (August 2009)

After the Waterfront Festival in Menominee I stayed home for a few days before heading out on the road. I was traveling to the southern part of my district to Gladwin, Michigan, 375 miles from Menominee. As usual, I traveled alone and I would join up with my regional staff person. The staff person and I would then meet with local officials, the media, organizations and hold town hall meetings. My RTL brown accordion folder traveled with me throughout northern Michigan; it was becoming a permanent part of me.

As I parked my car before heading into the local Gladwin newspaper office, my Chief of Staff Scott Schloegel called and asked if I would be available for a call from the President. I would certainly make myself available for a call from the President; I told Scott that I would begin my newspaper interview and would interrupt it to receive President Barack Obama's call.

At the start of the interview I advised the reporter that I would need to interrupt our interview around 11:00 a.m. to take a call from Washington, DC. It was of course no problem and we informally discussed health care, the Energy and Commerce Committee markup, my "No" vote on the markup, and the Stupak Amendment. As the interview continued, my phone began to vibrate. I excused myself and walked out to the outer lobby to answer the call. It was the White House operator asking if I could take a call from the President. I walked out to the parking lot and climbed into my car to secure better reception and to gain some privacy as I spoke with President Obama.

The President's call was cordial and we discussed my August schedule with all my public events. I advised the President that I was being interviewed by the local paper and would report back anything he wanted me to say on his behalf. The President just chuckled and said to tell them "Hello" and that he would be addressing the nation on health care when Congress came back after the August recess. The President went on to say that he understood my concerns on federal funding for abortion and he was not going to change the law. I was encouraged by his comments and asked if he would support my position and he said "...just listen closely to what I have to say during my speech on that subject in September." I did not push the issue with the President since he had already stated in June that he did not intend to change the law on abortion coverage.

I told the President that I would listen to his speech but health care reform would not pass if there was federal funding for abortion and if the Hyde Amendment was not going to apply to health care reform. The President again said to listen closely to what he had to say and promised that I would be pleased with his comments.

While I did not have a commitment from the President that he would support the Hyde language in health care reform, I thanked him for his call and said that I would see him in September. He wished me a good recess and I advised him of our son's wedding on Mackinac Island. He said congratulations and to give our son and daughter-in-law his best wishes. Once my conversation with the President ended, I returned to my interview and wrapped it up by declaring that I had a brief discussion with the President and I expected him to address the nation in September on health care reform. The reporter was grateful for the scoop on my conversation and the President's upcoming address to the nation.

I viewed the President's call as an acknowledgement that there was an issue that needed to be resolved before health care could move forward- not that he agreed with the Stupak Amendment. I immediately felt that despite Speaker Pelosi's warnings that she would not allow amendments to the House health care legislation, I had made headway after months of being stonewalled. Then again, this was a conversation with President Obama without his Chief of Staff, Rahm Emanuel, who was doing a great job of keeping the President out of the abortion debate. I imagined that Rahm was probably listening in on our phone conversation.

I travelled heavily throughout my district until August 25, when I shut down and joined my family to celebrate Ken's marriage to Cristina Yamakawa. The marriage was held on Mackinac Island and I took the week off. Mackinac Island holds a special place with our family and we were pleased that Cristina and Ken wished to be married at Ste. Anne's Catholic Church.

Laurie had done a magnificent job in planning the wedding, along with Cristina, Ken, the Yamakawa family, Ste. Anne's Catholic Church, Father Jim Williams, and the Grand Hotel staff. The icebreaker party that Laurie had planned was a huge success in bringing our newest family members and the bride's friends into our life and faith. Earlier that summer, Cristina had been baptized into the Catholic faith, received her First Holy Communion and was accepted into our church community through the spiritual guidance of Ste. Anne's parish priest, Father Jim Williams.

My niece, Stephanie (Stupak) Bennett and her husband Brad had also arranged to hold their daughter Harlie's Baptism at St. Anne's that weekend with Laurie and I serving as godparents. It was truly a spiritual and blessed time for our family and friends.

As requested, I extended the President's congratulations to the newly wedded couple, and Ken and Cristina flew back to California as August came to an end.

It was time for me to return to my duties as congressman and deal with the numerous requests for town hall meetings. I also wondered if the research that I requested from my staff on past abortion votes by Democratic Members of Congress had been completed.

CHAPTER 29

★ ★ ★

Televised Town Hall Meetings (September 2009)

I set up two televised town hall meetings in an effort to communicate with my constituents who truly wanted to learn about health care. These town hall meetings covered all the Upper Peninsula and most of Lower Michigan and were exclusively devoted to health care and the proposed House legislation, HR 3200. The live "call in" town hall meetings provided individuals with an opportunity to call in questions, which were screened by college political science students from Northern Michigan University and Central Michigan University. The calls were not screened because of the Tea Party callers but because many of the questions were similar and the students would consolidate them into more coherent questions. This saved time and allowed me to address more questions in the hour allotted for the town hall meeting. Public television allowed me sixty minutes for the program and the studios did an excellent job of advertising that I would appear live to answer questions on health care. In all honesty, I was surprised that public television was willing to offer me the time on the air to discuss health care. Then again, it was a great public service to have the sitting congressman appear and hold a live town hall meeting on such an important issue.

My first public television town hall meeting occurred on September 2, 2009, at WNMU on the campus of Northern Michigan University in Marquette, Michigan. As I did at every town hall meeting on health care, I defined the issue, my involvement in addressing the issue, the proposed solution to the issue and my position on the proposed legislation. Specifically, I made sure to mention in my opening comments that I was committed to protecting the sanctity of life and that my amendment in committee had been accepted and then rejected by only one vote. Furthermore, I promised to push the Democratic leadership to allow an amendment that maintained the current law stipulating no use of taxpayer funds for abortions.

After the ten- to fifteen-minute introduction, the town hall meeting was opened up for questions, starting with one from the moderator. I saved some of my best facts and statistics for my answers to the questions that I was sure I would receive. Because I had already held numerous town hall meetings throughout August and had received thousands of comments from my constituents, I had a good understanding of what would be asked in these televised town hall meetings.

For instance, in Michigan from 2000 to 2007, the annual family health insurance premiums rose 78.2 percent. Yet, workers' wages only rose 4.6 percent. Families, businesses and government could no longer keep pace with the rapidly rising costs of health insurance premiums.

As mentioned earlier, the average family health insurance policy cost $13,375. In Michigan's First Congressional District, the median household income was $38,771, which meant that thirty-four percent of a family's income was spent on health insurance premiums.

State and federal taxes, social security, and FICA ate up another third or approximately $12,923.67 of the family's income. So, after paying mandatory taxes and $13,375 in yearly health insurance premiums (in which you still must pay an out of pocket amount before your insurance coverage kicks in), the average family had just over $7,000 for rent or mortgage, utilities, car payments, and food. In my congressional district, no matter how you cut it, the numbers did not add up. A family could not afford to pay taxes, buy family health insurance and still expect to have money for housing, utilities, food and transportation. As I stated, American families, businesses and government could no longer afford the cost of health insurance.

Another shocking statistic that I used to explain my support for health care was an American Journal of Medicine report that found that sixty-two percent of all bankruptcies in the United States in 2007 were linked to medical expenses. An incredible seventy-eight percent of those people who filed for bankruptcy had health insurance. There was one small county near my district in which every bankruptcy filed within the previous year was due to medical expenses.

I did not let up on my arguments as to why our nation needed to pass health care reform now. Those individuals who had health insurance often did not care if their neighbor did not, until I reminded them that on average a family with health insurance was paying $1,017 more each year in premiums to cover the cost of treating those without. My constituents had no idea that they were paying an extra eighty-five dollars per month on their health insurance premiums to cover the uninsured.

My constituents believed that the uninsured lived in other congressional districts and not in the First Congressional District of Michigan. Still, my constituents all knew someone who was hedging their bets by not taking health insurance at work. People did not realize that these health risk-takers numbered 82,000 individuals, or that one out of every nine of my constituents was uninsured. When I mentioned this fact, I could see the wheels turning in their minds, for everyone knew someone who was running bare. Perhaps a child, a relative, or even they themselves were uninsured. I would follow up these comments with the statistic from the Harvard University study stating that 45,000 Americans died every year because they lacked access to basic health care.

This was a statistic that haunted me throughout the health care debate. Each time I would argue with a colleague, a reporter, or a constituent that we must protect the unborn child, my moral compass would spin me back to the fact that if I prevented health care from coming to the floor for a vote because I did not get my amendment, 45,000 Americans would *needlessly* die. If I really believed in the sanctity of life, then how could I allow so many American lives to be lost? Even Right-to-Life's abortion policy includes an exception for the life of the mother. If it was necessary to abort the child to save the life of the mother, then is abortion okay to save an existing human life? If so, was it okay to pass health care legislation to save 45,000 Americans without having statutory language which stated that there would be no federal funding for abortions, knowing full well that any American could use their own money to personally pay for an abortion? How then could I continue to deny 45,000 living, breathing Americans continued life over that of an unknown and unborn child? These questions continued to trouble me throughout the debate on health care.

Contrary to what people may have thought, the Stupak Amendment would not have stopped all abortions. The Stupak Amendment would have only prevented taxpayers' money from being used to pay for abortions. How could I let 45,000 Americans die every year because they did not have access to basic health care? My insistence on the Stupak Amendment was personally and professionally very important to me, but so was providing a basic human right of access to health care for all Americans.

During the public television town hall meetings, the abortion issue would enter into our discussions. As always, I was comfortable discussing the issue and I would succinctly explain how the Pitts-Stupak Amendment to prevent federal funding for abortion was defeated in committee by one vote, after the Amendment had already passed by three votes. I would then explain that I remained committed to the Hyde Amendment and would insist that we have an "up or down" vote on the Hyde Amendment during consideration of the health care legislation. As was my practice, I spent very little time on abortion because I was not going to change anyone's stance on the issue and my constituents knew my Pro-Life position.

After my public television town hall meeting on WNMU Public Television in Marquette, I flew down to Mt. Pleasant in the Lower Peninsula of Michigan to hold my second public television town hall meeting at Central Michigan University.

Overall, the televised town hall meetings were a great success. My constituents who wished to participate and listen to a serious discussion on health care were rewarded with the orderly manner in which the televised town hall questions were presented and answered. The Tea Party could not interrupt, shout at me or hurl insults at individuals who asked questions or were brave enough to support health care reform. The public television town hall meetings on health care were an orderly presentation on the greatest social issue that was being debated in our country since the vote on Social Security in the 1930s. I also considered my upcoming vote on health care to be the most important vote of my legislative career, as it would directly affect present and future generations and every man, woman, and child, including the unborn.

After Labor Day, I flew back to Washington, DC satisfied that my constituents who truly wanted to participate in the discussions on health care had had numerous opportunities to question me during the 2009 August recess. I accomplished what I had hoped to and felt confident that I could support health care reform, force a vote on the Stupak Amendment, and that Congress would finally pass national health care legislation. Personally, I was elated that my televised town hall meetings had foiled the Tea Party's constant attempts to disrupt my discussions and did not dampen my enthusiasm for national health care.

Back in Washington, I looked forward to hearing President Obama's address to the nation on health care reform. The speech would be delivered from the House of Representatives chamber, much like a State of the Union address. I had an additional interest, as the President had personally told me that he would address the abortion issue in his September speech. I needed him to make the case for health care reform to the nation, and his upcoming speech afforded me an opportunity to determine whether he was sincere when he said I would be pleased with his comments on abortion. I also wanted to determine if the President would keep his word to me; I reflected on our telephone conversation in August and replayed the interview in my mind.

Yes, it had been a good August for me personally and professionally but now I wanted to know if the research was complete.

It was time to begin my diplomatic efforts to gain commitments from my colleagues to support the Stupak Amendment. At the beginning of September, I had no idea how a House vote on the Stupak Amendment would turn out. If the research was accurate and if I could be persuasive enough with my colleagues, the Stupak Amendment had a chance of passing. It was September and it was time to listen to the President's speech on health care and how he would handle the abortion issue.

Throughout August, as I plotted my next attempt to attach the Hyde Amendment- now known as the Stupak Amendment- to the House's Public Option health care plan, I constantly replayed the Energy and Commerce Committee markup and my comments over and over in my brain. I believed that my best strategy for passing the Stupak Amendment was to keep my argument very simple, and find a better example as to why the amendment was needed. In Committee, Pro-Life arguments centered on the fact that if Congress remained silent on the issue then the Courts would rule that abortion was a covered benefit. While this argument was true, I still needed a simpler, more cogent argument that Members of Congress could relate to. I believed that perhaps Joe Pitts, Lee Terry and I had gotten too much in the weeds trying to parse the words and intent of the Capps Amendment. I had to do better.

Sometime during the August recess, I realized that under the Public Option Plan, the number of Community Health Centers would be greatly increased to provide Americans with greater access to health care. There was nothing in the legislation or in the Capps Amendment that would prevent Community Health Centers from performing abortions. At the time that I made my arguments in committee, the Hyde Amendment was still in effect. However, it would only remain so until September 30, the end of the fiscal year- only thirty days away. Because the Hyde Amendment is not permanent law, it must be renewed annually in the appropriations bills. Since the election of Barack Obama as president, Speaker Pelosi had not allowed the traditional RTL riders, including the Hyde Amendment, to be added to the following year's appropriations bills, which would begin on October 1. There was no indication that the Speaker would allow a renewal of Hyde. Therefore, under the Public Option, women could obtain abortions at Community Health Centers since there would be no prohibition against it. I believed that just about every congressional district included at least one Community Health Center with many of their patients on Medicaid. Without a specific prohibition on the use of federal funds to cover them, these clinics could perform abortions. I became convinced that every Member of Congress could understand the argument and that I should focus on this rather than whether public or private monies were used to pay for abortion services.

If Erika and April had compiled my scorecard as I requested, then the question became simply whether taxpayer funds should be used to pay for abortions. I had a concrete example in the Public Option Plan to demonstrate to Members of Congress that in fact, as written, abortions could be performed at Community Health Centers without the passage of a restrictive amendment such as Hyde, now known as the Stupak Amendment. I believed I had my simple explanation in keeping with my mantra of KISS: Keep It Simple Stupid. I looked forward to returning to Washington and trying out my Community Health Center argument on Members of Congress and forcing a vote on the Stupak Amendment.

CHAPTER 30

★ ★ ★

President Obama Addresses the Nation (September 9, 2009)

Labor Day was the latest it could be, September 7, 2009, and the next day I boarded my flight back to DC. As much as I love northern Michigan and our home on Green Bay (Lake Michigan), there were times that August when I was eager to return to Washington. It was also true that there were many occasions when I dreaded going back to DC because I'd had such a wonderful time with my family and friends in Michigan. However, on September 8, 2009, I was looking forward to returning to the capital to finish the Energy and Commerce Committee markup on health care and to listen to President Obama's speech to the nation. I hoped the President would sell health care to the skeptics and articulate a compassion for the health care needs of all Americans that had been missing in our deliberations.

The president of the United States has the greatest soapbox from which to lead the nation on any issue. I was afraid that President Obama had already used up his good will allowance with Congress and the American people. In the months since his Inaugural Address, President Obama and the Democrats had been non-stop in bringing forth and passing controversial legislation. The President signed the

Economic Stimulus Package, completed the 2009 Appropriations, the House passed climate change legislation and finalized the loans to the auto industry. The President had a very productive first eight months in office, but one of the complaints of the Tea Party was that the President was moving too fast and needed to slow down. The problems facing this president, America, and indeed the world with the global financial meltdown did not allow President Obama to take his time to explain all his actions to the American people. The situation called for action and all we got from the Republicans was rhetoric and distortions of the President's program. In American politics, the minority party should always play the role of "loyal opposition," but this was not opposition to the President's program- it was vitriol loaded with deceit peppered with racism.

Despite the deceitful Republican tactics, Democrats knew we had to move forward to lend a helping hand to our American families, the US domestic auto industry, and the world economy. The health care table had been set for President Obama and now he had to deliver it to the American people. The three House committees with jurisdiction over health care had passed and recommended the legislation to the full House for passage. Never had either the House or the Senate ever passed health care out of a committee, let alone gotten through three committees and had the legislation poised for debate on the House or Senate floor.

While the House Committees had come a long way in their ability to move health care legislation, its passage by the House was far from certain. Members were still smarting from having to walk the plank on climate change when leadership knew full well the Senate would not take up the legislation.

The question was: would the President's speech on health care challenge Members of Congress to become partners with the Administration in providing health care for all Americans, or were we just there to provide the needed votes to pass the President's signature program? Were Members of Congress going to have some ownership in the health care legislation and buy in and defend the initiative, or be left with joining the opposition and criticizing another expensive new social program? Each Member of Congress looked forward to the President's speech on health care to determine if we would be partners or victims of another poorly executed but well-intended program.

When I landed in DC on September 8, the first scheduled meeting was a taped interview with the Christian Broadcasting Network to preview the President's address to Congress on health care. We had votes at 6:30 p.m. and then we had our weekly Fellowship. It would be good to catch up with the guys at C Street since I had not seen them for five weeks.

On Wednesday, September 9, like just about every morning when I was in DC, I set my alarm for 6:30 a.m., go downstairs from my room at C Street, grabbed a banana and walked the three blocks to the House gym. At the gym, I worked out on the elliptical or with free weights and then showered and was ready for my first meeting, which began at 8:00 a.m. Besides the health benefits of a daily exercise, my workouts were also good for my mental health. As the pressure was mounting on me to pass the Hyde Amendment, the House gym became more and more of a sanctuary for me, as it had been following B.J.'s death. The House gym was a great place to hide, to think through the issues of the day and to keep the focus on my personal, professional and spiritual life. The value of the House gym cannot be overstated; I could work out in solitude or join in a game of basketball or encourage others to join P-90X.

Congressman Paul Ryan had introduced P-90X to Members in the House gym. After watching Paul do the program, I joined him in the workouts. By the fall of 2009 and most of 2010, we had convinced several other Members of Congress to join us in our early morning sessions; we set up a daily schedule for Members to follow and continue their regimen even when they were not in DC. Our workouts started promptly at 7:00 a.m.; Paul and I would arrive and set up the equipment we would need for our routine that day. When either Paul or I could not make an early morning session, the other would cover and have the equipment ready to go so Members had no reason *not* to complete their workouts.

Speaker Paul Ryan has since advanced to the extreme versions of the program. Paul and I built a working and personal relationship through our workouts; we are both fitness nuts, devoted to our Green Bay Packers, and love to hunt whitetail deer.

Even more important than the health and mental health benefits, our daily workouts enabled Members to get to know one another not as Democrats or Republicans but as friends with common interests, which broke down stereotypes and united us. Congress would work so much better if it had mandatory gym class for all Members.

Shortly before 8:00 p.m. on September 9, 2009, Members of the House and Senate gathered in a Joint Session of Congress for President Obama's address to the nation on health care. The President began his speech; I could immediately see that some Members of the Republican Party were starting to squirm as he outlined the problems facing our nation and how he was going to work with Congress to address the growing health care crisis. The President stated that every day, 14,000 Americans lose health care coverage and one in three Americans go bare- without any health insurance coverage- during any given two-year period.

The President talked about letters he had received from ordinary Americans who either had lost their insurance or were wrongly denied coverage. He brought up the cases that I had highlighted in my Oversight and Investigations hearings on health insurance companies improperly denying Americans their coverage when they needed it most- when they became seriously ill. The hearing I held on rescissions had been especially painful and the President highlighted two cases:

> "One man from Illinois lost his coverage in the middle of chemotherapy because his insurer found that he hadn't reported gallstones that he did not even know about. They delayed his treatment, and he died because of it. Another woman from Texas was about to get a double mastectomy when her insurance company canceled her policy because she forgot to declare a case of acne. By the time she had her insurance reinstated, her breast cancer had more than doubled in size.

> That is heartbreaking, it is wrong, and no one
> should be treated that way in the United States
> of America."

The President explained to the nation that the only reason for rescinding these insurance policies was that the individuals were about to undergo expensive medical treatments. American lives were apparently worth pennies compared to the thousands of dollars the insurance company saved by canceling (rescinding) health insurance policies.

The President went on to explain how the insurance industry would sell policies to small businesses. When an employee got sick, the insurance company would raise the premiums so high that the small business owner could no longer afford the policy. The small business owner did not have a big enough employee pool to spread the increased costs over a large number of employees to keep the health insurance affordable for all in the company. As the President stated,

> "Insurance executives don't do this because they're
> bad people; they do it because it is profitable. As
> one former executive testified before Congress,
> insurance companies are not only encouraged
> to find reasons to drop the seriously ill, they are
> rewarded for it. All of this is in service of meeting
> what this former executive called "Wall Street's
> relentless profit expectations."

When I called the health insurance executives to testify before the Oversight and Investigations Committee, I asked each executive to review the company's application for health insurance. I then asked each executive the meaning of some of the medical conditions and terms that were listed on the applications. Not only did I have difficulty pronouncing the terms, I had no idea what the terms meant. Surprisingly, neither did the health insurance executives. Still, these executives reserved the right to cancel an individual's health insurance policy based on terms and medical conditions that even they could neither explain nor understand. Under then-current standards, policyholders could face cancellation of coverage when they became ill and needed expensive medical treatment, even for unintentional nondisclosure of an unknown preexisting condition. As the President said, the insurance companies were placing profits over people.

About half way through his address, the President emphatically addressed the claims of the Tea Party and some Republican Members of Congress when he said,

> "Still, given all the misinformation that's been spread over the past few months, I realize that many Americans have grown nervous about reform. So tonight, I want to address some of the key controversies that are still out there."

The President was reassuring the American people that under his Health Care plan there would *not* be bureaucratic death squads to kill off seniors. Then the President pivoted to illegal immigrants when he said:

"There are also those who claim that our reform efforts would insure illegal immigrants. This, too, is false. The reforms—the reforms I'm proposing would not apply to those who are here illegally."

Suddenly, a Member from the Republican side of the House Chamber shouted, "You lie!" The Members present in the Chamber immediately booed the declaration.

The President paused and I could see him clench his teeth in anger, but he kept his cool. A loud murmur vibrated through the House chamber. The President stared in the direction from which the insult had come.

I thought to myself, "Welcome to our August town hall meetings with the Tea Party, Mr. President." In my seventeen years of attending joint sessions of Congress to hear our national and world leaders, Members of Congress had always conducted themselves in a professional, polite manner. This was the first time a Member of Congress had shouted out an insult to the president as he was addressing the nation.

President Obama was making a point that he would not sign into law a health care bill that covered illegal aliens; the ignorant person who shouted the comment had never even seen the proposed legislation or voted on any such legislation. At that point, the House committees had only passed the proposal out of committee and sent it to the Rules Committee, which had not yet even met on health care.

President Obama's next statement was, "It's not true." Then it appeared that he went back to his prepared remarks and mentioned abortion. I sat up a little taller and took down his words.

"And one more misunderstanding I want to clear up—under our plan, no federal dollars will be used to fund abortions, and federal conscience laws will remain in place."

I was pleased to hear the President's remarks on abortion but I realized we had different interpretations of "no federal dollars." The President wanted to set up an accounting mechanism whereby individuals or insurance companies would pay for abortions under the health care plan. My problem with the President and Congresswoman Capps's proposal was that under the Hyde Amendment, federal insurance policies could not support, encourage or promote abortions. The Capps Amendment allowed abortions to be paid for by a third party through an alternate funding source and recognized abortions as an essential medical benefit under the health care law. Allowing abortions in the health care law not only promoted but also encouraged abortions by providing a non-federal entity to pay for the procedure. While my Democratic colleagues stood up and applauded the President's statement on abortion, I saw no reason to stand for a federal government policy that would allow abortions in its sweeping health care law. I also feared that under the health care law there would be no more Appropriations RTL riders because the funding for health care would come from individuals and taxes on insurance companies. How the money was spent left great discretion to the Secretary of HHS and the Secretary would not need to rely on Congress for funding or determine which benefits would be paid for in the Exchange. Even if a woman was totally opposed to abortion, her insurance premium payments into the Exchange would pay for abortions. If she received a subsidy for payment of her health insurance, she could rely on benefits paid by the federal government to include coverage for abortions. HR-3200 and the President's proposal on abortion were contrary to Hyde and would not be accepted by the Pro-Life community.

The President also invited Members of Congress who had ideas and serious proposals on health care to meet with him. "My door is always open," the President reminded us.

The end of President Obama's speech was directed right at us Democrats when he mentioned the late Senator Ted Kennedy. Diagnosed with a terminal illness, Senator Kennedy penned a letter to the President asking that the letter be shared only after his death. A true humanitarian, Ted Kennedy expressed that health care was the "great unfinished business of our society." Ted Kennedy shared his belief with the President and all present by reminding us, "What we face is above all a moral issue; at stake are not just the details of policy, but fundamental principles of social justice and the character of our country."

The President ended his address calling on the better side of all of us and implored us not to kick the can down the road but to pass health care now.

CHAPTER 31

★ ★ ★

Disrespect Leads to Disorder (2009–2010)

A day or two later, Joe Wilson (R-SC) was positively identified as the Congressman who shouted, "You lie!" Even after admitting that he had screamed at the President, Joe Wilson stubbornly refused to apologize. Leaders of both parties urged Joe to reconsider and apologize to President Obama and Congress but he ignored their requests.

The fallout from Congressman Joe Wilson's "You lie" comment to the President became a rally cry for the Tea Party as the US House of Representatives brought forth a Resolution of Disapproval against Joe Wilson.

On September 15, six days after President Obama's address to Congress and the American people, the US House of Representatives passed H Res. 744, Resolution of Disapproval, by a vote of 240-179. Through my correspondence, I explained my affirmative vote disapproving of Congressman Joe Wilson's outburst: "I voted for the Resolution because there are rules and decorum in the US House of Representatives that we, as Members of Congress, are charged to uphold. We do not have the right to set our own rules, decorum, or traditions when it suits our purposes."

However, even before the Resolution of Disapproval was formally presented to the US House of Representatives for debate and deliberations, Joe Wilson's campaign set up a fundraising web site to reward his unprofessional outburst at the President. It is reported that Wilson raised over a million dollars for his campaign with his website. I believe that Wilson's outburst was planned for fundraising purposes. Unfortunately, unprofessional behavior continues to be rewarded in politics. Whatever happened to ethics and civility in the US Congress?

I often ask myself, "When does disrespect become disorder?" The answer to this question would play out during the weekend of March 20-21, 2010, as the Democratic Members of Congress walked arm in arm from the Cannon Building over to the Capitol to cast their votes for the Affordable Care Act.

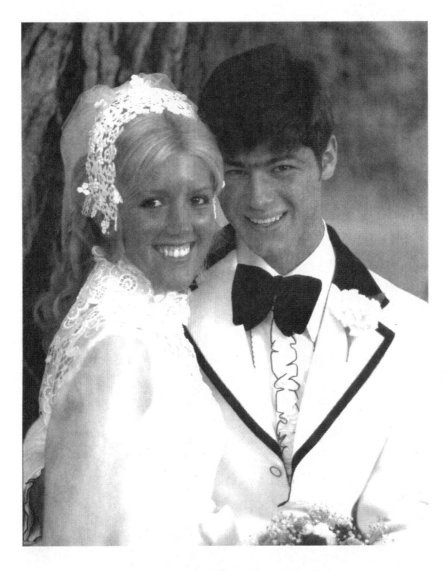

Bart and Laurie (Olsen) Stupak on their
Wedding Day, June 21, 1974

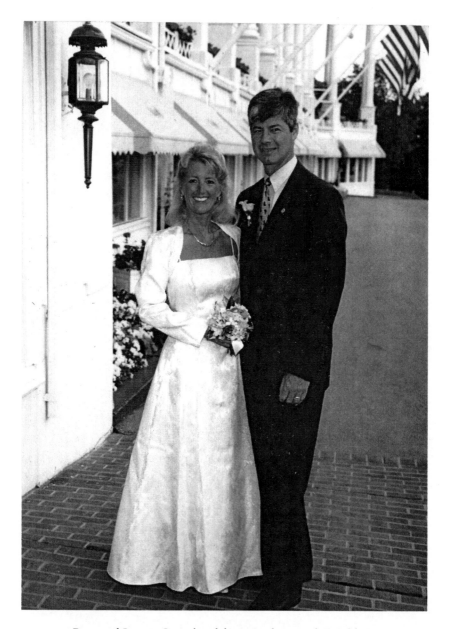

Bart and Laurie Stupak celebrating their 25th Wedding
Anniversary, Grand Hotel, Mackinac Island, MI

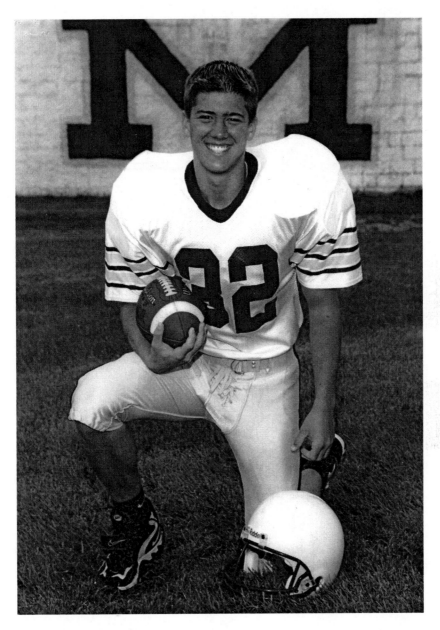

Bartholomew Thomas Stupak, Jr. (B.J.) age 17

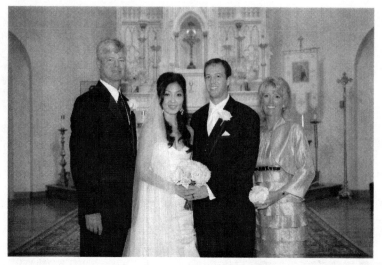

Bart, Laurie, Ken & Cristina (Yamakawa) Stupak, Ste. Anne's
Catholic Church, Mackinac Island, MI August 29, 2009

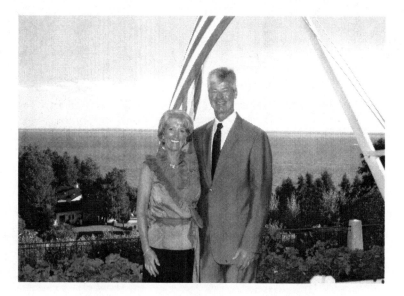

Bart & Laurie Stupak, Front Porch Grand Hotel,
Mackinac Island, MI August 2010

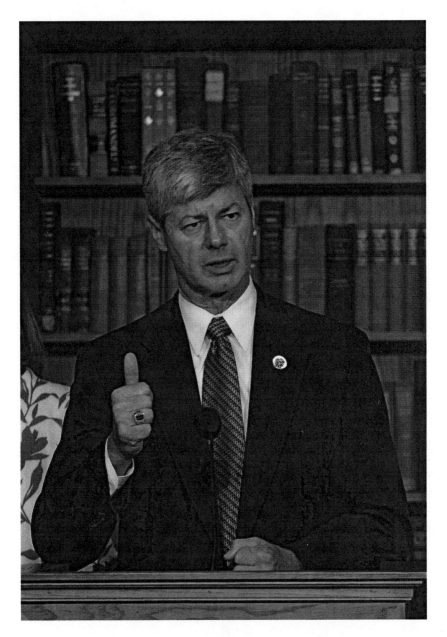

Congressman Bart Stupak's Press Conference
explaining the agreement on the Executive Order and
pledging support for the Affordable Care Act

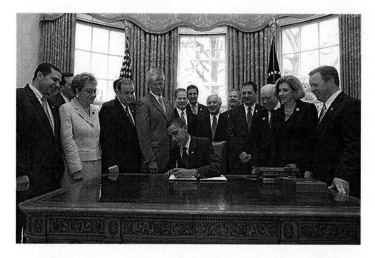

President Obama signing the Executive Order March 24, 2010

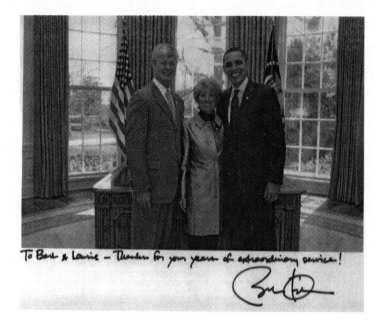

To Bart & Laurie – Thanks for your years of extraordinary service!

Bart & Laurie Stupak with President
Barack Obama March 24, 2010

CHAPTER 32

★ ★ ★

One-Man Whip Team (2009-2010)

By September, the health care legislation was becoming more and more unpopular with Democratic Members. There was pressure from the Tea Party activists, inconsistent statements from the Senate leadership on how they would develop their health care legislation, and a growing concern that President Obama was not fully engaged in the health care debate. While I had my own dealings with the Tea Party over the August recess, I came away unscathed and even more determined to pass health care.

However, throughout the country the Tea Party activists made the August recess miserable for Democratic Members who attempted to communicate seriously with their constituents on health care. No matter what a Member of Congress said, the ridiculous claims against the health care legislation by the Tea Party drowned out an honest, logical explanation of health care to the voters. No matter how Members demonstrated that the Tea Party claims were wrong, they just insisted that the Member of Congress lied and the health care legislation called for death panels, which would pull the plug on Grandma and then the IRS would level a death tax against her estate. The Tea Party claimed that with passage of the health care bill, 35,000 IRS agents would be hired to track down and audit income taxes to make sure taxes were paid. The Tea Party convinced voters that if they did not have health care coverage, the taxpayer would be placed in jail.

The Tea Party insisted that Members of Congress received a special deal under the health care legislation where they would enjoy a free "Cadillac Health Care Plan." Again, not true. Members of Congress were entitled to the same health care benefits offered to all federal employees under the Federal Employees Health Benefits Plan.

The Tea Party activists resurrected the yearly Internet rumor that Members of Congress did not pay federal taxes, Social Security, or Medicare taxes. The Tea Party took the tax rumor one step further to claim on the Internet that more than sixty Members of Congress were delinquent in their federal taxes and owed the government millions of dollars in back taxes. As always, there was not a shred of truth to their false, malicious attacks, but some people liked to believe the worst of Members of Congress. Voters may not have believed that their own Member of Congress owed the federal government back taxes, but the remaining 434 Members of the House sure in Hell were guilty. It was a difficult August back in the congressional districts, and Members of Congress were beginning to believe that it might be easier to vote against health care legislation than to vote for it.

The rise of the Tea Party began with the Wall Street Bailout in the fall of 2008. In late September, the Bush Administration came to Congress and asked for an open checkbook to bail out Wall Street. Treasury Secretary Henry Paulson met with Members of Congress and warned of a great worldwide depression if Congress did not give him and the Bush Administration complete authority to purchase the bad assets to reduce the uncertainty of the value of remaining assets held by financial houses and America's biggest banks. Paulson also wanted to use the US Treasury, if necessary, to recapitalize the financial system in case of total collapse. In other words, Secretary Henry Paulson, Federal Reserve Chairman Ben Bernanke, SEC Chairman and Former Congressman Christopher Cox, and the President asked Congress for a minimum $700 billion to one trillion dollars to stabilize the markets and put the full faith and credit of the United

States at risk to insure the value of the troubled Wall Street assets. While asking for this unprecedented authority and money from the taxpayers to bail out the bad decisions made by Wall Street, no one was being held responsible or accountable. When the American citizen makes a bad investment, he suffers the consequences. The citizen cannot come to Congress and demand that the American taxpayer cover his bad investment. I did not vote to allow Paulson and the Administration the keys to the US Treasury.

As Chairman of the Oversight and Investigations Committee, I always felt that individuals and companies must be held responsible for their actions and no one was being held responsible in this crisis. Each time the Emergency Economic Stabilization Act of 2008 or congressional appropriations supporting the Stabilization Act came up for a vote, I voted No. During my 2008 congressional campaign, the Tea Party applauded me every time I stated in candidate forums that I voted against the Wall Street Bailout. President Obama is often blamed for spending money on the Wall Street Bailout, but he was not president at the time of the crisis, nor when Congress approved the bailout. President Obama had to follow through with America's commitment once Congress passed the Emergency Economic Stabilization Act in early October 2008.

The Wall Street Bailout had mobilized the Tea Party, but former Republican Majority Leader Dick Army set up Super PACs to organize, mobilize, and fund the movement. The number one priority of the Super PACs was defeating national health care, the Democrats, and President Obama. The Tea Party made and funded the propaganda and the wild claims of health care death squads, that citizens would be jailed for not having health care and that illegal immigrants would receive free health care under the Democratic proposals. These claims were all untrue, but well-funded Super PAC advertising turns a lie into a truth in the minds of the uninformed.

A wise man once said that in war, truth is the first casualty. The Democrats who were trying to reform our nation's health care system were in a war with the Tea Party but they did not realize it. I was in my own struggle with the Democratic Party as I tried to protect the sanctity of life and create a right for Americans to access quality, affordable health care. I believed that health care was a right and not a privilege reserved only for those who could afford it. My two principles of life and health care were at war and I knew it.

I struggled to determine the best way to convince Members of Congress to join me in voting against the Rule and for inclusion of the Stupak Amendment in the health care legislation. As I reviewed my vote scorecard, I consciously broke down my list of Democratic Members of Congress into three categories. This RTL scorecard was neatly tucked into the front of my brown RTL accordion file as I set out to persuade Democratic Members of Congress to vote against the Rule accompanying America's Health Choices Act of 2009 if the Stupak Amendment was not made in order.

There were those Members of the US House of Representatives who had decided to vote against health care; Members who would definitely vote for the health care legislation; and, lastly, a group of Members who were truly undecided on their vote. Each group of Members of Congress presented a unique challenge on how I would frame my argument and ask him/her to vote against the Rule and for the Stupak Amendment.

The problem with my approach was that if a Member was determined to vote against the health care legislation, then that Member of Congress could possibly vote against the Rule and for the Stupak Amendment but then vote No on health care. I might win the battle but lose the war.

If a Member of Congress was going to vote for the health care legislation, then he or she would be very reluctant to vote against the Rule and for the Stupak Amendment, which was opposed by House leadership.

Then, there were Members of Congress who remained uncommitted in their vote on the health care legislation. These Members of Congress would be most challenging because they had to be convinced that there was an equal or greater moral justification to vote for the Stupak Amendment and health care vote.

While my friends like Mike Doyle thought that I was nuts and tilting at windmills, I quietly went about my business, pressing Democratic Members for their commitment to vote for the Stupak

Amendment and to vote against the Rule if I did not have a chance to offer my amendment. I was publicly pressing the staunch pro-choice Democratic leadership to grant my amendment during the House's consideration of health care reform. Mike may have been right. I may have been tilting at windmills but then again as Laurie says, I may not be the smartest person she has ever known but I am the most determined.

It wasn't just windmills that I saw when I examined the score-card. I believed that it was possible to include and win a vote on the Stupak Amendment in health care reform. I approached Democratic Members of Congress based on their previous votes, not on labels. I did not label Members as conservative or liberal, right-to-life or pro-choice, but rather as individuals who held beliefs that were revealed in their voting records, their statements back home in their congressional districts, and a sense of fair play. I also knew from my leadership position in the congressional RTL caucus and from whipping RTL issues for seventeen years that some of the most liberal members of the Democratic Caucus always voted for the Hyde Amendment.

While I was pleased with the President's speech, within a week I started to lobby individual Democratic Members of Congress to include the Hyde Amendment in health care reform. The Democratic Members that I targeted were taken from a scorecard that I had asked to be compiled by my staff person, Erika Smith, and Congressman Chris Smith's RTL staff person, Autumn Christensen. This score-card listed Democratic Members who had voted for the Hyde Amendment in the past. We also considered any public statements that Democratic Members may have made concerning abortion in health care reform. Then we added other significant RTL votes for each Democratic Member on our scorecard. It really wasn't a score-card that we assigned a numerical score to, but we charted critical votes cast by each Democratic Member to determine who may be sympathetic to my request and consistent with their past votes. My scorecard revealed that some Members of Congress were very consistent throughout their careers in voting for Hyde even though they were considered Pro-Choice Members of Congress. This scorecard developed by Erika and Autumn was critical to determining which Members to focus on, for I was a "one-man" Whip team.

I explained to these pre-selected Democratic Members that I needed them to vote No against the Rule if I did not get my amendment. Then, if I did receive my amendment, to vote Yes on the Stupak [Hyde] Amendment to the health care legislation. I also reminded them that none of our traditional RTL riders had been approved or included in the appropriations bills in this Congress as they had been over the past thirty years. The Democratic Members agreed that I deserved an up or down vote on the Stupak Amendment but then would quickly add, "Nancy said there would be no amendments." I would simply say, "I know, but I have not given up and I need you to stand with me."

Some Democratic Members did not wish to vote to defeat the Rule even if my amendment was not made in order. When I convinced Members to vote with me on the Stupak Amendment, they insisted that our discussions were confidential and that I could not tell or leak their names to the press or Democratic leadership. I kept my promise. The conversations and the names of Members who promised to vote for the Stupak Amendment were never publicly mentioned and never revealed to the Speaker or the Democratic Leadership. I kept these names confidential from my staff and from Erika Smith who I did not trust to keep her mouth shut.

My lack of trust in my health care advisor, Erika Smith, had been building for some time, as she had been a disruptive force in my DC and district offices. Erika thought she was better than anyone else in the office. While my staff would be busting their butts to get the constituent mail answered, she would not lift a finger to help. She was critical of other staffers and berated them. She was a complete ass to other personnel but was a charmer to me and to Scott Schloegel, my Chief of Staff. Erika insisted that she only handle one issue, health care, and other related issues on the Energy and Commerce Committee. Erika was hired to assist me with health care but that did not mean she could set herself apart from my other congressional personnel and not be full part of the Stupak team. As health care came into focus for the Democrats, Erika became more and more assertive and disruptive. Unfortunately for me, Erika Smith was also committed to the sanctity of life but she had become co-opted by the RTL organizations and the Catholic Bishops.

As I lobbied Democratic Members to vote against the Rule and for the Stupak Amendment, I could not afford to have Erika telling the RTL groups or Republican staff members how Democratic Members might vote on the Rule and the Stupak Amendment. By October of 2009, the abortion issue had become a national one and was causing problems for me within the Democratic Party. I did not need Erika, who tends to rub people the wrong way and say things to draw attention to herself, stirring the pot behind me. Health care was not about me or about Erika; it was about providing the American people access to quality, affordable health care. I had to keep the Members' trust and confidence, otherwise my amendment and I were doomed.

After the President's speech, I took up his offer to sit down with Members as he had an open door for serious proposals. My concern over the abortion language certainly was serious. I had won the vote in committee until one Member was persuaded to change his vote. Therefore, I drafted a letter to the President asking for a meeting and enclosed two Congressional Research Service Memos detailing how funding for the Public Option and the premium subsidy program would not require future congressional appropriations to operate. Without future appropriations, there was no opportunity to apply the Hyde language. Without Hyde, thirty years of precedent of not using taxpayer dollars to pay for, promote, or encourage abortions would be overturned.

The President never replied in writing to my correspondence, but I did receive an earful from his Chief of Staff, Rahm Emanuel. Most conversations with Rahm are fairly one-sided. As he bitched and cussed at me, I kept talking over him and he kept yelling, "You have to follow regular order to get your f_____ amendment!" I tried to explain to Rahm that I had followed regular order but the Speaker had not allowed one RTL rider at all in this Congress for the first time in thirty years; that I had won the vote in full committee until Waxman received a reconsideration of the vote and pressured

Members to change their vote; and that the Speaker had already declared that there would be no amendments to health care. "So tell me Rahm, who is following regular order?" He responded by insisting that the President would not get involved in the House's internal fights and that I needed to work things out with Speaker Pelosi. I shot back that the Speaker would not even meet with me, "So how in the Hell are we going to work this out?"

I ended each conversation with Rahm the same way: "Rahm, if you want health care, we [RTL Democratic Members] had better get a clean up or down vote on Hyde or we will defeat the Rule." It was September and Rahm did not believe me. In September, I quite frankly would not have believed me either but I was warning him of what was going to happen if we were unable to solve the abortion issue.

The reason my threat was not taken seriously by the Administration in September was that the health care legislation had not yet been finalized or presented to the Rules Committee. It was still early in the legislative process, but I felt it was important to keep the Stupak Amendment in the mix of outstanding issues that needed to be addressed before health care could move forward. Further, two CRS memos claimed that after health care passed, there would no longer be an opportunity to insert traditional RTL appropriations riders on the health care legislation. The principle of no public funding for abortions would then be buried under a national health care plan that was self-funded with an individual's premiums covering the essential health package as determined by a Pro-Choice Secretary of Health and Human Services, Kathleen Sibelius.

CHAPTER 33

———— ★ ★ ★ ————

First Live Town Hall Meeting
(September 25, 2009)

On Saturday, September 25, 2009, I held my first of several town hall meetings that Fall focused entirely on HR-3200 in Negaunee, Michigan at the local high school gymnasium. The Negaunee town hall meeting was the first time that I had ever used a Power Point presentation in a town hall meeting. On Friday, I asked my staff to set up and conduct a run-through to make sure that the presentation would work. The meeting had been advertised extensively and I was expecting a large crowd in this solidly Democratic area of the Upper Peninsula.

I was very pleased with the turnout and I was thankful that we had chosen the high school gym to accommodate the crowd. I spent approximately twenty minutes going through the presentation on HR-3200, then opened the meeting for questions. The attendees were very interested and asked good questions. We had a few Tea Party folks there but they did not attempt to take over the meeting or shout insults. The Tea Party knew that I enjoyed strong support in this area and many of my friends and supporters were in the crowd. After the meeting, I stayed another forty-five minutes, answering questions individually with constituents on health care and on other issues.

The questions from my constituents centered on the geographic disparities in Medicare reimbursement from one region of the country versus another region and the reimbursement differences within states.

Most of the town hall attendees had health insurance through their Steelworkers contract with Cleveland Cliffs Mining Company. They were satisfied with their insurance and did not want to lose it or have it replaced with a government-sponsored plan. They liked their doctors and wanted to make sure they could keep their current providers.

While the town hall meeting participants wanted to make sure that the health care legislation would not adversely impact their union health insurance, the steelworkers also understood the need to provide health insurance for the uninsured. I was amazed at how many individuals confided in me that they or a family member were without coverage.

While I raised the issue of abortion coverage in my Power Point presentation, it was not raised in questions from the audience. The abortion issue was brought up only in the private conversations I had with my constituents after the town hall meeting, and was usually a compliment for my strong RTL position and voting record.

My first live town hall meeting went well and the presentation that my staff and I had spent hours developing guided the discussion on health care. It was also very convenient to answer a constituent's question by flipping back to a slide highlighting the point I was trying to emphasize in my answer. I hoped that all town hall meetings would go as well as the Negaunee town hall meeting, but I knew better.

CHAPTER 34

$\star\star\star$

Meeting After Meeting
(September–November 2009)

On Monday, I received a call from the Speaker's office inviting me to meet with Nancy Pelosi in her office the next day on the health care legislation. My calls to Rahm, my public statements and the efforts of my "one-man Whip team" were beginning to pay off. In fact, the previous day I had authored and sent a letter to Speaker Pelosi signed by twenty-five Democrats and 158 Republicans, which stated, "We urge you to allow members of the House to vote their conscience with regard to abortion and health care reform by allowing consideration of an amendment to prohibit government funding of abortion."

With this correspondence, I felt Speaker Pelosi had received another opportunity to defuse the abortion issue, and she failed to take it. I surmised that this correspondence had caught the Speaker's attention and prompted the meeting. The letter contained 183 signatures stating that the signers would vote against the Rule on health care legislation that did not include an amendment preventing funding for abortion. I only needed thirty to thirty-five more Members to sign the letter and I could effectively block health care reform from coming to the floor without my amendment.

The Speaker did not waste time in addressing the abortion issue. She asked, "You are not really going to stand in the way of passing health care, are you?" I quickly responded, "No, I want health care reform to pass as much as anyone." In 1992, I ran on the principle that health care was a right of all Americans and not just for the privileged few who could afford it. Then she asked me why I thought public funds would be used for abortion. At that time, the House bill included the Public Option Health Insurance plan.

I told the Speaker that the CRS memo confirmed that once health care was passed, there would be no opportunity to attach the Hyde language to prevent public funding of abortion. The Speaker claimed that she still did not understand the problem, to which I responded that she had not allowed any of the traditional RTL riders on the appropriations bills. Since she had not allowed any of our riders, I had no reason to believe that she would allow the Hyde Amendment to become part of the health care legislation now or in the future. Therefore, I had to insist that the Stupak Amendment be made in order as an amendment to HR-3200.

The Speaker asked if I had met with Rules Committee Chairperson Congresswoman Louise Slaughter regarding my amendment. I laughed and said, "No, Chairperson Slaughter will not grant my amendment. She had not yet granted one RTL amendment this year." Further, I told Speaker Pelosi that she determines which amendments would be made in order, not Chairwoman Slaughter. Speaker Pelosi encouraged me to speak with Chairwoman Slaughter. As disingenuous as this request was, I promised that I would seek a meeting. The Speaker ended our conversation by stating that there would be no amendments to the health care legislation. I responded by stating that if there are no amendments then the health care legislation may never come to the floor.

During the meeting, Speaker Pelosi acted like she did not understand how abortions would be financed with taxpayer funds under the House Public Option health care legislation. I provided the simplest example. Under the Public Option, the number of the federally financed Community Health Centers was greatly expanded to provide Americans with greater access to health care. I explained that there was nothing in the legislation or in the Capps Amendment that would prevent federal money from being used to pay for elective abortions. The Speaker responded that the Hyde Amendment was still in effect. I said that it was, but the Amendment would only remain in effect for three more days, as it is not permanent law but must be renewed annually in the appropriations bills. And that Madam Speaker had not to date allowed any of the traditional RTL riders, including the Hyde Amendment, on this year's appropriations bills.

The Speaker then argued that Hyde was not necessary, as the Capps Amendment would allow individuals to buy an insurance policy under the Public Option plan that did not include abortion. I countered that the Capps Amendment allowed health insurance plans to receive federal funding to pay for abortion services, but required those funds to be labeled as private contributions. I explained that RTL organizations, the Catholic Bishops, and the Congressional RTL caucus viewed the Capps Amendment as nothing more than an accounting gimmick. The Speaker then turned to her Health Care Advisor Wendell Primus, who said that my understanding of Capps was wrong and there would be no public funding for abortion.

I then asked Wendell if he disputed the fact that under the Public Option the Secretary of HHS could mandate abortion as an essential benefit as had been done in the past. He said he could not speak for the Secretary of Health and Human Services but he doubted that abortion would be considered as an essential benefit. I countered that the courts had consistently ruled that if Congress failed to explicitly ban abortion coverage in health care services, then it was considered a covered benefit. The Pelosi meeting ended cordially.

I kept a cool head in the meeting and was respectful of Speaker Pelosi and Wendell even though they were wrong on the facts. I had a firm grasp of the issue and spoke in a quiet, confident tone. I was surprised that I did not get a response from the Speaker when I stated that the health care legislation would never come to the floor if I did not get a vote on my amendment. Then again, I figured that the Speaker was gauging my sincerity and commitment to the principle of no public funding for abortion in health care.

I then headed to the Rayburn Building for my meeting with Chairman Waxman and Congressman Doyle. Waxman had Doyle at the meeting for the sole purpose of convincing me to drop my demand for the Stupak [Hyde] Amendment. Waxman's logic was that the Energy and Commerce Committee had voted down my amendment and the issue was decided. I was ready for Waxman's argument.

First, I stated that the funding of abortion services in the health care legislation was a major concern that should be addressed by the entire House and not just the Energy and Commerce Committee. I assured Chairman Waxman that the Hyde Amendment had been the law for thirty years and RTL Members of Congress, the Bishops, and RTL groups were not going to abandon it at this critical time in the health care debate. Further, if Members of the US House of Representatives were given the opportunity to vote up or down on a clean Hyde Amendment, it would pass the House. I ended my rebuttal to Chairman Waxman that even President Obama recognized that Hyde had been an "historic tradition of not financing abortions" and he was not looking to change it. Plus, three weeks ago in his speech to Congress the President had stated that there would be no federal funding for abortions. All I was doing was following up on the President's promise.

Waxman countered that the Capps Amendment did not allow public funds for abortion. I simply responded by saying that I disagreed on whether Capps funded elective abortions with taxpayer money but either way Capps violated Hyde language by promoting and encouraging elective abortion through federal policy.

I thanked Chairman Waxman and Congressman Doyle for their time but told them that we disagreed on this issue and I would continue to press for my amendment. I ended the conversation by stating, "Let's just put up the amendment and allow Members to vote their conscience. If I lose the vote, so be it. But you cannot deny us an opportunity to vote on this very important issue."

Chairman Waxman said that Speaker Pelosi would not allow my amendment. I responded by saying, "Then Speaker Pelosi will not be able to pass the health care legislation."

CHAPTER 35

★ ★ ★

September, Come October (2009)

After our September 23, 2009, Energy and Commerce Committee markup on HR-3200, the remaining amendments were sent to the Rules Committee. The longest and strangest markup I was ever involved with started in late July and was finalized on September 23. Now, it was anyone's guess as to when the Speaker would call up the health care bill for a vote on the House floor. However, before she could bring the legislation to the floor she had to have the votes to pass the Rule. As September gave way to October, the Speaker did not have the votes for the Rule and even fewer votes for health care.

The Speaker was having trouble securing votes for health care from the New Democratic Network, the Blue Dogs, the RTL Democrats, and the southern Democrats. Speaker Pelosi was focused on securing enough votes for passage and did not seem too worried about securing votes for the Rule. I believed she assigned Chairman Waxman and Congressman Doyle to rein me in and convince me to drop my opposition to the Rule and the underlying legislation. Waxman, Doyle and Speaker Pelosi knew that I wanted to pass health care but they were not sure how long and hard I would push for the Stupak Amendment. Despite the "shot across the bow" in

July, Speaker Pelosi never dreamed or seemed to believe that I could actually take down the Rule.

If the Speaker had remembered her history, she would have recalled that I was part of the freshmen class that took down six Rules and upended floor action numerous times in the 103rd Congress (1993-1994). Speaker Pelosi probably did not realize that I was one of a handful of Members who had attended a Parliamentary Class conducted by then-Majority Whip Congressman David Bonior (D-MI) and Congressman Barney Frank (D-MA) in 1995. The informal Parliamentary Classes were David Bonior's effort to teach some of us freshmen Members how to handle ourselves on the floor as we fought the White House on NAFTA (North American Free Trade Agreement). Congresswoman Pelosi had been part of the anti-NAFTA group opposing President Clinton's trade pact with Mexico and Canada.

Then, when the Democrats lost control of the House in 1995 after their forty-year control as the Majority Party, it became imperative to always have a Democratic Member observing the floor proceedings and special orders. The Democratic Members who volunteered to monitor the floor were required to understand the parliamentary rules contained in the 1,488-page Jefferson Manual.

I had learned that a Member may have the best-intended piece of legislation but it may never come to the House floor for consideration if the Rules of the House are not explicitly followed. I had witnessed more than one well-meaning amendment derailed by the parliamentary proceedings in the US House of Representatives.

One might think that the men and women elected to Congress would observe unfailingly rational and ethical standards of decorum while on the Floor. Unfortunately, that is not always the case. For example, I once had to use my parliamentary knowledge to challenge and rein in Congressman Dan Burton (R-IN) during his Special Order arguing that Clinton White House Counsel Vince Foster had been murdered by someone with close ties to the Clinton Administration. Congressman Burton discussed how he conducted his own experiment in his back yard by shooting into a watermelon, which was supposed to represent Vince Foster's head, to demonstrate that Foster could not have committed suicide. Burton's theory and arguments on the floor crossed the line of ethical behavior and I called him on it. Congressman Burton weakly apologized, but his conspiracy theory exists yet today.

As the Speaker suggested, I scheduled a meeting with Rules Chairwoman Louise Slaughter for October 1. I walked over to the Rules Committee Room in the Capitol and waited in the reception area at least fifteen minutes before the meeting began. It was not really a meeting so much as a one-sided lecture.

After I requested that Congresswoman Slaughter consider making the Stupak Amendment in order to the health care legislation, she denounced it as leading back to the days of back-alley abortions. Congresswoman Slaughter claimed that she personally knew a young woman who had died from a back-alley abortion and "…we are not going back to that." Louise Slaughter did not have to say anything more. There was no way she would even entertain the idea of making the Stupak Amendment in order. I knew the meeting would be useless, but since the Speaker instructed me to meet with Slaughter, I did. I did not want the Democratic leadership saying that I was not going through "regular order" even though they themselves were not.

After the Slaughter lecture, I did not get angry. I just became more determined to push my amendment and increased my outreach to the Members on my scorecard. I knew any response I would give to Slaughter would be meaningless. I realized that the help I had given her via my legislative and negotiation skills, which had allowed her GINA legislation to become law after a twelve-year stalemate, was history. Realizing that my counterargument to Slaughter's speech would have only inflamed the situation, I decided to thank the Chairwoman for her time. I did tell Slaughter that I knew that she would not give me my amendment but I was meeting her at the request of the Speaker so no one could say that I did not follow regular order.

I am sure that Congresswoman Slaughter viewed me as a RTL zealot. But then again, I viewed her as a very ungrateful Pro-Choice zealot who was unwilling to even consider the Pro-Life position. It was no wonder that her legislation was tied up for twelve years, given that she would not even try to see the other side of the argument. At least Speaker Pelosi heard me out on the issue; Slaughter did not give me the time of day or even a moment to explain what the Stupak Amendment meant to the passage of heath care. I never asked Congresswoman Slaughter to agree with me, but she could have behaved with more professional courtesy.

In the meantime, Waxman and Doyle set another meeting in Waxman's office on October 7. Nothing new came from that short meeting other than we agreed to keep the lines of communication open. Plus, after the Slaughter lecture, I was in no mood to continue worthless meetings. I pulled my scorecard from my brown accordion file and reached out to twelve more Democratic Members on my list.

Ten of the twelve Members said they would stand with me and vote for the Stupak Amendment. I was starting to secure enough commitments that I could comfortably win the vote on my amendment if every Republican would stand with me and every Democrat followed through on his/her promise to do so. The Democrats who committed their vote for the Stupak Amendment were solid Members and their word was good with me. I was confident of victory. I just needed an opportunity to offer it for a vote.

My outreach to Members occurred when we were walking over for votes, on the House floor, outside of committees, in the House gym, or at Democratic caucuses. The caucuses were occurring almost daily as Speaker Pelosi brought in guest speakers to explain the health care legislation and convince caucus members to support HR-3200. I discussed my RTL strategy with my targeted Democrats whenever and wherever I could find a quiet moment alone with no staff present.

CHAPTER 36

———— ★ ★ ★ ————

End of RTL? (October 2009)

In the meantime, as our Oversight and Investigations hearings were wrapping up and Members were clamoring for a vote, Speaker Pelosi continued to ignore the RTL Democrats. When asked about the abortion issue, the Speaker would simply respond that the President had assured us in his September speech that there would be no public funding for abortion coverage in the health care legislation.

The President and Speaker Pelosi were correct in their assertion that the underlying proposed Public Option Health Care legislation did not specifically include public funding of abortion. However, the three House committees that had jurisdiction over the proposed health care legislation: Ways and Means, Education and Labor, and Energy and Commerce, (Medicaid, Medicare, CHIP, and all health care related issues and programs) had all narrowly voted to include Pro-Choice amendments adding funding for abortions. The way the House Public Option Health Care stood now, abortion would be a benefit allowed and paid for under federal law. I could not simply stand by and permit this to occur.

October flew by and the fighting between our respective political camps on abortion continued with no respite. I would do an interview and then Diana DeGette or another Pro-Choice Representative would counter my position. If I wasn't doing a press interview, I was meeting with RTL Members of both parties urging them to stick together and to push for a vote on our amendment. The RTL meetings were non-stop as Chris Smith requested constant updates and I attempted to keep our core group informed. Many of us RTL Democrats wondered if the US Conference of Catholic Bishops truly wanted to pass the Stupak Amendment or just wanted an audience to preach to while I tracked down the votes to defeat the Rule.

The media demands were constant and I urged Jim Oberstar (D-MN) and Dan Lipinski (D-IL) to help me by taking some of the interviews, as I could not keep up with all the requests. The group felt that it was better if we had just one spokesperson giving interviews so we could stay on message. Unfortunately, the group insisted that I continue to be the sole spokesperson for the Stupak Amendment, formerly known as the Hyde Amendment.

The US Conference of Catholic Bishops' lobbyists were demanding meetings with House leadership on the Stupak Amendment. The Democratic leadership had no desire to meet with them because they had no intention of allowing the amendment. Richard Doerflinger, the Associate Director of Pro-Life Activities for the US Conference of Catholic Bishops, was especially persistent with his demands. The Bishops, with the permission of my health care Legislative Assistant Erika Smith, chose my congressional office as their home base from which to operate while working the House of Representatives. I was forced to put my foot down and instructed my Chief of Staff, Scott Schloegel, that when I came back to my office, I did not want staff members conducting meetings in my personal office or in the legislative room. In addition, my staff was being overwhelmed with phone calls and faxes urging me to support the Stupak Amendment.

I found it interesting that callers did not realize which office they were calling. When the staff person answered, "Congressman Stupak's office," the caller apparently did not realize that they were urging the congressman after whom the amendment was named to vote for his own amendment. Did they really think it was necessary to overwhelm my office with phone calls, faxes and emails asking me to support the Stupak Amendment?

It seemed like everything was spinning out of control. Erika Smith behaved as though she thought *she* was the congressman and kept setting fires for me, which I was then obliged to drop everything to put out and smooth over hard feelings with other Democratic Members. Unfortunately, Erika overplayed her role and her own self-importance.

Erika did not ask for meetings with the Democratic leadership- she demanded them. Because of the position that I held in the bi-partisan Congressional Right-to-Life Caucus, Erika demanded that Members of Congress and their staffs do exactly as she dictated on Pro-Life issues. I would get angry calls from Members willing to support the Stupak Amendment but vigorously complaining that Erika angered their staff with her pompous attitude. By late October, I had lost all faith and confidence in Erika to represent my interests and those of the Right-to-Life movement. Still, despite Erika Smith, I managed to secure a last-minute meeting between the Bishops' lobbyists and Majority Leader Steny Hoyer.

Steny Hoyer represented our last best chance to discuss allowing the Stupak Amendment to be made in order under the Rule. Rumors were persistent that health care would be voted on and passed by the end of October. The rumor was fueled by the fact that the US House of Representatives voting calendar listed our targeted adjournment date of October 30, 2009. All the Members knew that October 30 was not realistic and we would be voting into November. However, on the way to the targeted adjournment date, the Speaker did not have enough votes to bring the Rule to accompany health care to the floor of the US House of Representatives.

Always a gentleman, Steny Hoyer agreed to meet with me along with the Bishops' representatives: John Carr, Richard Doerflinger, Jayd Hendricks, and Nancy Wisdo. We met Steny in the ornate Majority Leader's office in the Capitol. Steny was attempting to be polite as he wolfed down a sandwich. In late October, the Members most deeply involved in finalizing the health care legislation did not have many chances to eat or sleep.

Steny heard us out on the reasons why Leadership should allow a vote on the Stupak Amendment. Steny simply said that he appreciated the visit, but whether the Stupak Amendment would be made in order or not was out of his hands. I appreciated his honesty and asked him to relay the message to the Speaker that she would not have enough votes to pass the Rule for health care without the Stupak Amendment being made in order. Steny acknowledged my request and said that I had the Speaker's attention. Still, the Speaker was insisting that there would be no amendments to the health care bill because if she gave in on one then she would have to allow numerous amendments that could possibly take down the health care bill. I told Steny that I understood the Speaker's predicament and that that was even more reason to incorporate my amendment in the Manager's Amendment.

As the name implies, the Manager's Amendment is offered at the beginning of the House floor debate on a piece of legislation. The Manager may accept amendments friendly to the underlying legislation for incorporation, which saves time and effort. Usually an amendment included as part of the Manager's amendment is non-controversial. There are occasional times when the Manager's Amendment is very contentious. Leadership relies on the strength of the Chairman of the committee with subject matter jurisdiction to incorporate the controversial amendment to quell any controversy and pass the underlying legislation. The Majority Party may also insert a provision in the underlying bill to try to hide an amendment and not draw attention to the provision inserted between the time the legislation leaves the Rules Committee and is ready for floor debate.

The Minority Party must review and understand the Manager's Amendment and be prepared to challenge the provisions that were not in the original legislation when it left the committee of jurisdiction. Provisions inserted in the legislation without following regular order of committee hearings and markup usually required the consent of the Chairman of the committee with subject matter jurisdiction and the Speaker.

I did not realize it then, but my suggestion to Steny Hoyer of inserting my amendment in the health care legislation through a Manager's Amendment would be agreed to and then withdrawn by the Speaker within the next several days.

Steny said that no matter what his personal feelings were on the issue, Nancy Pelosi was not going to give in and she would roll me on my amendment. I said fine: just give me a clean vote and we will see who rolls whom. Then, Richard Doerflinger decided to give his dissertation on the history of the Hyde Amendment. I cut him off after five minutes because neither Hoyer nor anyone else in the room needed to hear his lecture yet again.

As we departed the Majority Leader's office, I told the representatives of the US Conference of Catholic Bishops, "If I know Steny, he is probably talking to the Speaker right now. He knows that I don't bullshit. If I said I have the votes to block the Rule, I have the votes to block the Rule." Steny also knew how to count votes. Before becoming Majority Leader, he had served as the Democratic Whip. He knew what I knew: the Democratic leadership needed to deal with me, that time was running out, and that they were short of votes.

As we started to walk back over to my Rayburn office, Richard Doerflinger spoke up and said, "You know the whole Right-to-Life movement is counting on you. If you do not win this fight, it will be the end of the Right-to-Life movement." I told Richard that I doubted that the whole Right-to-Life movement rested with me and that the movement had greater problems in the Senate than in the House. Doerflinger repeated his statement and added that if I didn't pass the Stupak Amendment in the House, the issue would never get to the Senate and the Right-to-Life movement would be dead.

Richard was trying to tell me that the US Conference of Catholic Bishops had put all their marbles on the Stupak Amendment. I looked at Doerflinger and said, "You should not be spending your time on the House; you had better get your butt over to the Senate. I can neither control nor take responsibility for the Senate. I will get my amendment one way or the other because Pelosi cannot pass the Rule or health care legislation without my support."

Doerflinger then asked for my list of Members that I was counting on to vote with me on the Rule. I politely told him that was not possible because I gave Members my word that their names would not be disclosed to anyone, including the Bishops. Doerflinger was a little taken aback. I explained that it was nothing personal but I had credibility with those Members of the House that had been built up over seventeen years and I would not betray their confidence. It would be because of their trust that I would win the vote on the Stupak Amendment. My problem was getting the Stupak Amendment made in order.

I was convinced that Nancy Pelosi had enough votes to pass health care even if she had to rely on the votes that she carried in her pocket. Each Speaker carried "votes in their pocket." It meant that Members, usually of the Speaker's party, did not wish to vote for the legislation under consideration because it was not popular with the voters in the Member's congressional district. However, these Members promised the Speaker that if the legislation was within a couple of votes of passage they would not vote against it. On occasion, I had given the Speaker my vote to carry in her pocket. Speaker Pelosi may have had the votes to pass health care, but she did not have the votes to bring health care to the floor under a Rule dictating that there would be no amendments. If you don't pass the Rule there is no legislation as stated in the Jefferson Manual, which I had studied carefully years before national health care became a possibility.

I excused myself from the Bishops' group and slowly walked back to my office on this beautiful fall day in DC. I wanted to call Laurie for an update as my mother-in-law, Elaine Olsen, was headed to the hospital in Escanaba. When I called Laurie, her mother was still consulting with the doctors but it looked like she would be spending the night at St. Francis hospital in Escanaba. St. Francis is the only hospital located in Delta County. It is a Catholic hospital run by the Sisters of the Third Order of St. Francis. The Sisters have operated and served our area for over a hundred years, and we are thankful for their continual commitment to health care and our community.

I went back to the issue at hand. How could I convince the Democratic leadership to make my amendment in order? The fact was starting to sink in that the Speaker really could not bring health care to the House floor because she did not have enough votes to pass the Rule. The question was whether Speaker Pelosi understood this reality.

CHAPTER 37

———— ★ ★ ★ ————

Ellsworth Amendment (October 2009)

I was looking forward to returning home for a few days to escape the pressures of DC. My district travel was light; I had a couple of congressional events around my hometown of Menominee so I did not have to travel throughout my massive district. I wanted to stay close to home while my mother-in-law underwent colon cancer surgery. In between phone calls with Laurie, I managed several press interviews before heading home.

As I was finishing up the last votes of the week on the House floor on Friday, I was hanging along the back rail checking in with some of the Blue Dogs and making sure everyone was good with my strategy. As I made my way back toward the Pennsylvania corner, Congressman Brad Ellsworth of Indiana grabbed me and said that he had worked out an agreement with Speaker Pelosi on the abortion language. Ellsworth also stated that the women's groups would support his amendment. I asked why he did not include me in his discussions; Congressman Ellsworth said the discussions just sort of happened but that I would be pleased with his amendment.

I was not really surprised by Brad's strategy of trying to resolve this issue by himself, as he was now running for the US Senate. Brad wanted to be the hero that worked out the abortion amendment.

He wanted to please both sides of the issue so he could ride into the Senate. Congressman Ellsworth was solidly Right-to-Life and a former Sheriff in Evansville, Indiana; I had actually helped recruit him to run for Congress. Once he was elected to the House in 2006, I was assigned to mentor him, although Brad really did not need any mentoring: there were all kinds of people willing to help a young, good-looking sheriff from Indiana. Brad was voted one of the most beautiful people in Congress and he had no trouble getting media attention. Congressman Brad Ellsworth was "hot" right now and he was running for US Senate.

I knew that Brad meant well but I had seen this before and I knew that he was being played by the Speaker and the women's groups. Brad did not know the history of Right-to-Life issues in the US Congress, the significance of his amendment, or how his amendment would undermine the Stupak Amendment. At least he had enough sense to mention it to me before he put out a press release and introduce an amendment that the Right-to-Life movement could not support. I believed I still had time to pull him back from the brink before he angered both sides of the issue.

Ellsworth also said that Right-to-Life and the US Conference of Catholic Bishops were reviewing his amendment and he thought they would sign off in approval. I thought that Ellsworth was in over his head and I asked him for a copy of his amendment. He said it was being drafted as they had just agreed to the concepts but he would be happy to share it with me as soon as he had it in hand. I appreciated his honesty and said that I would be happy to work with him. I just had the feeling that this was going to divide the RTL Democrats. If Ellsworth had an agreement with the Speaker it would take the mounting pressure from the leadership and White House off the RTL Democrats. I did not know how long I could keep the Members continuing to support my strategy of forcing a vote on the Stupak Amendment. Even though no one had seen the Ellsworth proposal, Brad was telling RTL Democrats that he had a deal with the Speaker and the women's groups. The idea of the Ellsworth Amendment would have a considerable appeal for Members. It was Friday afternoon, October 30, 2009, and the written version of the

Ellsworth amendment would not be available until after all of us left Washington, DC for the weekend.

I tried to look on the bright side. If Brad's amendment was acceptable to everyone, my job was complete. The two principles that had been tearing me apart and keeping me awake at night would finally be in harmony. If there was agreement in providing national health care without government funding of abortion, I could vote for health care and retire. I headed to the National Airport to catch my plane home.

My plan was to deal with Ellsworth next week. I just wanted to board my flight from DC to Detroit, then on to Green Bay, Wisconsin. I looked forward to the peace and quiet of the one-hour drive from the Green Bay airport to my home in Menominee, Michigan.

Somehow, Congressman Brad Ellsworth's amendment had been leaked to the press. I could almost hear the uproar as I flew home 28,000 feet above the earth's surface on my flight from Washington, DC to Detroit, Michigan.

CHAPTER 38

★ ★ ★

Endurance Week (October 30, 2009
through November 5, 2009)

The week of October 30 through the fifth of November was a true test of mental and physical endurance. It was also a week of sadness and loss, which began in Washington, DC and ended in Escanaba, Michigan with the unexpected death of my mother-in-law, Elaine Olsen. All week long I battled with a pushy Committee Chairman Henry Waxman, a persistent Congressman John Dingell, Pro-Choice friend Diana DeGette, and the good humor of Congressman Mike Doyle. All of this while the Stupak coalition was slowly falling apart.

As I boarded my flight to Michigan on Friday, the thirtieth, my mother-in-law had just undergone surgery to remove a blockage in her colon, Congressman Brad Ellsworth had floated a proposal that drove a wedge between the Pro-Life Democrats, and my legislative assistant was being a pompous ass to other Members of Congress. I just wanted to go home, check on my mother-in-law, support my wife, and then return to DC as quickly as possible to hold my coalition together. If I could keep it from falling apart, I could secure my amendment even though the Speaker made it very clear that there would be no amendments to the Health Choices Act of 2009, H.R.

3200. Without the Stupak Amendment, congressional Democratic and Republican Pro-Lifers would vote against the Rule to accompany the bill, H.R. 3200. The national health care bill could not be brought to the floor without Democratic Pro-Life votes.

The Rules Committee changed the name and bill number for the health care legislation while it was en route from the Energy and Commerce Committee to the Rules Committee markup. HR-3200 was now HR-3962 and the name was changed from America's Health Choices Act to Affordable Health Care for America.

Throughout my career, I had constantly reminded Pro-Life Groups, Catholic Bishops, clergy, and constituents that no Right-to-Life Legislation could ever pass without the support of Pro-Life Democrats. The Republican Party never had enough votes in the House to pass RTL legislation on strictly a party line vote. Depending on the issue, the critical thirty to thirty-five Democratic RTL votes were required to pass Pro-Life legislation. Now, I was asking these Democratic and Republican Members of the US House of Representatives to join with me to block legislation from coming to the floor that would break the thirty-year truce with the Pro-Choice groups on the Hyde Amendment.

Earlier in 2009, the truce had already been broken with the constant denial of traditional RTL riders on the appropriations bills. The Democratic leadership, backed by a Pro-Choice president, simply believed that it could ignore repeated requests for our RTL riders and pass any legislation despite our RTL objections. Now, with the greatest legislative goal in more than fifty years poised for a vote on the House floor, the Speaker was beginning to realize that she had a problem with the RTL Democrats who vowed to defeat the Rule and derail health care.

There was nothing more I could do. I had repeatedly warned Leadership that we would defeat the Rule. We had already demonstrated that we could back in July with the DC Appropriations. The DC Appropriations bill was the warning shot across the bow to the Speaker that we had the votes necessary to defeat the Rule on the health care legislation. I do not know why, but Speaker Pelosi did not seem to take our warning seriously. By the end of October, I had quietly done my homework and I was ready to battle the Speaker if she forced my hand.

I was well aware that the Speaker had more tools to work with and could deliver plum assignments, legislative policy initiatives, or important projects to Members of Congress who supported her agenda. The bottom line was that the Speaker and the leadership had great leeway to give in to Members' demands on critical issues such as the upcoming vote on the Rule accompanying the Affordable Care Act of 2009. A Rule vote is viewed as a meaningless vote to constituents in the district, but it means everything to the legislative process in the US House of Representatives.

All I could offer a Member of Congress was an opportunity to stand up for the unborn child and not use taxpayer money to pay for abortions. While these are noble principles, noble principles usually do not win very many votes in Congress. I had a personal relationship with these Members of Congress, which was developed over seventeen years of working together on RTL issues. Each Member I spoke with and asked to stand with me, to stand on a principle, were willing to do so because somewhere over the past seventeen years, I had stood with them.

The Members knew that I was fighting for a firmly held belief and they respected that; I had credibility with these men and women on Right-to-Life issues. They were willing to stand with me because they trusted me, which is why it was extremely important that I kept their confidence and did not disclose their names to Leadership or to the press.

My research had shown that sixty Democratic Members of Congress repeatedly voted to exclude taxpayer funding of abortion when provided an opportunity on an "up or down" vote. Still, as strongly as these Members may have felt about taxpayer funding for abortion, most of them were unwilling to vote against the Rule because the Rule did not directly address taxpayer funding for abortions. As far as I could determine, these Members had never been faced with the question of voting against a Rule to force a vote on a RTL amendment. I was attempting to convince them to go one step further by voting against the Rule and the Democratic leadership.

Some Democratic Members were also adamant about the fact that "No Amendments" meant "No amendments, no exceptions," including the Hyde Amendment, no matter how noble the cause. I had to use every persuasive argument I could think of to keep Members voting with me against the Rule. Speaker Pelosi was doing an excellent job of convincing Members to vote for the Rule and every day my coalition was under tremendous pressure. However, because I kept my promise of confidentiality to RTL Members regarding their promised votes, Speaker Pelosi did not know which Members to pressure. Of the sixty Members who stated that they would vote for the Stupak Amendment, only about thirty said they would be willing to vote against the Rule if I did not receive my amendment. By the end of October, the thirty had shrunk to just over a dozen. I still had enough to defeat the Rule, but my numbers were dwindling.

I was asking Members to play inside baseball against Leadership on one of the most sweeping and controversial pieces of legislation to come before the House of Representatives in over fifty years. All I could argue was that each time I asked for a Pro-Life rider or amendment in the past year, I was denied. The health care legislation was too important not to allow us Right-to-Lifers a chance to vote our conscience. Just give us a vote. If RTL Democrats stuck together I would get my amendment only because the Speaker needed our Democratic votes to pass the Rule.

In November of 2009, there were 257 Democrats and 178 Republicans in the US House of Representatives. No Republican Member of Congress would vote for the Rule, so Speaker Pelosi could afford to lose thirty-nine Democratic votes. In July, nineteen of us Pro-Life Democrats wrote to the Speaker, warning, "we cannot support any health care reform proposal unless it explicitly excludes abortion from the scope of any government-defined or -subsidized health insurance plan." If Speaker Pelosi could secure the votes of all the remaining Democrats for the Rule accompanying HR-3962 except for the nineteen who had signed the letter, she did not have to allow the Stupak Amendment. But as with any piece of legislation, Members will not vote for the Rule if they are opposed to the proposed underlying legislation. Members of Congress opposed legislation based on constitutional, philosophical, or congressional district opposition to the proposed legislation. There were also several Democrats who already declared that they were not going to vote for the health care legislation and thus would not support the Rule accompanying the underlying legislation.

I repeatedly told Speaker Pelosi and White House Chief of Staff Rahm Emmanuel that if they had the votes to go ahead and bring the health care bill to the floor with its Rule without the Stupak Amendment. I was confident that we would defeat it. Or better yet, if they just allowed my amendment, they could pass their Rule- and let the votes fall where they may on the Stupak Amendment. But Speaker Pelosi would only say NO- there would be no amendments. I believed Speaker Pelosi knew that I would have the votes to pass the Stupak Amendment. The interest groups on both sides of the abortion issue were bombarding House Members to either support or defeat the Rule and then defeat or pass the Stupak Amendment. It was going to be a miserable week or two until the issue came to a vote.

For me the Rule vote was going to be the easy one. The more difficult vote would be on health care if the Stupak Amendment were to be defeated. The Democratic leadership constantly called caucus meetings during the week to whip members and paid personal visits to Members to persuade them to vote for the Rule. I was locked in meeting after meeting with leadership and other well-intentioned senior Democratic Members asking me to explain my foolish ways and demanding to know why I would want to kill health care reform. I remember calling the White House Chief of Staff, Rahm Emmanuel, saying, "Rahm, just tell the Speaker to allow the amendment and we can pass this legislation onto the Senate. I have the votes to block it and I do not want to stop health care reform." Rahm would only say, "You have to work this out." He would not offer any help to resolve the issue.

The Democratic Whip team led by my friend, Majority Whip Jim Clyburn was conducting a two-question whip count. The first question asked by the Whip team was, "Will you vote for the Rule without the Stupak Amendment?" The second was, "Will you vote for the passage of HR-3962, Affordable Health Care for America?" By all counts, the Whip count was short on the Rule.

The bottom line was that Speaker Pelosi did not have the votes for the Rule. Speaker Nancy Pelosi, her House leadership allies, the President, Cabinet Members, Senator Harry Reid and the proponents of health care were trying mightily to secure the last few votes needed to pass the Rule to allow HR-3962 to come to the floor for a vote. These last few votes needed to secure passage of the Rule were proving more challenging than the Speaker imagined. Nancy Pelosi remained unsure of how many votes I was holding to vote against the Rule.

The Democratic leadership was confident that they had the votes for the health care bill but they could not bring it to the floor without the Rule. Each day the pressure became greater and greater on me and on the RTL Democrats refusing to support the Rule without the Stupak Amendment. The pressure was especially great on known Right-to-Life Democrats because leadership knew who they were based on their past votes. While I kept my promise not to disclose to House leadership who was standing with me in voting against the Rule, the leadership team was doing a good job of determining who was in favor of the Stupak Amendment. I pleaded with Members to stay strong and not cave into the Speaker. We had to take a stand. If we were unsuccessful, the Pro-Life movement could be destroyed once and for all as Richard Doerflinger predicted. It was critical that the RTL Democrats continue to stick together.

I finally arrived home in the early evening of October 30 and Laurie was preparing dinner. I came through the front door talking on the phone. Immediately, I could see that Laurie was not happy. When she realized that I was talking to a Bishops' representative, she was *really* unhappy with me. In retrospect, I should have stayed in the car and finished my call but I wanted to see Laurie and see how she was holding up with her mother having difficulty coming out of her surgery.

The Bishops' representative was demanding that I call Congressman Brad Ellsworth and convince him not to offer his amendment. The Bishops and the RTL groups were totally opposed to the Ellsworth Amendment. I was trying to explain to the Bishops' representative that I had just arrived home and I was going to spend a few minutes with my wife and I would call Ellsworth later. As always, the Bishops wanted me to do what they wanted and they wanted it done immediately. I told the caller that I would get in touch with Ellsworth tomorrow morning and nothing more was going to be accomplished tonight. Further, I added that if the Bishops were upset with the Ellsworth Amendment then they should call him and tell him. Apparently, the Bishops had tried to contact Ellsworth but he was not returning their calls, which only infuriated them. I again told the representative that we should all step back and deal with Ellsworth in the morning; we were all exhausted and needed a break.

Laurie's report on her mother was not good. I could see that she was stressed and exhausted. She had spent all day at the hospital with her father, who was eighty-eight and really did not understand what was going on with his wife. Ken Olsen relied on his only child, Laurie, to make sense of it all. He was a strong man and a World War II combat veteran who had survived three bouts of cancer and could not understand why his wife was not up and talking to him. Ken was also hard of hearing and had refused to purchase new hearing aids after losing one while mowing his lawn several years earlier. It was a taxing and stressful day for Laurie, who had just arrived home shortly before me from St. Francis Hospital in Escanaba, an hour's drive north from our home.

Laurie explained that her mother's colon cancer surgery was quite extensive but that the doctors were confident they had removed the tumor and all the cancer. Laurie's mother would have a long recovery and right now was not doing well as she was still bleeding internally. The doctors were having trouble stabilizing her. We both agreed that we all needed a good night sleep and we would head back up to Escanaba in the morning to be with Laurie's mother and father.

Over dinner we discussed how Laurie's mother had never really been sick and generally refused to go to the doctor. She was a very modest, private person and never sought to have a colonoscopy. While Elaine complained of stomach problems and discomfort, she never sought out medical advice and only occasionally saw her old-time "female doctor." We discussed how best to take care of her father while her mother was recovering and rehabilitating from colon cancer. We both agreed Laurie would be spending a lot of time in Escanaba taking care of both of her parents.

A few hours later as we said good night and offered an extra prayer for Elaine and Ken Olsen, we both fell asleep exhausted.

Morning came quickly and I was up early on that Halloween Day reviewing emails and calls that had come in from Friday night. Laurie was also up early and we had a light breakfast before heading up north to Escanaba and St. Francis Hospital. Escanaba is on Eastern Time and our home in Menominee is located in the Central Time Zone, so it was an hour later in Escanaba. Laurie had already talked to her father by phone and we agreed to meet him at the hospital.

We had a full evening of activities scheduled back in Menominee, so it was important that we arrive early in Escanaba to catch the doctors making their rounds, spend time with Laurie's mother and get back home by the afternoon. Before we knew about Elaine's surgery, we had scheduled the unveiling of my portrait, which had been commissioned by local businesses and was to be hung in the local public library. My brother, his wife, his son and daughter-in-law were coming down for the portrait hanging and then dinner at our home. It was going to be a long day and a busy evening.

We spent all day at the hospital. Laurie's mother was very uncomfortable from her colon cancer surgery and when the doctors administered pain medication her blood pressure would drop. Throughout the day, Laurie spoke to the doctors and different attempts were made to stabilize her mother's vital signs. Laurie and I were able to see and talk to her and we communicated through written notes; she was on a ventilator and unable to speak. Laurie spent most of the day sitting by her mother and I kept her father entertained. Periodically, I would go out to our car and answer emails and place phone calls back to DC. It was a painfully long day for all of us.

By late Saturday afternoon we left Laurie's mother and made sure that her father arrived safely back at his home. Laurie and I headed back to Menominee for a quick stop at home to change our clothes and start dinner preparations.

We arrived at Spies Public Library a few minutes late and greeted our guests and friends who were involved in commissioning the portrait. The local artist, Kay Eaton, was there with her family. Although the small gathering of family and friends at Spies Library was extremely warm and friendly, Laurie and I were a little on edge about her mother. A small ceremony was held and my comments were brief. I usually do not give long speeches and I apologized for being especially brief as our thoughts and prayers were with Laurie's mother who was struggling. After the ceremonial unveiling of the portrait, I personally thanked everyone who was involved in commissioning the project. Laurie and I spent a few extra minutes with Nancy Douglas, who had raised the funds to pay the artist and coordinated every aspect of the portrait and the ceremony. We left the library and headed for home. As we entered the house, Laurie said that she wanted to call the hospital and check on her mother.

Laurie was finally connected with the intensive care nurse that was responsible for her mother's care. The nurse was alarmed as she had been trying to contact Laurie's father and he was not answering his phone. The nurse stated that Laurie's mother had taken a turn for the worse and urged us to drive up to Escanaba immediately. We dropped everything and headed for Escanaba.

I drove as Laurie called her father and told him to meet us at the hospital. We called and cancelled dinner with our guests and drove through the dark to Escanaba, not knowing that death was knocking on Elaine Olsen's door.

At the hospital, the doctor convened a family meeting and basically said that Laurie's mother would not make it through the night. They could not stabilize her blood pressure and her vital organs were beginning to fail. Unfortunately, the extensive surgery was too much for Elaine to handle; she was in great pain and her body was shutting down. It was decided that the doctor should make her comfortable, since there was nothing more that could be done to save her life. We gathered in her hospital room and prayed as mother slipped away around 10:30 p.m. on Halloween night.

I drove Laurie's father back to his home and he seemed to be in shock. I am not sure he understood that his wife of sixty-four years had died. From that night forward, Ken Olsen never mentioned Elaine by name. While he lived for another five years after his wife died, Ken Olsen would ask who that person in the pictures was, and why did she die so young? While in assisted living and the nursing home, Ken insisted on wearing his wedding ring and became upset when the ring slipped off his withered finger and he could not find it. He had truly loved his wife and her death was too much for him to handle. Immediately after Elaine's death, we realized that Ken Olsen suffered from dementia and that Elaine had covered for him. Ken and Elaine had complemented one another and Laurie and I did not realize how progressed Ken's dementia was. We would move Ken to the Menominee area so Laurie could spend time and care for him. Laurie was an only child and all care and comfort for her father fell to her, which she graciously and dutifully carried out even as the disease took away her father's mind.

Elaine Olsen died late Saturday evening, October 31. We called our son, Ken, the next day and on Monday we went to make funeral arrangements. Laurie's father was stoic and the funeral arrangements fell to his only daughter. Needless to say, I did not head back to Washington DC immediately after Elaine's death but that did not prevent Washington, DC from coming to me. While I wrote Elaine's eulogy my home phone and cell were both ringing constantly, to the point of irritation. The calls interrupted serious family conversations and we were spending a lot of time in Escanaba with Laurie's father.

In addition to writing an unexpected eulogy, I was attempting to keep my RTL coalition together from a thousand miles away. The Ellsworth Amendment was being attacked from all sides. The Bishops wanted me back in DC but my presence was needed more in Menominee. Ken and Cristina flew in on Tuesday; the wake and funeral would be Wednesday afternoon and internment on Thursday morning. The earliest I could travel back to DC was Friday. Some of the RTL Members believed that my Friday, November 6, 2009 arrival back in DC would be too late to hold together a large enough number to defeat the Rule on health care, if that was still our strategy. During this sad week and between family gatherings, I called all the key Members of our coalition and Chris Smith, the Republican Co-Chair of the Bipartisan Congressional Right-to-Life Caucus.

The Democratic RTL members wished to have a meeting on the status of my discussions with the Speaker and what our strategy would be heading into the weekend.

CHAPTER 39

★ ★ ★

Friday, November 6, 2009

I called Congressman Jim Oberstar and asked him to convene a meeting of the RTL Democrats on Friday morning, November 6, 2009. I told Jim that my staff would send out the notice but I needed him to conduct the meeting, as I would be flying back to DC that morning. I advised him that I had a layover in my flight to DC and I would call in from Chicago O'Hare airport. I had been away for the past week with my mother-in-law's passing and funeral and I wanted to let the Democrats know that it was critical to stick together so we could force a vote on the Stupak Amendment.

My staff sent the meeting notice to all the RTL Democratic Members of Congress. The plan was for Erika Smith to call the meeting to order and immediately turn it over to Congressman Jim Oberstar. I would be on the phone to encourage the Members present to hold firm, as the Speaker insisted that the House of Representatives would vote this weekend on the Health Choices Act of 2009.

As is often the case, my flight from Green Bay to Chicago arrived late and I hustled to make my connecting flight to Washington, DC. I was one of the last passengers to board the flight and my cell phone rang. It was Congressman Jim Oberstar and several of the RTL Democrats complaining about my staffer, Erika Smith. Erika did not immediately turn the meeting over to Congressman Oberstar and instead dictated assignments to the Members of Congress present. The Members on the phone call made it clear that they would work with me but not Erika. I quickly told them that I would deal with Erika when I arrived back in DC but it was important that we stick together and force a vote on the Stupak Amendment. The Members expressed concern that Congressman Brad Ellsworth was still trying to shop his version of the Hyde Amendment and he was splitting the RTL Democrats. I explained that I had a meeting scheduled with Brad once I landed in DC. I urged the RTL Democrats to continue to stand with me as I would be in DC around noon for the scheduled vote on legislation on the House floor and would discuss strategy with them then.

I leaned back in my seat and wondered what Erika had done now to upset the RTL Democrats. I had so many "irons in the fire," I really did not have the patience or the time to deal with a rogue staffer. According to an email I received, Erika started the meeting and never turned it over to Congressman Oberstar. She ran the discussion and told- not asked- Members of Congress what they would do in support of the Stupak Amendment. Once in DC, I discussed the meeting with Members and learned that Congressman Oberstar demanded to know who Erika worked for and who had given her the authority to dictate legislative prerogatives to Members of Congress. The exchange between Erika and Congressman Jim Oberstar was not very pleasant and several Members walked out of the meeting. Once again, Erika overstepped her position and angered the Members with whom I had been working to support the Stupak Amendment.

When I landed at National Airport in Washington DC, my Chief of Staff, Scott Schloegel, picked me up and whisked me off to the Capitol. Votes had already been called. Scott quickly filled me in on the pending votes and dropped me off at the steps leading up to the House Chamber. Because of my mother-in-law's funeral, I had missed several days of votes and neither of us wanted me to miss any more. I sprinted up the steps and entered through the ornate brass doors to the Capitol. I then passed the elevators and the Capitol Police and Sergeant at Arms personnel guarding the East door entry to the House floor. I swung open the door, bounded up the two steps onto the House floor with my voting card in my hand, and literally ran right into Speaker Pelosi.

We both had surprised looks on our faces as we bumped into each other and Nancy Pelosi said, "We have to talk." I responded, "Let me vote first." I stepped onto the floor and inserted my card in the voting machine to electronically record my vote. I then stepped down the two steps to the outer rail of the House floor where the Speaker was waiting for me. Speaker Pelosi asked how Laurie was doing with the unexpected loss of her mother. I thanked her for her concern and her phone call to Laurie and me earlier in the week. Next, the Speaker said that we needed to talk and that she would make some time late that afternoon. I responded that we definitely needed to discuss matters; Speaker Pelosi said that her staff would call my office later in the day with a time for the meeting.

Before I could meet with Pelosi, I needed to discuss matters with Congressman Ellsworth and the rest of my team. As the Speaker and I departed, I headed for the Pennsylvania corner to check in with my colleagues. The Members of Congress who congregated in the Pennsylvania corner knew Laurie and they expressed their condolences. The Members in the corner were our friends and they were sincere in their expressions of sympathy. Mike Doyle put his arm around me and said it was good to have me back and asked if I was ready to pass health care. I quickly responded, "Only with the Stupak Amendment." Mike just laughed and said, "He is back!"

Speaker Pelosi never stated why she wanted to meet with me and she did not have to; we both understood that I had the votes to block the Rule to the Health Choices Act. Before I could meet with Speaker Pelosi, I needed to meet with Congressman Ellsworth to discuss his amendment and huddle with the RTL Democrats. Since several votes had been called, I remained on the floor voting and discussing strategy with the RTL Democrats back in the Pennsylvania Corner. I informed the RTL Democrats that I would be meeting with Speaker Pelosi later that afternoon, but I was scheduled to meet with Congressman Ellsworth first. The RTL Members urged me to find a solution to the impasse on the Rule so they did not have to vote against the Rule and Speaker Pelosi.

I stopped briefly at my congressional office in the Rayburn Building to pick up my RTL file. My RTL file contained the Stupak Amendment, my personal whip count, personal contact information for key Democrats, and the proposed Ellsworth Amendment. Then, with my red file in hand, I headed to Ellsworth's office in the Cannon Building.

The Cannon Building is my favorite of the three US House of Representatives office buildings. I love its classic architectural style, high ceilings and third floor Cannon Caucus Room. My original office, which I occupied during my first four years in Congress, was 317 Cannon. One of the previous occupants of the three rooms that comprise my suite was Congressman John F. Kennedy.

The third floor of the Cannon Building circles around the open second floor, revealing the Cannon Rotunda below. The third-floor balcony circling the rotunda looks down over the main entrance off Independence Avenue. I did not realize it at the time, but an Associated Press photographer snapped my picture from the third-floor balcony as I crossed the Cannon Rotunda with my red file in hand. I was all alone in the frame. The photo graced the cover of the National Journal magazine and was published on the front page of one of the Capitol Hill newspapers. For me, that picture came to symbolize my struggle and the weight I was carrying as I fought to protect the sanctity of life while desperately trying to pass quality affordable health care for all Americans. These two conflicting principles fit so neatly in my brown accordion file but they gnawed at my heart and mind as I struggled to reach an acceptable compromise.

I did not wish to have any staff with me for this meeting with Congressman Brad Ellsworth. The logical staffer to join me in the Ellsworth meeting would have been Erika but I did not have time to deal with her immaturity right now. When I was on the House floor earlier in the day I received an earful from the RTL Members who had attended the earlier meeting with my wayward staffer; Erika had caused enough problems for me for one day and my meeting with Brad was not going to be pleasant. I needed to inform Congressman Ellsworth that the remaining Members of the Stupak coalition would not accept or support his amendment.

CHAPTER 40

★ ★ ★

Ellsworth Meeting (November 6, 2009)

I was back in DC to prepare for the debate on health care, pass the Stupak Amendment, and if necessary defeat the Rule. Right now, it was time for Brad to drop his proposed amendment, get on board and fully support the Stupak Amendment. Ellsworth had overplayed his hand and had damaged his reputation within the RTL Caucus and National Right-to-Life. It was obvious that Brad had tried unsuccessfully to make the Stupak Amendment the Ellsworth Amendment to claim RTL support throughout Indiana in his upcoming Senate race. The Ellsworth Amendment had been soundly rejected by National Right-to-Life, the US Conference of Catholic Bishops, and the bi-partisan Congressional Right-to-Life Caucus. Brad's closest friends still supported his legislative efforts, but he had no authority to negotiate with Speaker Pelosi on behalf of RTL Democrats. Further, Speaker Pelosi was adamant that there would be no amendments to the health care legislation. Without the full support of the RTL Democrats, Brad was checkmated. Congressman Ellsworth had served fewer than three years in Congress and did not have the credibility or the trust of the RTL Democrats. While Brad had worked in good faith on his amendment, I had already secured commitments from RTL Democrats to vote for the Stupak

Amendment and to vote against the Rule if the Stupak Amendment was not made in order by the Rules Committee.

The meeting with Congressman Ellsworth and his staff was tense. There were just three of us in Brad's inner personal office. The lighting seemed darker than normal. I must have had a furrowed brow. After a brief greeting, Brad immediately asked his staff person to explain his amendment. The staff person started the conversation with how he believed the Ellsworth Amendment provided more protection for the unborn child than the Capps Amendment.

I immediately interrupted the staffer and stated, "The purpose of our efforts over the past four months has been to preserve the Hyde language, not modify the Capps language." The staffer countered that the women's groups "…were supporting the amendment and Indiana Right-to-Life has looked favorably upon the amendment." I asked, "Is Indiana Right-to-Life going to endorse it?" To his credit the staffer said that no final decision had been made. I shot back that it really made no difference what Indiana RTL thought because National Right-to-Life, the Bishops and all the RTL support groups were against the Ellsworth Amendment.

I apologized for interrupting and the staffer turned his presentation into a legal argument that made no sense to me. I sat quietly and the staffer seemed to run out of enthusiasm for the amendment and closed his explanation by declaring once again that Indiana RTL supported the Ellsworth Amendment. Brad quickly added that he was hoping I could secure the Bishops and National Right-to-Life support for his amendment.

My response was swift and succinct. "The Ellsworth Amendment is nothing more than the Capps Amendment with different wording but the same result: government promotion of and funding for abortions. The Ellsworth Amendment fails to prevent abortions from being performed in federally funded health clinics, which would be greatly increased in number under the health care law. Further, the Ellsworth Amendment promotes a policy in which the federal government supports abortions, contrary to Hyde and the Stupak Amendments," I argued.

I made it very clear that the Stupak Amendment was the only amendment that National RTL, the Catholic Bishops, and the bi-partisan congressional RTL caucus would support. I did not question the motives behind the Ellsworth Amendment. His proposal was too little, too late and offered limited protection for the unborn child. The Ellsworth Amendment would not be accepted and Brad would be viewed as offering an amendment counterproductive to RTL efforts. While Speaker Pelosi and the women's groups may have supported the Ellsworth Amendment, the rest of us would not.

I asked, "Brad, will the Speaker make your amendment in order?" "No," he answered, then quickly added, "But the Speaker could include my amendment in the base bill or in the Manager's Amendment." I simply responded, "Brad, that is wishful thinking." I further explained to Brad and his silent staffer, "If the Speaker made your amendment in order she would only garner one more vote. Your vote, Brad. If the Speaker made my amendment in order, which is supported by National RTL and the Bishops, she would get the handful of votes that she needs."

Speaker Pelosi could not and would not start granting individual Members of Congress their own amendments to garner support for the Rule and health care. The time for individual Members to insert their personal concerns or amendments in the health care bill had long since passed. The only issue remaining was the vote on the Rule and the Stupak Amendment.

I knew I had Brad on the defensive, so I lowered the tone of my voice, leaned forward in my chair and said, "Brad, I understand what you are trying to accomplish but the RTL Democrats will not support the Rule. Your amendment will not even be made in order. If all the RTL Democrats stick together with the Republicans, then we, not the Speaker, control the process. Why don't you join us?"

Next, I asked Brad if he had the Republicans lined up to support his amendment. Once again Brad said no, and that he was hoping I could line them up for him. I then asked, "Have you sent your amendment over to Congressman Chris Smith for his review?" Once again, Brad simply said, "No." Finally, I explained to Brad that he had to decide whether he would stand with us RTL Democrats or stand alone. If he insisted on pursuing his own course, he and his amendment were not going anywhere.

I sensed that Brad did not want to answer my last inquiry and that he had no idea what his next move would be, so I offered him an out. I offered Brad, "If you will drop your amendment and place your support behind the Stupak Amendment, I will add your name to it." I explained that the Stupak Amendment would be presented to the Rules Committee as the Stupak-Pitts Amendment but I could rename it the "Stupak-Pitts-Ellsworth Amendment." With caution I explained, "I need to check with my Republican colleagues, but I will ask them to sign off on having your name added as the second or third name on the Amendment."

Without conferring with his staff person, Brad said that he would appreciate having his name added to the Stupak Amendment and that he would not vote for the Rule if the Stupak Amendment was not made in order. We shook hands and I left to call Congressman Joe Pitts and Chris Smith to secure their permission to add Brad Ellsworth as a sponsor of the Stupak Amendment.

When I returned to my office, I filled Scott in on the day's activities and my meeting with Ellsworth. Overall, it had been a good day. I was exhausted, as I had been up since 4:00 a.m. to catch the flight back to DC.

I called my Republican colleagues Chris Smith and Joe Pitts and they had no problem with adding Brad Ellsworth's name to the Stupak Amendment. Another hurdle crossed. What was next? I had the votes to defeat the Rule on health care and the Speaker had to come to terms with that fact. I still had not heard from the Speaker. Maybe she believed she had enough votes to pass the Rule. No, the Speaker had overplayed her hand and she knew it. She needed to negotiate as she indicated when I saw her on the floor a few hours earlier. Tomorrow would be another long day whether we voted on health care or not.

I was finally able to look over the paperwork that was stacked on my desk and attempted to get caught up after being away for the past week. I no sooner started to go through the pile when Rachel Stevenson, my scheduler and executive assistant, came in and informed me that the Speaker's office had just called and I was to immediately go over to her office for a "mandatory meeting." I wasn't aware of *mandatory* meetings with the Speaker; Members are generally *invited* to meetings with the Speaker. Rachel said that the Speaker's staff insisted that I attend the meeting and immediately. I grabbed my brown RTL accordion file and headed to the Speaker's office in the US Capitol building.

CHAPTER 41

★ ★ ★

Speaker Pelosi Agreement
(November 6, 2009)

The Speaker's spacious wing of offices located on the second floor of the US Capitol overlooks the National Mall. The spectacular view from the balcony is one of the most coveted in Washington, DC. This balcony is a premier spot from which to witness presidential inaugurations, the lighting of the Capitol Christmas tree, political protests and demonstrations for and against wars and legislation. Marriage proposals, legislative negotiations, and cool drinks on warm summer nights have also taken place on the Speaker's balcony, or so I've heard; I personally have never been invited by any Speaker to join them on their balcony for a drink or a discussion. During my time in Congress, I often brought visitors here during business hours and stepped out on the balcony so they can take their tourist pictures of the monuments and buildings lining the National Mall. It is truly a fabulous view.

I knew the meeting with Speaker Pelosi would not be pleasant so I squeezed my constant companion, my brown accordion RTL file, a little tighter under my arm and picked up my pace. My accordion file had been with me since the end of July and it was starting to look a little ratty. The sun was setting earlier and earlier as fall had settled over Washington, DC. Autumn is usually my favorite time of year; this year, however, fall had not been so great and there was little time left to enjoy it now. I did not expect to enjoy my meeting with the Speaker, either.

As I walked, I wondered who else would be attending the meeting. I was sure that Chairman Waxman would be there and possibly Wendell Primus. George Kansarious, the Speaker's Parliamentarian, would also probably be in attendance to advise me that I could not block the Rule based on some arcane rule found in Jefferson's Manual. Damn, I should have brought my copy of the Jefferson Manual as I had already marked the pertinent parts with little yellow sticky notes. Since I was alone, I was certain that the Speaker would attempt to overwhelm me with her perceived facts and logic that the Capps Amendment adequately addressed all my RTL concerns. Pelosi would claim that I was being an obstructionist to national health care. I told myself to be strong, not raise my voice, and to be prepared to use my strongest argument that federally funded health clinics could perform abortions under the language contained in the Capps Amendment. I was prepared make my argument on the clinics; I was comfortable with my position and confident that I had the votes to block the Rule to health care.

I expected the Speaker to turn on the charm in an attempt to persuade me to drop my demand to include the Stupak Amendment. I expected her to claim that national health care would be the greatest legislative accomplishment in the past fifty years. The Speaker would remind me that for almost a hundred years, presidents had implored Congress to pass a national health care plan that covered all Americans. How could I continue to stand in the way? The Speaker would claim that the democratically controlled Congress had been provided with both the opportunity and the responsibility to do what no other Congress had done before: create a national health care program that would cover all Americans. Speaker Pelosi would remind me that she already had enough votes to pass health care and I was standing in the way of history by insisting on my amendment. She would also claim that she had repeatedly stated that there would be no amendments to the health care legislation and she simply could not allow mine without allowing many other well-meaning ones. She would then say that she knew me and she knew that I really did not want to be remembered as the person who killed national health care. She would say that it was time to give up my crusade.

These thoughts raced through my mind as I climbed the narrow, 150- year-old spiral stone staircase to the second floor. I entered and moved past the numerous meeting rooms along the back corridor, where I bumped into Richard Doerflinger, John Carr and Nancy Wisdo from the US Conference of Catholic Bishops. I was surprised to see Richard and his team emerging from a meeting. I asked, "What are you doing here?" Richard answered, "We had a meeting with the Speaker's staff and nothing has changed. They will not allow your amendment."

Richard inquired, "What are you doing here?" I replied, "I am going to a mandatory meeting with the Speaker." He wished me luck. I said, "Why don't you join me? After all, I am sure my meeting is about the Stupak Amendment." He responded, "What do you think? Will the Speaker allow us in your meeting?" I said, "There is only one way to find out."

We approached the receptionist and I explained that I had a meeting with the Speaker and I asked if representatives of the US Conference of Catholic Bishops could join me. We were told to take a seat and the receptionist left to inform the Speaker that I was present. John Carr quipped that he felt like he was being called down to the principal's office and that he had done something wrong. We all chuckled but John was right- we *were* being called into the principal's office.

A few minutes later we were escorted into the Speaker's large meeting room in the southeast corner of the Capitol. Energy and Commerce Chairman Henry Waxman was already in the room along with Majority Leader Steny Hoyer. The Speaker was not present. There was an awkward silence while we all sat and waited for Speaker Pelosi.

When Nancy Pelosi entered the room, I was quite surprised to see my good friend, Congressman Mike Doyle, with her. As surprised as I was to see Mike, the Speaker was even more surprised to see Richard Doerflinger, John Carr and Nancy Wisdo, the main lobbyists of the US Conference of Catholic Bishops. I explained that I had asked Richard and the group to join me when I bumped into them coming out of a meeting with the Speaker's staff. I further explained that if we were going to try to reach an agreement on the Stupak Amendment, we might as well have all the critical people at the table. The Speaker cut my explanation short and said that they, the Bishop's representatives, were invited to join the meeting.

The Speaker asked us to explain why the Capps Amendment did not satisfy our concerns over abortion, since she believed it was consistent with the Hyde Amendment. Before anyone could even answer, she launched into a stern lecture of how we were denying health care rights to women and that women just could not support the Stupak Amendment.

Nancy Pelosi did not stop there. She spoke about being a Catholic and reminded us that she represented the City of St. Francis [San Francisco], repeating some of the points she made when she had addressed the Democratic Caucus the evening before being elected Speaker almost three years ago. I looked at Mike- we had heard this speech before- but he did not acknowledge me. Nancy Pelosi added a new wrinkle to her speech as she told us she graduated from Trinity University here in Washington, DC and expounded on her Catholic credentials. As a practicing Catholic, she could accept the Capps Amendment and could not understand why we could not. Everyone around the table listened intently to the Speaker as we formulated our responses.

John Carr was the first to speak and told the Speaker that the Stupak Amendment maintained the status quo that had existed for years. John explained that even federal employees could not pur-chase abortion coverage in their health care plans because the Hyde Amendment prevented federal funds from being used to pay for abortion coverage. The Speaker remained silent.

I chimed in that the Capps Amendment was not even close to the Hyde Amendment. Hyde not only prevented taxpayer funds from being used for abortion, it went even further and prevented the federal government from encouraging or promoting abortions through its actions or policies. Under the Public Option health care legislation, the House would greatly increase the money available for federally funded health centers and there was no prohibition on abortion in the federal health centers. Finally, I said that the language on the conscience clause in the Public Option was not as strong as it should be and was not in keeping with the Weldon language.

The Speaker countered that she had discussed the Capps Amendment with Cardinal George and if the Bishops' representatives would just tell Cardinal George that the Capps Amendment was an acceptable compromise, Cardinal George would withdraw his opposition.

That statement was too much for Richard Doerflinger and he began to lecture the Speaker on the imperfections of the Capps Amendment, assuring her that Cardinal George and the US Conference of Bishops would never accept the Capps Amendment.

The Speaker did not directly respond to Richard but stated that under Medicaid, taxpayer funds could not be used to pay for abortions, so my earlier statement about federally funded health centers was unfounded. I responded that under the proposed House Public Option Health Care Plan, individuals receiving coverage were not necessarily on Medicaid but could receive a subsidy to buy health insurance. I also reminded the Speaker that since she had not allowed our traditional RTL amendments, the prohibition on Medicaid paying for elective abortions did not apply. Therefore, there was now an even greater need for the Stupak Amendment. I was polite, firm and forceful in my counterargument. Speaker Pelosi did not respond immediately.

Chairman Henry Waxman swung the discussion back to the Capps Amendment and offered that if the House accepted the Stupak Amendment for this Congress (2009 and 2010), we could fight about the Amendment in the next Congress. I quickly rejected that idea because there was no guarantee that we would even get a vote in the next Congress on either the Hyde or Stupak Amendment. Henry Waxman said, "I am only focused on this Congress and not the next Congress. Plus, any legislation that this Congress passed could be changed by the next Congress." I retorted, "I agree with your assessment as to the next Congress, but whether it is this Congress or the next, we should be given the opportunity to vote on Hyde, now the Stupak Amendment. But we are not even given an opportunity to vote on the Amendment in this Congress. Therefore, there is no reason for me to vote for the Rule on health care."

The discussion then turned to the RTL riders and the fact that for over the past thirty-plus years, all Speakers had allowed the traditional RTL amendments. However, Nancy Pelosi, as Speaker, had not allowed any RTL amendments at all this year. The Speaker responded that when the bills made it to conference between the House and the Senate, the RTL amendments would be added. I told the Speaker, "I respectfully disagree with your assessment, as no RTL Democrat will be part of the conference committee and the President will not insist on our RTL amendments. Therefore, we have no voice in the conference committee and thus the Hyde language will never be considered in conference."

Once again Waxman asked, "Would you be willing to add the Stupak Amendment to this year's appropriations bills instead of adding it to the health care legislation?" I responded, "The health care legislation is self-funded so it does not rely on the annual appropriations from Congress for funding. We need the Hyde language in the appropriations bills and the Stupak Amendment in the health care legislation."

Chairman Waxman stated that there was no way he could convince the Democratic Caucus to accept my suggestion of putting the Hyde language back in the appropriations bills *and* the Stupak Amendment in the health care legislation. I responded that all I wanted was a vote on the Stupak Amendment. I would deal with the appropriation bills as they came to the floor just like I had on the DC Appropriations Bill.

I then reminded the Speaker and Waxman that my effort to bring down the Rule on the DC Appropriations Bill earlier in the year was simply to demonstrate that if push came to shove on health care, I had the votes to block it. I suggested that if they didn't believe me, they should just schedule the vote. Congressman Mike Doyle just shook his head, as he knew how stubborn I could be.

Chairman Waxman was obviously the idea man, as he continued to offer different scenarios and compromises to the Capps Amendment. I was dug in on the Stupak Amendment or nothing. Richard Doerflinger and Waxman went around and around on the merits of the Stupak Amendment; I listened closely but kept quiet and tried to figure out how we could reach some type of compromise.

Nancy Wisdo and Steny Hoyer said very little. Nancy Pelosi kept getting up and going into another office off the conference room. It was obvious to us that the Speaker was conferring with the Pro-Choice faction in the outer office.

An hour had passed and we were going nowhere. It did not appear that we would be able to reach an agreement. Steny Hoyer would just roll his eyes whenever Richard spoke. I believe that it was Steny or Speaker Pelosi who in exasperation claimed, "Now you know why bishops and priests should keep their noses out of politics!" Without missing a beat, John Carr shot back, "This is why politicians should keep out of theology, even if they attended a Catholic University."

The Speaker, Waxman, and I entered into a discussion on the timetable for implementing parts of the health care legislation. While the health care legislation would become law immediately upon passage, certain parts were to be phased in over a three- to four-year period. We concluded that under the House's Public Option health care plan, 2013 would be a critical year for implementation of the new law. The Speaker then proposed that for 2009 and 2010 she would allow all our traditional RTL amendments on the appropriations bills. And in the health care legislation she would write in the Stupak Amendment.

In other words, the Stupak Amendment would automatically become part of the health care legislation for the duration of the 111th Congress. The Speaker made it very clear that the Stupak Amendment would be included in health care for ONLY two years, 2009-2010. Starting in 2011, the House would be guaranteed an opportunity to vote on including the Stupak Amendment in health care on a yearly basis. The outcome of the vote on the Stupak Amendment would determine whether taxpayer funds would be used to pay for abortion. We discussed the conscience clause and federally funded health centers and again the Speaker said that if they were covered in the Stupak Amendment, then they were part of the agreement.

So, for the next fourteen months, which included the two fiscal years that remained in the 111th Congress, the Stupak Amendment would automatically be included in the health care and appropriation bills. Starting in 2011, the Members of the US House of Representatives would be guaranteed a vote on the Stupak Amendment as it pertained to health care.

I looked at Doyle and then Doerflinger. Mike said, "Bart, this is the best deal you are going to get. You would be guaranteed a vote on your amendment in every Congress. You have to agree to this deal." I did not respond to Mike; I instead turned my attention to Richard and asked what he thought.

Richard said, "The US Conference of Catholic Bishops wished to have the Stupak Amendment written into law." The Speaker shot back, "The Stupak Amendment would be written in the law for the next two years, plus RTL would be guaranteed a vote every year thereafter on the Stupak Amendment." Speaker Pelosi correctly told Richard that RTL was not currently guaranteed a vote every year. Plus, there were years when RTL did not have enough votes to sustain the Hyde Amendment.

The proposal put forth by the Speaker and Chairman Henry Waxman was forward-looking. I believed the Speaker thought that if Democrats passed national health care legislation, then the Democrats would increase their House Majority and would defeat any future attempts to add the Stupak Amendment to health care.

In exchange for this agreement, the Speaker demanded that a letter be distributed to all Members of Congress, signed by the US Conference of Catholic Bishops, stating three things: the Bishops supported the agreement reached with the Speaker on the Stupak Amendment; the Bishops urged the Members of the House to vote for the Rule and, lastly, that the letter must state that the Bishops supported the health care legislation and encouraged House Members to vote for the legislation. With this compromise agreement and letter from the Bishops, the Speaker turned the Bishops' opposition into support of health care. Everybody would win.

While I was mentally examining the impact of the Speaker's offer, Richard Doerflinger continued to lecture on the history of the Hyde Amendment. Mike Doyle was staring at me and signaling me to cut off Doerflinger. I looked at Speaker Pelosi and her eyes were starting to glaze over as Doerflinger droned on. Finally, I started to kick Richard under the table to cut him off. He was oblivious and continued to hold his hands over his stomach and drone on.

Steny Hoyer stood up and said, "Hey, after you beat us, it is time to leave." Steny left the meeting. Finally, I butted in and said, "We accept your proposal Madame Speaker. The Stupak language will be in the health care legislation for the next two years and then each year thereafter we are guaranteed a vote on the language in the funding of health care." Speaker Pelosi said, "Yes, that is the agreement." We all rose and shook hands. Richard was still talking as the Speaker and I summarized the agreement and he stood and belatedly shook hands with Speaker Pelosi and Congressmen Doyle and Waxman.

The Speaker told the bishops' representatives that she needed the letter tonight. John Carr and Nancy Wisdo said that they would have to place a conference call to Cardinal George and the rest of the bishops on their committee. Nancy Pelosi encouraged the bishops' representatives to act quickly as she wanted the letter tonight for distribution to all House Members, Democrats and Republicans.

As we rose to leave the meeting, the Speaker said to Mike and me, "Now, I need you two to do me a favor." Mike and I said, "Sure, what do you need us to do?" The Speaker said, "Now, I want you to call all of your supporters and tell them that we have a deal and they must vote for the Rule tomorrow." I stated, "It is after 7:00 pm on a Friday night and the Members are no longer in their offices." The Speaker responded that her staff would provide the cell phone numbers of all the Democratic Members if we did not have their numbers. The Speaker again repeated her request that Mike and I call the Democratic Members in my coalition. Pelosi stressed that it was critical that we call the Members who were poised to vote against the Rule accompanying the health care legislation.

Richard, John and Nancy left the meeting and the Speaker's staff showed us to the phones in the reception area of the Speaker's office. Mike and I made calls advising the Democratic Members that an agreement had been reached with the Speaker and that they should vote for the Rule tomorrow. Mike had no idea who to call as he did not know everyone in my coalition. I had my brown RTL accordion file with most of the cell phone numbers of my group of RTL Democrats. Still, there were one or two cell phone numbers that I did not have. The Speaker's staff had those private numbers, which should not have surprised me. While we were making calls, Speaker Pelosi said she had to meet with and sell the agreement to the women Members of Congress.

I called Heath Shuler, John Tanner, Nick Rahall, Joe Donnelly, Jim Oberstar, Steve Driehaus and several other Members. Mike also made calls to the Members who congregated in the Pennsylvania corner. Together, we personally spoke with about twenty Members of Congress, who were elated that we had reached an agreement and agreed to vote for the Rule the next day.

We left a voice message for the Members who we did not personally speak with, asking them to vote for the Rule accompanying the health care bill. I was unsuccessful in my attempts to contact Congresswoman Kathy Dahlkemper (D-PA) and Marcy Kaptur, but left the message that we had reached an agreement with the Speaker. After an hour or so, Mike and I finished our calls and headed for the Democratic Club for a celebratory beer and dinner.

The Democratic Club is both a restaurant and bar located three blocks northeast of the Capitol and next to the Democratic National Headquarters. It is a private club with its membership consisting of Members of Congress, lobbyists, Democratic staff persons, and other card-carrying Democrats. On this Friday evening, the Democratic Club was fairly quiet, as the regular after-five crowd had already left.

I was hungry and exhausted. Mike and I sat down at a table and ordered a beer while we examined the menu. We toasted the agreement and ordered a steak dinner. It was going to be a quiet, enjoyable evening. Mike was laughing about Doerflinger and how the guy would not stop talking during our meeting with the Speaker. Mike said Richard had to learn when to shut up, declare victory and go home. Mike was laughing because he knew I was kicking Doerflinger under the table while he kept talking.

We had not even finished our first beer when my cell phone rang. It was Speaker Pelosi. The Speaker simply said, "The agreement is off. The women's group rejected the agreement." I retorted, "You are the Speaker; what do you mean the agreement is off? We shook hands on the deal. You insisted that we call my coalition members to tell them that we had an agreement!"

The Speaker asked if my amendment was at the Rules Committee and I told her that it was. She responded that I had better get over to the Rules Committee and ask that my amendment be made in order. I asked if she would allow my amendment and she just insisted that I go to the Rules Committee.

During the call, I stressed that the Stupak Amendment must be made in order since she [the Speaker] had reneged on the agreement. The Speaker replied that she did not know if my amendment would be made in order but I had to get over to the Rules Committee before they finished taking testimony on the Rule. Again, I stressed that my amendment had to be made in order or I would take down the Rule. The Speaker would not give me any indication how she intended to deal with the Stupak Amendment, and I never received an answer from her on the reasons why the Democratic women rejected the agreement we had negotiated.

The Speaker then asked if I had enough votes to pass my amendment. I told her that I did but now I was unsure because I had told my supporters that we had an agreement. Again, Nancy Pelosi urged me to return to the Capitol and present my amendment to the Rules Committee.

I went back and told Mike about the call as our dinners were being served. Mike said he could not believe that the Speaker would go back on her word and that I had better go over to the Rules Committee. I immediately called Congressman Joe Pitts, the co-author of the Stupak Amendment, who was already at the Rules Committee. Joe indicated that the Committee was taking testimony from the Chairmen of the three committees with jurisdiction over the health care legislation, and urged me to immediately come over because after the Chairmen finished their testimony, Energy and Commerce Committee Members were scheduled to testify. Since both Joe and I were Members of the Energy and Commerce Committee and Joe had been present at the committee hearing, we should be up to testify next.

Mike stayed to finish his dinner and I headed for the third floor of the Capitol where the Rules Committee was meeting. I checked in with the Staff Director for the Rules Committee and advised him that both authors of the Stupak-Pitts Amendment were present and wished to testify in support of the amendment. The Staff Director confirmed that our amendment was properly filed along with the required sixty-four copies. Rules Committee staff assured us that we would be next up to testify. It was now after 9:00 p.m. Although it was repeatedly stated that no amendments would be made in order, the small Rules Committee room was packed with Members of Congress offering amendments to the proposed health care legislation.

As is common, the Rules Committee melded together the three bills that came from the committees with jurisdiction over health care. The Rules Committee assigned a new name and bill number to the House Public Option health care legislation. The bill number and the name of the health care legislation was now HR-3962, Affordable Health Care for America Act.

Joe and I sat in the Rules Committee room believing we would be called upon to present testimony in support of the Stupak-Pitts Amendment. Chris Smith came over to the Committee and joined us. Chairwoman Slaughter systematically recognized Members of Congress and invited them to come up to the front tables and present their testimony in support of their proposed amendments. Joe and I sat there as Chairwoman Slaughter recognized the Members of the Energy and Commerce Committee, Ways and Means Committee, and Education and Labor Committee. However, Chairwoman Slaughter passed us over and failed to recognize Joe and me.

I went back to the Majority Staff Director and asked why Joe and I were not recognized when the other Energy and Commerce Committee Members presented their amendments. I was told that the Chairwoman was aware of our amendment and she would call on us at the appropriate time.

Democratic Majority Leader Steny Hoyer came by the Rules Committee around 10:00 p.m. I asked Steny what was going on, as the Rules Committee still had not recognized me and I had been there for more than an hour. Steny just said they would get to me. I then asked if the Stupak Amendment would be made in order and he said he did not know. I asked Steny, "If no one knows whether my amendment will be made in order, then it is obvious that Slaughter is going to make me wait all night in hopes that I become frustrated and leave so that she can deny my amendment." Steny just said that I had to stay and offer my amendment but he did not know if it would be made in order.

After learning from the Speaker's staff that the agreement had been rejected by the women's groups, John Carr, Richard Doerflinger, and Nancy Wisdo came by to see what was happening in the Rules Committee on the Stupak Amendment. The Bishops had presented the Speaker with their letter of support for health care legislation and the Speaker insisted on one change. In the letter of support, the US Conference of Catholic Bishops thanked me for my courage and leadership. Speaker Pelosi insisted that the Bishops also thank Mike Doyle for his leadership in resolving our disagreement. I had no problem with the Bishops giving Congressman Mike Doyle credit in their letter. However, the letter was never distributed to Members of Congress because Speaker Pelosi was forced by the Democratic women of Congress to call off the agreement.

As we were all standing outside the Rules Committee, I told Steny that I couldn't believe he did not know whether my amendment would be made in order, as he would be running the floor debate on health care. Steny would just say that the decision was not up to him. I countered that I could not believe that no one in leadership could tell me what the hell was going on!

I was fuming, "I had an agreement with the Speaker, which she reneged on. You're the Majority Leader who runs the floor and you cannot tell me if my Amendment will be made in order? The Chairwoman of the Rules Committee has refused to allow me to testify in support of my Amendment." As I made each point, my voice was getting a little louder. I was getting angry.

I was seething with questions. "Why can't anyone tell me whether my amendment will be made in order or whether I will even be allowed to testify in the Rules Committee? Why was the agreement with the Speaker called off? Why am I being treated like dirt when I have tried for months to work with everyone to avoid a fight over abortion in health care? It seems to me that the more I try to resolve our differences, the worse I'm treated. Hell, I should just block the Rule and be done with health care." Steny listened patiently as I let off steam. I knew that if I walked out of the Rules Committee, Pelosi and Slaughter would claim that I never offered my amendment. It was clear that Chairwoman Slaughter was doing everything she could to make my evening miserable.

Steny motioned for me to walk down the hallway with him as there were other people standing outside the Rules Committee room. Side by side, Mike, Steny, and I walked down the third-floor corridor. Steny tried to calm me down and assured me that the Stupak Amendment would *probably* be made in order since the Speaker told me to go offer the amendment. I asked him, "Then why have I not been recognized to testify?" Hoyer had no good answer but insisted that I stay at the Rules Committee and not give Slaughter an excuse to reject my amendment. I then asked Steny, "In other words, Slaughter will call on me last. And she is hoping I leave so she does not have to recognize me or my amendment?" Hoyer never answered. He asked whether I had the votes to pass my amendment. I told Steny I did before Mike and I called Members telling them we had an agreement with the Speaker. Now I was not sure what to tell Members and it was a little late to try to rally support for an amendment that might never be made in order.

Steny ended the conversation by saying, "Make sure you have the votes to win your amendment tomorrow." Steny left and Mike and I and the Bishops' representatives went back into the Rules Committee to watch the parade of Members presenting their amendments.

Finally, well after midnight, Chairwoman Slaughter asked Congressman Jim McGovern (D-MA) to take the chair. The only people present were committee staff, a few reporters, Joe Pitts, Chris Smith, and I, waiting to testify on the Stupak-Pitts Amendment. While we were waiting, we were joined by Kathy Dahlkemper and Marcy Kaptur. As Chairman McGovern called us up to speak in support of the amendment, the remaining Democratic women on the Rules Committee, Chellie Pingree and Doris Matsui, walked out of the hearing.

Joe Pitts, Chris Smith, Kathy Dahlkemper, Marcy Kaptur and I asked that our statements in support of our amendment be made part of the record. With our statements admitted in the official record of the Rules Committee, we each said a few words in support of the amendment. When we completed our testimony, Chairman McGovern simply said, "Thank you."

Congressman Doc Hastings (R-WA) said to the five of us at the table presenting the Stupak Amendment, "I understand why the Congressmen are here but why are you women here?" The comment seemed innocent enough, but after the long, emotional and frustrating situation we had just been through, Doc's comment was not well received. Congresswoman Kathy Dahlkemper just stared at Hastings. Then she lit into him.

Kathy explained to Hastings that she was solidly Pro-Life and that no one should ever question her Pro-Life credentials. Kathy explained that she was probably the only person in Congress who had a child out of wedlock and had received food stamps to help feed her baby. She could have aborted her child, but instead she chose Life. She gave birth to a son. Her son has given her a grandchild whom she loved very much. She just didn't talk about being Pro-Life, she lived it. There was complete silence in the Rules Committee.

The remaining Republicans on the Rules Committee praised our amendment and said it should be made in order. Everyone in the Committee Room knew that only Speaker Nancy Pelosi could make the Stupak-Pitts Amendment in order and she was not present.

I was grateful to Congressmen Joe Pitts, Chris Smith, and Mike Doyle, who stayed with me throughout the evening and into the early morning hours of November 7, 2009. Later that evening, I was joined by Congresswomen Kathy Dahlkemper and Marcy Kaptur, who also testified in support of the Stupak Amendment. I am grateful to both of them as well and I commend Congresswoman Dahlkemper for having the courage to share her very personal story about her strong commitment to Life.

Once again, I felt like the Democratic Party was punishing me for believing in and advocating for the sanctity of life. I know the Democratic women had rebuked Kathy Dahlkemper and Marcy Kaptur for their strong commitment to Life earlier that evening when Speaker Pelosi met with the Democratic women and they forced the Speaker to renege on her agreement with me. We witnessed the pettiness, the intolerance and the abuse of power by lawmakers. The long evening and the negotiations with the Speaker only served to reinforce my commitment to leave Congress when my term ended in December 2010.

As I look back on that tumultuous day, I am reminded that in Washington, DC there are those with power and those who know how to use power. The way I was treated throughout my last term in Congress made it much easier for me to leave elected office. The weeks leading up to the vote on the Stupak Amendment truly tested my faith, my endurance, and my determination.

CHAPTER 42

★ ★ ★

Saturday November 7, 2009

I t was 1:30 a.m. when Mike and I arrived back at C Street. I wondered out loud whether my amendment would be made in order and Mike reassured me that it would. My last comment to Mike was, "Well, then why wouldn't Steny or anyone else give me any assurance that it would?" Mike said, "Because they don't know what to do with you and your amendment."

I was hoping that Mike would say that the Speaker told him that she would make my amendment in order because I really needed a good night of sleep. It had been weeks since I had slept soundly and woke rested in the morning. I knew that I would spend yet another restless night wondering if my amendment would be made in order. As I jumped into bed, I reviewed the day's events starting with leaving my home at 4:30 a.m. to catch my flight back to Washington DC. I had been awake over twenty-one hours. Even though I was exhausted, I could not shut down my brain. I read, prayed and recited the rosary; I tried everything I could think of to take my mind off the Stupak Amendment and my own health care hell. Unfortunately, I rehashed every interview and every discussion with colleagues. I examined my scorecard in my head and thought about how to approach Members and convince them to vote for my amendment. In my little bedroom back at the house on

C Street, I could find peace and quiet. However, my overly active brain kept whirling with thoughts and ideas. Once again, I had very little sleep.

I could never have predicted how often I would ask B.J. whether I was doing the right thing. What was I failing to see? How could I protect the sanctity of life and still provide access to quality health care for all Americans? Finally, I would ask B.J., Jesus, and now my mother-in-law to turn off my brain and allow me to get some sleep.

I finally fell asleep for a little while but awoke at 6:00 a.m. It was Saturday, November 7, 2009, and I did not need to get up so early. The Whip Report on the Rule accompanying the health care legislation would not be out for a couple of hours; I tossed and turned and finally got up at 8:00 a.m. I looked at my Blackberry and found that the Rule accompanying HR-3962, The Affordable Health Care for America Act, had been filed at 2:26 a.m.

I quickly examined my Blackberry. Sure enough, the Stupak Amendment was listed and it would be debatable for twenty minutes, equally divided between both sides. Speaker Pelosi had finally granted my amendment. I needed to make sure the Stupak Amendment would pass and my brain started to race.

Last night Mike and I had called most of the Members of Congress in my coalition and told them that we had reached an agreement with the Speaker. There would be no Stupak Amendment and we should all vote for the Rule. Now, I had to ask them to vote for both the Rule and the Stupak Amendment.

On Saturday morning, very few of my supporters knew that the Speaker had reneged on her agreement. Members of Congress were not aware that the Democratic Women had rejected the agreement that the Speaker had negotiated in good faith to avoid a showdown between the Pro-Life and Pro-Choice Members of Congress. Now, I had to get the word out.

I was excited and had work to do to ensure passage of the Stupak Amendment. After all these months of meetings, warnings, and threats to bring down the Rule without my Amendment, my Amendment was made in order. I wanted to let out a scream but I did not want to wake up Mike in the next room. I sat on the edge of my bed and felt that I had won a major victory but no one knew it yet. The Speaker had blinked. Now, the opposition only gave me a few hours to marshal enough votes to pass the Stupak Amendment. If I could get the word out to my supporters and RTL colleagues it could be a major victory. As Richard Doerflinger said, the whole RTL movement depended on passing the Stupak Amendment. I guess Richard was right but I still had a lot of work to do. Sitting on the edge of my bed in my pajamas, I felt euphoric but anxious, as I had to round up at least 218 votes for the Stupak Amendment within a few hours.

I got up, dressed, and quickly headed for St. Peter's Catholic Church on the corner of Second Street and C Street, less than a block from my C Street boarding house. I often visited St. Peter's to think and pray. I slipped in the back door of the church, quickly said a prayer of thanks for the amendment and asked God for assistance and strength to prevail on the upcoming vote on the Stupak Amendment. I then headed for the Capitol and the floor of the US House of Representatives.

The session of the House of Representatives was scheduled to begin at 9:00 a.m. I wanted to pick up a copy of the Union Calendar, located on the table behind the House Floor, to make sure my amendment was listed. Also, the Whip's Notice said that there would be ten one-minute speeches and I wanted to see who was lined up to speak. Once again, I needed to ask Democratic Members to support the Stupak Amendment on the House Floor.

By now the formal name of the Stupak Amendment was the Stupak, Pitts, Ellsworth, Smith, Kaptur, and Dahlkemper Amendment. It was the only amendment allowed to the US House health care legislation, The Affordable Health Care for America Act. I fought for seven months to make this amendment permissible under the Rule and now I needed to deliver the votes to pass it. Once again, I thought of Richard Doerflinger's warning that the entire RTL movement depended on the passage of the Stupak Amendment. I quickly put Richard out of my mind and headed to the House floor.

I arrived at the House floor and picked up the Union Calendar. There it was, the Stupak Amendment. I was elated but frightened.

I had about twenty minutes before the debate on the Rule and the Stupak Amendment would start. I had to contact about sixty Democrats and over 170 Republicans, and had very little time to make sure the Democrats would now vote for the Rule and the Stupak Amendment. How was I going to get the word out? I decided to start with the Democratic leaders in the RTL Caucus; I would have to personally contact about twenty Democratic Members to get their final commitment to vote for the Stupak Amendment. Now, after all the statements, pleas, and challenges I had made to the Democratic leadership to just put up my amendment and let the votes fall where they may, it was time to meet the challenge head on.

I quickly called and left messages for the sponsors of the Stupak Amendment informing them that the vote was on for today and asking them to pass the word amongst our known supporters. I asked them to call me later with the names they needed me to whip. In my call with Congressmen Chris Smith and Joe Pitts, I asked them to keep all the House Republicans voting for and supporting the Stupak Amendment.

Members of Congress were lining up on the floor to present their one-minute speeches and I noticed that not one of the Democratic speakers would be supporting my amendment. I stepped back out into the Speaker's Lobby to make my way over to my Rayburn office.

In the lobby, I was confronted by a couple of reporters asking about my amendment. They questioned whether I had enough votes to pass it because the Pro-Choice groups claimed I did not. I assured them that the Pro-Choice groups were incorrect and that I had enough votes to pass my amendment. They also questioned me about how many votes were needed; I responded with minimal information and informed the reporters that I would receive at least 220 votes for my amendment and 218 were needed for passage. The reporters continued to challenge me by stating that not everyone I thought would vote for my amendment would actually vote for it and it sounded like I could not afford to lose any of my supporters. Once again, I tried to explain that I had enough votes. The reporters then asked if they could see my whip count and I told them that I did not have a whip list. They asked, "How can you be so confident in passing the amendment when your own count has just enough votes to squeak through?" I simply said that I was confident. Their next question was, "How many Democrats will vote for your amendment?" I answered, "Around forty." The reporters asked where I was getting the extra votes since there were only thirty-five reliable RTL Democrats. I finally said that I looked forward to the vote on my amendment. If the Pro-Choice groups believed that I did not have enough votes, then let us vote right now and see who was correct.

Despite their many probing questions, I was not going to give the reporters the names of the Members who would be voting for the Stupak Amendment. I intentionally low-balled the number of Members who had promised to vote for the Stupak Amendment, as I did not wish to have the Pro-Choice groups badgering Members of Congress who might be viewed as sympathetic to my amendment. There was simply not enough time for the one-man Whip team to reach out to all sixty Democratic Members who said they would vote for the Stupak Amendment. I needed to contact as many Democratic Members as possible, but it was Saturday and many offices were not fully staffed on the weekend.

While I was speaking to the reporters, Congressman Joe Pitts was on the House floor giving his one-minute speech, in which he stated:

> "...I went last night with my colleagues Bart Stupak, Chris Smith, Marcy Kaptur, and Kathy Dahlkemper before the Rules Committee after midnight. The final outcome is this: There will only be one Pro-Life amendment offered on the floor today. It will be the Stupak, Ellsworth, Pitts, Smith, Kaptur, and Dahlkemper amendment that will prevent Federal funds from funding abortions in both the public plan or with affordability credits. It just codifies the Hyde Amendment for the two new programs."

"This actually preserves the status quo of our law today. No federal government funding for abortions. Just like SCHIP, Medicaid, DOD, FEHBP, and Indian Health.

This is a bipartisan amendment. The Pro-Life groups- National Right-to-Life, Catholic Bishops, and family groups- all support this. I urge the Members to support this amendment when it comes to the floor today."

Once again, Congressman Joe Pitts beat us to the punch. He was on the floor informing our colleagues that it was game on and only the Stupak Amendment enjoyed the support of all the RTL groups and the Catholic Bishops, regardless of what may be said during the debate on health care.

By the time I arrived back at my Rayburn office, Scott informed me that National RTL and the Catholic Bishops were looking for me. I told Scott that I understood they were looking for me but I needed some time to think strategy so I did not answer their calls. Scott and I discussed the late night, the last amendment to be recognized in the Rules Committee, the Democratic women walking out of the Rules Committee and the reporters badgering me on whether I *really* had the votes to support my amendment. I told Scott that I just wanted this whole thing to be over: let's vote on the amendment and health care and then go home. I had been back in DC for less than twenty-four hours and I wanted to go home, away from this madness and be with my family. My wife had just lost her mother. Our son and his wife of two months had come home from California for the funeral and were still with Laurie in Menominee.

While my heart may have been in Menominee with my grieving family, my head was in DC and the job I needed to do. It was time to return the calls from the US Conference of Catholic Bishops and Doug Johnson of National Right-to-Life.

The one-minutes were over and there were five suspension bills on the calendar that had been debated the previous day. Leadership called for the votes. Around 9:40 a.m. on Saturday morning, we started voting on five suspension bills. No doubt one of the reasons for the early votes was to determine who was present to vote. Leadership had repeatedly warned Members that votes would occur throughout the day and Members were expected to be present to vote.

Voting on the floor gave me an opportunity to discuss the Stupak Amendment with Democratic Members who I was counting on to vote for the amendment. The fact that I was willing to strike an agreement with the Speaker to avoid this vote was well received by Members. The realization that the Speaker was forced to renege because the Pro-Choice Women's Caucus would not agree to the deal only reinforced the Members' determination to vote in favor of the Stupak Amendment. For weeks, I had been pounded by Pro-Choice and women's groups as being inflexible and trying to kill health care if I did not get my amendment. No matter how many times I said it, my offer of allowing Members to vote their consciences on the Hyde Amendment always seemed to fall on deaf ears. Back in 1993-1994 with the Democrats in control, the House Members voted on the traditional RTL amendments and lost the vote. RTL Members accepted the fact that we lost but respected the fact that we were given the opportunity to vote our conscience on a principle we cared deeply about. I had negotiated a similar agreement with the Speaker and the Democratic women's groups had rejected it. To the Speaker's credit, she had allowed the Stupak Amendment. The Democratic women insisted they had the votes to defeat us; later in the day, we would see which side had the votes for and against the Stupak Amendment. As I left the floor I felt confident that Members understood that I had done all I could to avoid this showdown and that my coalition was determined to pass the Stupak Amendment.

Congresswoman Louise Slaughter, the absentee Chair of the Rules Committee, called up HR-903, the Rule accompanying The Affordable Health Care for America Act. The Rule was subject to one hour of debate, equally divided between the Democratic Majority and the Republican Minority. As Slaughter made her opening comments, you could see the Democratic women Members of Congress line up as she spoke. I knew this was trouble. I sat at my desk and watched as Congresswoman Slaughter individually yielded to each Congresswoman in line "…for a unanimous consent to the gentlewoman from [state of the congresswoman]."

Each Congresswoman in line would "ask and be given permission to revise and extend her remarks." The Congresswoman would then make a statement highlighting a positive principle in the health care legislation such as:

"Mrs. MALONEY. Mr. Speaker, I support ending gender discrimination in [health insurance] premium prices."

"Ms. LEE of California. Mr. Speaker, I support affordable health care and this Democratic bill so that domestic violence may never be used ever again as a preexisting condition."

"Ms. KILPATRICK of Michigan. Mr. Speaker, I support our House bill which will let women and doctors control their health decisions."

"Ms. ZOE LOFGREN of California. Mr. Speaker, I support the Democratic bill to let our kids in their twenties get insurance and keep healthy."

The Republicans would object as the unanimous consent is traditionally used to allow a Member of Congress to insert in the Congressional Record their statement in support of or in opposition to the legislation being debated. The Member is not supposed to give a short speech. In all, thirty-five Democratic Congresswoman asked for and received unanimous consent and made a short speech in support of the health care legislation. Each Republican objection to the unanimous consent was directed to the Speaker Pro Tempore of the House at the time. The Speaker Pro Tempore was John D. Dingell, Jr. of Michigan, the longest-serving Member in the House of Representatives and my mentor.

Speaker Dingell stated that it was his intent to allow all Members of Congress seeking unanimous consent. Whether they were Democrat or Republican, their request would be granted on this important, historic legislation.

"The Chair has a comment to make here. The Chair is going to request the Members on both sides of the aisle to respect the rights of the other Members. Members have the right, under the rules, to ask unanimous consent. If Members on one side of the aisle want their right protected, the Chair observes that they should then respect the rights of Members on the other side of the aisle. It will be the purpose of the Chair to try and see that all Members are heard at the proper time and fashion and to see that the rules are carried out. The Chair will also try to see that the debate is conducted with a measure of comity and grace and decency, and the Chair would request my friends on both sides of the aisle to respect that." (Congressional Record, November 7, 2009, p. H12601)

What each Democratic Congresswoman did was give a short speech highlighting a positive principle in the health care legislation. These speeches were orchestrated, positive sound bites on the virtues of the bill, and it drove the Republicans nuts. The Republicans on the floor were screaming for regular parliamentary order and the Chair, Congressman John Dingell, continued to recognize the Democratic Congresswomen. It was getting testy on the floor and not a good way to start off a long day of partisan debate on a very divisive issue.

As Speaker Dingell stated: "Looking down from the Rostrum here, the chair observes that the line to the Speaker's right [Democratic side] is getting shorter and that the time of the gentlewoman from New York [Slaughter] will shortly expire. That time will then move to the minority side, at which time Members of the minority may want to make the same requests that Members of the majority have made. The Chair is going to do his

level best to see to it all Members are protected in
their rights." (Congressional Record, November
7, 2009, p. H12603)

The Republicans continued to complain about the waste of time
the majority unanimous requests took up. When asked if she would
agree to an extra hour of time to debate the Rule, Congresswoman
Slaughter stated, "I am calling for regular order. I would like to really
get on with this bill." Democrats would not agree to extend debate
time on the Rule, and Slaughter continued to yield unanimous
consent to Democratic women over the repeated objections of the
Republicans.

Having witnessed this tactic before, I knew the Republicans
would then parade their representatives to make their negative comments on the Affordable Health Care Act. It was going to be a long
and bitter debate and we were only on the Rule.

In response to this denial for extra time, the Republicans lined
up twenty-one Members- eleven women and ten men- to speak out
against the health care legislation under their unanimous consent
requests. The Republican message on health care as espoused in their
unanimous consent statements were:

Ms. BACHMANN. "Mr. Speaker, I rise in opposition to the
job-killing bill that will cut $500 million from Medicare and poten-
tially collapse the economic economy".

Ms. MILLER of Michigan. "Mr. Speaker, I rise in opposition
to this job-killing, deficit-exploding government takeover of health
care system."

Mr. DAVIS of Kentucky. "Mr. Speaker, I rise in opposition
because of the tyranny that is being exercised by the majority to step
in between the American people and their freedom to make their
own health decisions."

Mr. GOHMERT. "Mr. Speaker, I rise in opposition to the
abuse of process in not allowing people to come to the people's
House and just make statements over eighteen percent takeover of
the US economy."

With the continual verbal exchanges between the Members of the Rules Committee over the unanimous consents, I became more and more concerned that I would lose my Republican support for the Stupak Amendment. I knew that Members of the Rules Committee worked until at least 2:00 a.m. and were now on the floor with probably four to five hours of sleep. I could see that their patience was in short supply. I was afraid that partisan emotion would soon overtake reason and the Stupak Amendment would be a casualty of partisan politics. If partisan politics prevailed, House Republicans would not vote for the Stupak Amendment, simply because I was a Democrat.

It was time to call the Bishops' lobbyists. I spoke with either Richard Doerflinger or possibly John Carr. As there were a number of phone calls back and forth between me, Richard and John that afternoon, I am not entirely clear as to what order I spoke with whom. Because Richard was the Director of Pro-Life Activities, most of my conversations took place with him. The first comment Richard made was, "Did you see what just happened on the House floor?" I told him that I had and that his concern was not unfounded, as I had seen too many inflammatory statements polarize the Members of Congress into a partisan, "Hell no, we will not vote for any Democrat or Republican amendment or legislation now!" Both sides were equally guilty of allowing their flame-throwing Members to turn a civilized debate into a partisan frenzy through their words and actions. I assured Richard that I could not pull back Chairwoman Slaughter nor could I dissuade the Republicans from retaliating with their lineup of Members seeking unanimous consent to extend their remarks in opposition of the health care legislation. It was going to be a long, emotional, heated debate. Richard was worried about the fate of the Stupak Amendment. I told Richard that I was going to call Doug Johnson and ask him to "score" the vote on the Stupak Amendment in an effort to hold the Republicans. Doug said that RTL would again send a letter to all the congressional offices stating that RTL would score the vote on the Stupak Amendment. We had come too far not to follow through on all the details of a strategy that was in constant flux.

Scoring a vote meant that an organization such as National Right-to-Life would consider this vote a critical one. When an organization decided whether to endorse a candidate in an election, they reviewed the incumbent's voting record and determined how he or she scored on the votes considered critical to the core mission of the organization.

Seldom did I ever receive a perfect score from National RTL. My score with them hovered around eighty percent because they "scored" some votes that had very little impact on protecting the sanctity of life. With the Michigan RTL scorecard, I had a perfect record because they only scored meaningful RTL votes. Unlike National Right-to-Life, Michigan RTL did not score the Republican budget bills. No matter what the budget contained, if RTL language was included in the bill, the Republican budget was usually scored.

Through the afternoon, rumors swirled that the Republicans were going to put up their votes for the Stupak Amendment and then immediately withdraw them before the gavel fell to announce the vote result on the amendment. This rumor was so pervasive that Richard Doerflinger called me again and insisted that I go over to address the Republicans who were caucusing on the Stupak Amendment. I had a difficult time convincing Richard that I as a Democrat could not simply walk over and address the Republican Caucus on the Stupak Amendment. I told Richard that with Chris Smith and Joe Pitts in the Republican Caucus, I was confident they would hold the Republicans together and vote for the Stupak Amendment. Richard was very insistent that I reach out to Chris and Joe, whom I had already spoken with earlier in the day. I assured Richard that I would follow up with them.

Later, I learned that Cardinal George had called Republican Leader John Boehner (R-OH) and told him that the Republicans had better not play games with the Stupak Amendment. Cardinal George and the Bishops were counting on the Republicans to "stand with Stupak." Boehner objected and said that some of the Republican Members were thinking of abstaining and voting "present" on the Stupak Amendment. Cardinal George told Boehner that if he thought the Bishops were tough on the Democrats who did not support the Stupak Amendment, the Bishops would be even tougher on the Republicans who did not vote with Stupak. Boehner told Cardinal George that he would communicate the Cardinal's message to his caucus.

Around 1:00 p.m., the debate on the Rule was complete and Congresswoman Louise Slaughter asked for a recorded vote. As Members arrived to the floor to vote, many of them checked with me for the latest development and asked whether they should vote for the Rule. Once I voted Yes on the Rule, the RTL Democrats followed suit and voted Yes as well. After I cast my vote, I doubled back to talk with the Blue Dogs and the Hispanic Caucus Leaders.

The Blue Dogs had no problem voting for the Stupak Amendment but that did not necessarily mean that they would vote for the health care legislation. Even though a couple of the Blue Dogs voted against the Rule, they still agreed to vote in favor of the amendment.

I had struck a deal with the Hispanic Caucus. Some of the Members were concerned with the Republican Motion to Recommit on the health care legislation. They feared that the Motion to Recommit would include language authorizing the deportation of families whose parents could not prove their citizenship. Most members of the Hispanic Caucus would only vote for the Stupak Amendment if the RTL Democrats voted against the Republican Motion to Recommit no matter what language the Republicans inserted on immigration.

The Hispanic Caucus feared that the Republicans would add language deporting all illegal immigrants and/or deny benefits to all men, women or children who could not produce proof of citizenship upon demand. The Hispanic Caucus was afraid that children would be deported because their parents could not produce proper paperwork and the children would be forced to leave the only country they had ever known.

I agreed with the Hispanic Caucus that if they voted for the Stupak Amendment, we would vote against the Motion to Recommit if it contained divisive immigration language. I reminded

Congressmen Solomon Ortiz and Joe Baca of our agreement as they voted on the Rule.

The Rule passed with 247 Yes and 192 No votes. It was time to move the debate in the US House of Representatives to HR-3962, Affordable Health Care for America Act. History was about to be made. After nearly a hundred years of presidents calling upon Congress to pass health care legislation, the US House had finally maneuvered a national health care bill to the floor for debate. While the debate raged for hours, both Democrats and Republicans strategized on how to secure the last votes to pass or defeat the health care legislation. Barring some unforeseen circumstance or crisis, each party knew that the historic vote on health care would occur later in the day, Saturday, November 7, 2009.

Before the debate began on health care, Majority Leader Steny Hoyer asked for unanimous consent to address the House. Hoyer asked the Members of the House to honor John Dingell, the longest-serving Member of the House, who had championed health care throughout his career. Congressman Hoyer said, in part:

> "…this is obviously a historic day. There were some of us who were for it and some of us who were against it, but I know that all of us, all 434 of his colleagues, are honored to serve with longest-serving Member of this House, who has committed himself to health care throughout his Life, as did his father. We honor him for the service he has given to our country.
>
> Ladies and gentlemen, let us stand in honor of JOHN DINGELL." (Congressional Record, November 7, 2009, pp. H12622-12623)

After this recognition and honor given by House Members to John Dingell, there was one more suspension vote before the health care debate could start in earnest.

The Rule debate had only served to increase the partisan tension on the floor between the Democrats and Republicans. HR-3962, Affordable Health Care for America Act, was strictly a partisan bill. Within the Democratic Caucus there was indignant divisiveness over the Stupak Amendment. Therefore, I thought it was ironic that the last suspension vote before the start of the contentious debate on health care was a bill "Recognizing the 20th Anniversary of the Ending of the Cold War." Hell, the Cold War was not over: it had simply moved to the House Chamber. Neither side was talking to the other; each side had claimed victory and promised to bury the other. Still, I worked and longed for détente.

Throughout the afternoon, I worked the phones and met with members of my coalition. Everyone was set to vote for the Stupak Amendment. Richard Doerflinger called me again and insisted that the Republicans were planning to hang me out to dry on the amendment. I again told Richard that everything was set; we just needed to get through the next four to five hours of debate on the health care bill. I tried to explain to Richard that the debate would not get out of hand on the Stupak Amendment, as only a few House Members would participate due to the fact that we were only allowed twenty minutes of debate time. I sensed that Richard was anxious and just wanted the vote on the Stupak Amendment over. I explained to Richard that it was unfortunately going to be a long, emotional night as final passage of the House Health Care bill, which the Bishops supported with the passage of the Stupak Amendment, would come late into the evening.

I told Richard that if either Democrats or Republicans played any games with the Stupak Amendment, I would urge my coalition members to vote "Present" on the health care legislation. To pass legislation in the US House of Representatives, the legislation under consideration must receive a majority vote of those Members present and voting. In this case, a "Present" vote is equivalent to a "No" vote.

I had no intention of voting "Present" nor was I going to direct other Members to vote "Present." My purpose in discussing the "Present" vote was to reassure him that I had thought through all legislative scenarios. Richard did mention that there were some Republicans who were rumored to vote No on the Stupak Amendment because they still believed that if it were defeated then the RTL Democrats would vote No on the health care legislation. This rumor was worth exploring and I called Chris Smith and asked for his assessment of whether the Republicans would abstain or vote for the Stupak Amendment.

Chris stated that some of the more conservative Members were discussing voting against the Stupak Amendment and that I should reach out to Congressman John Shadegg (R-AZ), Steve King (R-IA), and Todd Aiken (R-MO). These were the Republican Members who were urging Republicans to vote "Present" on the amendment. The logic behind this strategy was that these Republican Members did not trust the RTL Democrats to hold firm on protecting the sanctity of life and that the Senate would not support the Stupak Amendment. Chris and I agreed that I would personally discuss the amendment with these three or four Republican Members. I had another touchy issue that I had to discuss with Chris Smith and we agreed to meet on the House floor after the Rule vote.

Chris Smith and I met briefly on the floor with Todd Aiken (R-MO) and John Shadegg (R-AZ) and discussed their desire to vote "Present" on the Stupak Amendment. I implored them not to vote "Present" but to stand with us RTL Democrats and pass the Hyde (Stupak) Amendment. I explained that the Stupak Amendment was the Hyde Amendment that they had supported over the years. The only difference from the Hyde Amendment was a new name and that it was being offered by a Democrat. Other than these technical distinctions, it was the same amendment they had supported for years.

Aiken and Shadegg questioned whether there were enough Democratic votes to pass the Stupak Amendment. There were 178 Republicans plus thirty-five reliable RTL Democrats, which only gave me 213 votes. I needed 218 votes to pass the Stupak Amendment. I reassured them that I had more than thirty-five Democrats who would vote for the Stupak Amendment but added that I needed every Republican to vote with me. I further stated that the only reason Speaker Pelosi negotiated with me yesterday was because she knew she did not have the votes to pass the Rule. To pass the Rule, she had to allow the Stupak Amendment. Even though the women's groups were predicting victory in defeating the Stupak Amendment, their claims were in vain if we stayed united.

I needed every Republican vote and as many Democratic votes as possible to defeat a presidential veto and to encourage the Senate to include the Stupak Amendment in its health care legislation. The greater the Pro-Life vote total in the House, the more pressure it would place on the Senate to insert the Stupak Amendment into their health care legislation. The greater the number of votes for the Amendment, the stronger the position we would hold in the conference committee with the Senate.

John Shadegg was being Shadegg. Since the Stupak Amendment was not his idea, John was not inclined to support it, especially as it was a Democratic initiative. I spoke to John and asked that if he could not support us to at least not vote against us: to just vote "Present" if he had to vote at all. Todd on the other hand wanted assurances that if the President vetoed the health care legislation because of the Stupak Amendment there would be enough Democratic votes to defeat the veto. I assured Todd that there were not enough Democratic votes to sustain a veto and President Obama would not veto health care on the Stupak Amendment alone. I shared with him the President's statement to *CBS* when he said, "I'm Pro-Choice, but I think we also have the tradition in this town, historically, of not financing abortions as part of government-funded health care. My main focus is making sure that people have options of high quality care at the lowest possible price." Based on this statement, I was confident the President wanted health care more than he wanted this fight over abortion. He would not veto health care legislation solely because the Stupak Amendment was added to the legislation.

After answering Congressmen Shadegg and Aiken's concerns I felt confident that most, if not all, of the Republicans would vote for the Stupak Amendment. I had one more issue to discuss with Chris Smith as the time was drawing near to debate the Stupak Amendment.

I explained to Chris that my RTL Democrats had asked as gently as possible that the Republicans tone down the emotional rhetoric and not display the graphic photos of discarded fetuses during the debate on the Stupak Amendment. Further, I explained that many Democratic RTL Members wished to join in the abortion debate but were turned off by the graphic rhetoric and displays.

Chris defended the Republican tactics as necessary and important in educating the American people and the Democrats on the horrors of abortion. I responded that I understood his point but we needed the Democrats to vote for the Stupak Amendment. We could not afford to lose any Democrats and I feared some may vote against the amendment because of what was said and the photos displayed during the debate. As best as I could, I explained that health care was a very emotional, partisan issue. Tempers had been flaring throughout the day and it would not take much for the Democrats to walk away from the Stupak Amendment.

Chris looked a little perplexed at my request. I confided in him that he would be surprised with the number of Democratic votes that would be cast for the Stupak Amendment. He would be even more surprised when a number of liberal Democrats voted for the Stupak Amendment. When asked which ones, I mentioned David Obey and Richie Neal (D-MA) and he was shocked. I explained that these Democratic Members had voted for Hyde when it was a clean amendment. Since the Hyde Amendment was first passed in 1976, rarely had Members of Congress been afforded an opportunity to vote for the original purpose and intent behind the amendment, which simply stated that there would be no public funding for abortions.

I asked Chris not to say anything to other Members of Congress about Obey and Neal and to allow these two Members of Congress to quietly put up their votes for the Stupak Amendment. I asked him to especially not say anything about these two Members to the press. Then I added, "If you think I am wrong, check with Autumn. She and Erika have developed a master list of how Democratic Members have voted over the course of their careers on specific RTL legislation."

From the master list, I had made another list and targeted about ninety Democratic Members who I believed could be convinced to vote for the Stupak Amendment. Again, in confidence I told Chris that I felt that approximately sixty Democratic Members would vote in favor of the Amendment. Therefore, we had enough votes to prevent a presidential veto of the legislation over the Stupak Amendment. Chris was still denying that I would generate sixty Democratic votes and said if I did it would be the greatest RTL victory since Hyde. Chris became giddy! I swore him to secrecy on my vote count and asked him who would be speaking on the Republican side on the Stupak Amendment.

Chris went over the Republican list of speakers in support of the Stupak Amendment and I did not have any real problems except for Michelle Bachmann. Bachmann was viewed as a partisan hack and tended to turn Democrats off. Bachmann was also known for her wild, false allegations and personal attacks on Democrats. Chris tried to justify her speaking on behalf of the amendment because Bachmann represented the very conservative wing of the Republican Party and he needed her to speak. With only twenty minutes of debate equally divided by the two sides, the Pro-Life side only controlled ten, which would be split: five minutes for the Republicans and five minutes for the Democrats. The conclusion was that Bachmann and other Republican speakers would not have enough time to alienate the Democrats because each speaker would only have thirty to sixty seconds to speak. Congressman Joe Pitts, the co-author of the Stupak Amendment, would control the time for the Republicans.

The Democratic list of speakers on the Stupak Amendment would be me, Ellsworth, Dahlkemper, Lipinski and Kaptur. I had encouraged other Democratic Members to ask for unanimous consent to insert their remarks in the record. Chris said he also encouraged the Republican Members to submit their remarks for inclusion in the Congressional Record.

The debate on the Stupak Amendment took place at 8:00 p.m. on November 7, 2009, and the vote occurred two hours later. After the debate on the Stupak Amendment, the Republicans offered their substitute bill, Common Sense Health Care Reform and Affordability Act, as an amendment debatable for an hour.

Finally, at approximately 10:00 p.m., the Speaker Pro Tempore called for a recorded vote on the Stupak Amendment. As Members of the US House of Representatives made their way to the House Floor to electronically record their votes, I was flushed with emotion.

During my seventeen years in elected office, never had I tried harder to avoid a vote and never had I been more confident of the outcome of one. Still, I believed it was tragic that the focus of national health care came down to abortion. I had repeatedly warned my colleagues in committee briefings, hearings, and through correspondence, imploring the President and his staff not to allow abortion to be injected into the national debate on health care. My Pro-Choice friends broke the truce that had existed on the abortion issue for thirty years; Congresswoman Lois Capps had offered the Pro-Choice amendment in the Energy and Commerce Committee markup of the health care legislation. Now, the whole country was watching to see how the US House of Representatives would vote on the abortion issue, rather than to learn what benefits were contained in the health care legislation. No, they wanted to know where their Member of Congress stood on federal funding for abortion in health care.

CHAPTER 43

★ ★ ★

Vote for Life (November 7, 2009)

My head hurt; several days had passed since I had enjoyed a good night of sleep. The vote was being called on the Stupak-Pitts amendment to HR-3962, the Affordable Health Care for America Act. It was late and the press gallery was full of reporters watching this pivotal vote. I could not avoid the stares. I just wanted to be alone; I quickly disappeared into the little red copy room just off the Pennsylvania corner. I was confident that we would prevail on the Stupak-Pitts amendment.

There is an old saying that victory has many fathers, but I did not want to hear the congratulatory bullshit. I just wished to finalize the vote on the Stupak Amendment and then move quickly onto Final Passage of the Affordable Health Care for America Act, HR-3962. I ran over and checked with the Hispanic Caucus to make sure that they would be voting for the Stupak Amendment. Henry Cuellar (D-TX) and Joe Baca (D-CA) were voting and they asked if we still had a deal. I said, "Yes, I gave you my word." They responded okay and voted for the Stupak Amendment.

I moved to the back of the chamber by the cloakroom, where the computer was recording the votes simultaneously with the lighted electronic voting board on the East wall of the House Chamber. With the Republicans putting up their votes early, the Stupak Amendment quickly achieved 218 votes and was still climbing. The Pro-Choice proponents were in shock and disbelief.

As I walked down the center Democratic aisle to thank David Obey for his vote, the Speaker grabbed my arm and acknowledged that I had been right. Then she explained that after our meeting her staff had given her a closer review of my amendment. Upon closer review, it was determined that the Stupak Amendment was in fact needed to prevent elective abortions at federal health centers. I responded by saying that now we had to persuade the Senate to accept the Stupak Amendment. I also mentioned that Joe Cao (R-LA) would be voting for the health care legislation because of the Stupak Amendment; Speaker Pelosi said that was also her understanding. I then pointed out that her wish for bi-partisan support for health care legislation would be achieved; she smiled and said, "Thank you."

I continued my way down the aisle and thanked David Obey for his vote on the Stupak Amendment. I mentioned to David that the next vote for health care would be a bipartisan vote. I told him this was in honor of his sister. David said, "Thank you." and squeezed my arm. David's sister had died at young age from cancer that left her family mentally and financially drained. David's sister did not have good health care coverage and David had promised her that he would pass national health care. I headed for the Pennsylvania corner and the red copy room.

I stood stoically satisfied as the Stupak amendment passed the House with a 240-194 vote! Many of the women were shocked; I was satisfied. My months of quiet diplomacy had paid off. The Stupak Amendment received 240 votes, which meant that sixty-four Democrats had voted with me to protect the sanctity of life; one out of every four Democrats in the US House of Representatives had voted for the Stupak Amendment. As I stood and took in the vote total, I was moved to tears and headed for the little red copy room so I could be alone.

The Pro-Choice Members who had predicted my defeat were shocked as they began to realize that some of the most liberal Members of the Democratic Caucus had voted in favor of the

Stupak Amendment. In their arrogance, the Pro-Choice Members of Congress never stopped to consider the meaning behind it. They had failed to conduct their own due diligence; the Pro-Choice Members never researched how each Member of Congress had historically voted on public funding for abortions. They never understood the simple context in which I framed the question: should there be public funding for abortion, or not? The Pro-Choice forces had no idea that I had quietly whipped the question over the past few months. I do not believe the Pro-Choice Members realized that I had developed a coalition and that my amendment, like the final vote on the Affordable Care Act for America, would truly be a bipartisan vote. The Pro-Choice forces never engaged nor understood the personal implications of the Stupak Amendment for a Democratic Member.

After the August mark-up in the Energy and Commerce Committee, I realized I had to do a better job at explaining and keeping the Stupak Amendment simple. I had asked my staff to research each Democratic Member's personal history on public funding for abortions. For over two months, I had personally lobbied each Member who I believed would support the Stupak Amendment, quietly forming coalitions and holding the Republican Caucus close to earn their trust and support. I did my homework when no one else had; I understood how to frame the issue when discussing the amendment with Democratic Members.

I also realized that my work would also guarantee me a major challenge in the Democratic primary next year. I really did not care at all because I knew that I was not going to run again, although I could not tell Members of Congress that at this point in the game. If I did, I would lose my clout and influence. To me, the principle of standing up for the sanctity of life was worth more than any political opposition. My decision not to seek re-election allowed me to push forward without worrying about political fallout.

At about the same time the vote was called for the Affordable Health Care for America Act, my family called on my cell phone. I wanted to talk with them, so I slipped back into the little red copy room. It had been a brutal week; we had buried my mother-in-law, and I had left my family to push and force a vote on the Stupak

Amendment. I just wanted to hear their voices and then get some sleep.

I was pleased to hear the pride my family expressed in the passage of the Stupak Amendment and that it had won by such a large margin. I hoped the passage of the amendment erased the shortcomings that I had displayed since August, as my heart and soul were focused on securing and passing the Stupak Amendment against all political, legislative and personal odds. The call with my family brought tears to my eyes. Suddenly, Silky came in and yelled "Hey Stu, you have to vote! You can't miss this one! After all you're the guy that got us here! You okay?"

"Yeah, Silky, I am fine," I responded as I left the little red copy room to vote. "Silky" is Congressman Bill Pascrell, a Democrat from Paterson, New Jersey, one of my best friends, and a regular in the Pennsylvania Corner. During one of our first meetings with Bill, Mike Doyle mentioned that Paterson was known as the silk capital. Since then, Bill has been known as "Silky" to his congressional colleagues.

As I was voting and thanking the Members in the Pennsylvania corner, I received a hug from Mike Doyle and my phone started ringing. I hesitated to answer, because the last person I wanted to talk to was yet another reporter. Thankfully, it was my oldest brother Frank calling from a Catholic wedding in the Detroit area to congratulate me. Everyone at the wedding had watched the vote on the Stupak Amendment and was thrilled to see it pass. My brother told me that a huge cheer went up from the wedding guests as the Stupak Amendment passed and that I was their hero. Unfortunately, I also realized that I was now a shithead in the eyes of those who opposed my Amendment.

On the back pages of the Congressional Record there is the *Daily Digest,* which succinctly summarizes the day's legislative highlights in the US House of Representatives and the US Senate. For November 7, 2009, it states:

Highlights

The House passed H.R. 3962, Affordable
Health Care for America Act.

House of Representatives

Chamber Action

Stupak amendment (printed in part C of H. Rept. 111-330)
that codifies Hyde Amendment in H.R. 3962. The amendment
prohibits federal funds for abortion services in the public option. It
also prohibits individuals who receive affordability credits from purchasing a plan that provides elective abortions. However, it allows
individuals, both who receive affordability credits and who do not,
to separately purchase with their own funds plans that cover elective
abortions. It also clarifies that private plans may still offer elective
abortions (by a yea-and-nay vote of 240 yeas to 194 nays with 1 voting "Present," Roll No. 884).

I could not have said it better.

Naively, I did not realize the impact the Stupak Amendment
would have across the country nor the hatred it would bring to bear
on my family and me. I even convinced myself that the Senate now
had to accept the Stupak Amendment with its overwhelming support from House Democrats. Surely, Majority Leader Reid did not
want to go through what the House just went through on the Stupak
Amendment. I was also convinced that the Right-to-Life issue was
put to bed and that Democrats could now get back to expounding
the virtues of national health care. Yet, somehow in my heart I knew
my health care hell was not over.

CHAPTER 44

★ ★ ★

Dueling Press Conferences (November 7, 2009)

As I cast my vote for H.R. 3962, Affordable Health Care for America Act, I watched as Joe Cao (R-LA) voted with the Democrats to ensure the bipartisan passage of the historic health care legislation. It was truly a memorable night.

From out of nowhere appeared Chris Smith and Joe Pitts, who urged me to join them at a press conference. It was late and a press conference was the last thing I wanted to do. I initially declined their offer. They insisted that I join them and said that they were heading right up to the third-floor House Press Room. The Congressmen promised that the press conference would only take fifteen minutes. I felt that I owed Chris and Joe this small favor, as they had made sure the Republicans stood with me on the Stupak Amendment. We had to leave right then to start our press conference before Speaker Pelosi started her own. Their explanation sounded logical and we headed to the House Press Room.

On the way up to the pressroom Chris kept asking, "How did you convince the liberals to vote for Pro-Life legislation?" I tried to explain that I had done my homework and I knew that I had at least sixty votes. Chris was totally befuddled. As usual, Joe Pitts showed little emotion and simply said, "I did not believe Chris when he told me that you had sixty votes for the Amendment." All I could say to Joe was, "Ye of little faith!" We all laughed as we walked up the one flight of stairs to the third-floor House Press Room.

We entered the House Press Room and Chris' press secretary said that the reporters had left to cover the Speaker's Press Conference, but that they would be back afterwards. I said, "Fine, then there is no need for me to be here and I will leave the press to you." Chris again insisted that I stay, for we had the only bipartisan amendment and had to demonstrate our bipartisan commitment to life. Reluctantly, I stayed.

Suddenly, Michelle Bachmann showed up and I knew that this was not going to be good. Speaker Pelosi's press conference had already begun and she was joined by several of the Democratic Committee Chairmen instrumental in passing the health care legislation. As the long line of Democrats took to the stage, I knew this was going to be a long conference if everyone was going to speak. There is an old saying in politics that while everything has been said, not everyone has said it. True to form, each person at the Speaker's press conference had to speak and say the same thing over and over again. The US House of Representatives had been the first body to pass national health care and it was truly a historic night.

As we watched the Speaker's press conference, Bachmann and some of the other Republicans present started to pile on the Speaker with personal insults. Their comments about her clothes, her high heels and her "obvious" plastic surgery were over the top. They watched the press conference and ran down the Speaker. Their comments were not jokes; they truly detested her. Finally, I said, "You guys should get a grip." I went into a back office and watched the press conference by myself.

I was disappointed that John Dingell was given a minimal role in the Speaker's press conference. While everyone acknowledged John Dingell's lifelong commitment to health care, he was no longer Chairman of the Energy and Commerce Committee and he said very little. As John Dingell sat in a chair and leaned forward with his cane in front of his face, he looked like and reminded me of "Yoda" from

Star Wars. Like me, John looked like a fish out of water with the Republicans at their press conference. John Dingell was a Jedi Master and I but a mere mortal. My heart went out to him. He had fought his whole career for national health care as his father had before him. Now, John was resigned to a few words while Waxman received the praise for shepherding the health care legislation to the floor. To me it did not seem fair that John Dingell played a minor role in bringing health care to the House for a vote. I told myself that the final chapter on health care had not yet been written and the Democratic Leadership would need Dingell to work with Members of both the House and the Senate to pass health care.

Finally, the Speaker's press conference was over and a couple of the reporters came back and covered ours. I remember very little of it, as I was totally exhausted. I said that I was very pleased with the sixty-four Democrats who supported the Stupak Amendment and that we had enough votes to reject a presidential veto on the amendment. I stated that I did not expect a veto based on the Stupak Amendment. It was a strong vote and the President would realize his veto would be for naught. I also mentioned that with the strong House vote on the Amendment, the Senate should accept it also and avoid a divisive fight like the one the House had needlessly endured.

At around 1:00 a.m., I left the Capitol building and walked back to my room at C Street. I prayed for a good night sleep and thanked the Lord for delivering the necessary votes. As usual, I said my prayers and silently said good night to Laurie, Ken, Cristina, and B.J. I also asked B.J. to let me sleep tonight. In the silence of my room, my thoughts and tears turned to my deceased son.

CHAPTER 45

★ ★ ★

Home Town Flavor (November 2009)

I finally secured a restful night of sleep. It was not a long sleep, probably only six hours, but I felt good in the morning. It was Sunday, November 10, and instead of beginning my day with a workout, I hustled to the airport for my flight back home. As usual, the trip took approximately eight hours.

During the flight from Washington, I reviewed the Power Point presentation in preparation for my town hall meeting in Escanaba. I was returning home to my congressional district to sell health care legislation to an extremely skeptical public. I had promised my constituents that I would come back and hold health care town hall meetings in the areas that I was unable to visit during the August break. The editor of the local paper, the *Escanaba Daily Press,* had skewered me for not holding a town hall meeting during the August recess as demanded by Tea Party activists.

Now was the perfect time to squeeze in a town hall meeting. The House had passed the Public Option Health Care Plan and the Stupak Amendment had won easily. I was riding high. I was confident in my knowledge of the health care legislation and I was ready to match wits with the Tea Party antagonists who were planning to attend my meeting.

I knew the people in Delta County; I had grown up in neighboring Gladstone and Laurie was an Escanaba native. I began my law enforcement career as a City of Escanaba police officer. Between the two of us, Laurie and I knew just about everybody in Delta County. I enjoyed great political support there and I always won my elections with big margins. Delta County contained an active Pro-Life community that would be over the moon with my amendment. The citizens of Escanaba and Delta County were my friends and relatives, and I was looking forward to my town hall; I was their hero.

My health care Power Point slides had been updated to reflect the passage of the Stupak Amendment and contained a limited comparison of the House Public Option Plan along with the Senate's incomplete proposal, which focused on an insurance exchange program patterned after the Massachusetts state health care plan.

I could not have been more wrong on my optimistic assessment of mood of the large crowd that packed the theater at Bay de Noc Community College. To my surprise, the Escanaba Town Hall was the most contentious of the town hall meetings that I held in November and December of 2009. The hostile feelings of the crowd toward the proposed health care plan caught me off guard. While there were a few Tea Party activists doing their best to disrupt my presentation, I was most disappointed with the demeanor and comments of some of the participants who I thought were my friends and supporters.

Following my presentation, I decided to begin the questions with someone I knew and recognized and who I considered reasonable and respectful. I thought it was important to begin the questioning on a positive note and help diffuse the tension that I felt in the theater. The first person I recognized was the wife of a police officer and I called on her by name.

I will never forget her hostility and the exchange between us. Her question was really a statement damning me for voting for legislation that she was convinced would benefit illegal immigrants. She and her husband vacationed in Florida and, therefore, she was an expert on illegal immigration. She stated that she "would be damned if she was going to allow illegal immigrants to get another free benefit from our government."

In my response, I pointed out that section 347 in the health care bill explicitly prohibited federal subsidies for individuals who were not in the United States lawfully. In addition, I flipped back to a previous slide, which stated that under Section 1786 of the bill, medical coverage was prohibited for illegal immigrants under the Medicaid and Children's Health Insurance Programs. She did not believe me. No matter what I said, I was wrong. Her mind was made up: there was no way that this health care legislation could ever be enacted because taxpayers' money would provide health care benefits for illegal immigrants.

She denounced government-sponsored health care. She claimed that she and her husband had personally witnessed illegal immigrants accessing health care and living off the US taxpayers, and she was sick and tired of it. She just screamed at me. I realized then that she was a racist and a bigot. I felt sorry for her, and I wondered if there was a hidden story behind her outrage. Her husband, who had served in law enforcement with me, had suffered more than one heart attack and government-sponsored health care had pulled him back from the brink of death. Most of their medical expenses would have been covered by his insurance. I could not understand her hatred and bigotry.

She and her husband enjoyed their government-sponsored insurance and pensions, but she would be damned if anyone else should be able to access what she had. As she screamed down at me from the top row of the theatre, the Tea Party activists started to pile on.

It was a very long night at the Escanaba town hall meeting, and one I will never forget. I was shocked and disappointed by the lack of respect and decorum shown there. I was not only disappointed by the lack of respect given to me, but also the lack of respect and civility shown to friends and neighbors with opposing viewpoints.

As I was leaving the college, the editor of the paper who had accused me of ducking out on my constituents during the August break told me that no amount of money would be enough to get him to conduct a town hall meeting and he apologized for the unruly crowd. I discussed the Escanaba town hall meeting with the editor a few days later and assured him that not all town hall meetings were fueled by irrational and rude people.

On November 18, I organized a telephone town hall meeting and fielded questions from across the district's thirty-one counties. Like the public television town hall meetings, the tele-town hall means of communication provided a rational setting for constituents to ask questions and state their opinions both for and against health care. Even though the live town hall meetings remained difficult, I continued to conduct them. I felt that the live town hall meetings provided me with the greatest amount of feedback and I believed that it was incumbent upon me as congressman to keep my constituents informed on key issues. I felt it was important for me to continue conveying my long-standing position that health care was not just for the privileged few who could afford it, but for all Americans. It was time for me to make good on my promise.

When I returned to DC, I was bombarded by requests for interviews on the health care legislation and the Stupak Amendment. I conducted interviews with Fox News Radio, Fox and Friends, the Washington Post, Politico, the Escanaba Daily Press, Hardball with Chris Matthews, CBS Radio, and the Detroit Free Press. These interviews were all in addition to the local media covering my telephone town hall meeting on November 18, 2009.

I had the honor of meeting with Cardinal George, President of the US Bishops Conference. While I appreciated that the Cardinal stopped by the Capitol to thank and congratulate me for the passage of the Stupak Amendment, I thought it was odd that he did not meet me in my own office but asked me to meet with him in Congressman Chris Smith's office. In my conversation with Chris and Cardinal George, I tried to impress upon them that our job was only half done and that the Stupak Amendment would never pass the Senate. No matter how I outlined the difficulties the Stupak Amendment would face in the Senate, my concerns fell on deaf ears. At that point, I was the hero of the Right-to-Life movement and the US Conference of Catholic Bishops.

After four intense days in Washington, DC, I looked forward to flying back home to Menominee and spending some time deer hunting over the Thanksgiving holiday. This Thanksgiving would be very difficult as my mother-in-law was no longer with us. While I looked forward to going back home to Michigan, I knew that Thanksgiving dinner would never be the same.

CHAPTER 46

★ ★ ★

Clueless Bishops/Thankless Senate (December 2009)

As I stated earlier, the Senate is the place where good legislation goes to die. The Public Option Health Care Bill, H.R. 3200 was no exception. The Senate did not believe in the Public Option and it was dead on arrival. Senator Max Baucus, as Chairman of the Senate Finance Committee, had floated several trial balloons in hopes of crafting a bipartisan plan. Word was that he was leaning toward a bill similar to what the State of Massachusetts had implemented under Governor Mitt Romney. He felt that by designing national health care legislation based on the Massachusetts model, bipartisan support could be achieved. The Massachusetts plan was thought to be working well and considered a success, providing health care coverage to the uninsured citizens in that state.

I was not impressed with the rationale behind the Massachusetts plan, as it was based on incentives to private insurance companies to provide health insurance coverage. I had investigated the insurance industry in my role as Chairman of Oversight and Investigations and did not see how citizens purchasing their health insurance through the insurance exchanges would find affordable health insurance. I was also skeptical of the fact that necessary safeguards would not be implemented to prevent families from being underinsured or denied coverage when the policyholder suffered a serious injury or life-threatening diagnosis.

Even more important to me was the Senate's refusal to remove the antitrust exemption for the insurance industry. Removing the antitrust exemption and allowing the Secretary of HHS to negotiate lower prescription drug prices were two major principles in the House Public Option plan that created competition in the insurance industry and drove down the cost of prescription drugs. The Senate health care bill was not generating any support in the US House of Representatives.

The Senate worked through November and December of 2009 to develop health care legislation that could garner the required sixty votes in the Senate to invoke cloture, a process in parliamentary procedure aimed at bringing debate to a quick end. The Stupak Amendment also needed to generate sixty votes to overcome Senate obstacles, including a filibuster.

The House of Representatives returned after the Thanksgiving recess on December 2, 2009. I took an early flight back to DC, as I had been invited to address the US Conference of Catholic Bishops Executive Committee on the status of health care legislation and the Stupak-Pitts Amendment. I met with the Bishops' Executive Committee at their offices on the campus of the Catholic University of America.

I addressed the Executive Committee and cautioned that while the Stupak-Pitts Amendment had passed 240-194 with sixty-four Democrats voting for the Amendment, "...we had a long way to go to ensure that current law is maintained when expanding access to health care coverage." Further, I warned that both President Obama and Speaker Pelosi had publicly stated that they "...were willing to remove the Stupak-Pitts language in conference."

I stated that I was still working to secure a Democrat to offer the Stupak-Pitts Amendment to the Senate health care bill and that Senator Hatch had already proposed to offer the identical language of the Stupak Amendment on the Senate floor.

I closed my remarks to the Bishops' Executive Committee by stating, "It is not the time to sit back on our hands and hope for the best. We must push through to the finish line and ensure that any health care reform bill that moves forward maintains current law with regard to federal funds for abortion."

After my remarks, there was a question and answer period. The Bishops could not understand why Senator Casey would not offer and pass the Stupak Amendment. It was obvious to me that the Bishops had relied upon the House of Representatives to protect the sanctity of life and reach an agreement on acceptable language in the conference committee. It dawned on me that was why Chris Smith, Joe Pitts and Trent Franks (R-AZ) were always pushing the extreme Life positions in the US House, knowing that there was no support in the Senate for their extreme RTL positions and that reasonable RTL language would emerge from the conference with the Senate. Suddenly, the extreme RTL positions made sense knowing that the language would be rolled back by the Senate. They needed to be able to give up some language to achieve an agreement, even when the Senate was controlled by the Republicans. There simply was not enough strong support for RTL language in the US Senate, regardless of which political party was in control.

I thought it was telling that the Bishops had no idea or plan on how to deal with the Senate. While I urged an aggressive grassroots effort by all RTL groups to pressure the Senate into protecting the sanctity of life at all stages, my pleas fell on deaf ears. Flooding a congressional district with calls or mail to support RTL issues was relatively easy compared to mounting that pressure statewide. I had an uneasy feeling that even though the issue was out of my hands, it was being placed squarely on my shoulders. I was expected to see the Stupak Amendment all the way through to the end, regardless of the personal or political cost.

As Scott, Erika and I drove back to the Capital, I felt like one man on an island defending the RTL principle while at the same time advocating for passage of national health care. These two principles clashed and they were incongruent. I believed it made perfect sense for Democrats to be protecting the truly vulnerable infant in the womb while providing health care for those Americans living outside the womb. Was I alone in my beliefs?

CHAPTER 47

★ ★ ★

"I Will Deny We Ever Talked"
(December 2009)

The Senate began discussions on the Stupak Amendment in early December of 2009. While I had discussions with Democratic Senators Bob Casey (D-PA) and Ben Nelson (D-NE) and Republican Senators Tom Coburn (R-OK) and Orrin Hatch (R-UT), the outlook for including the Stupak Amendment in the Senate bill looked bleak. Senators Casey and Nelson and I spoke often on who would best handle and advance the Amendment; I was encouraging both Senators to withhold their support of the Senate health care bill unless the Senate included the Stupak Amendment. Because the Senate was dealing with insurance exchanges and not a public option, the Senators were trying to modify the Stupak Amendment to apply to private health insurance policies, which conceptually was more difficult for the Senators to accept. While the Stupak Amendment prevented private insurance companies from providing abortion coverage in the policies offered to federal employees, it did not prevent these same insurance companies from offering an abortion rider paid for by private, not taxpayer, funds. Even though I argued that the Stupak Amendment and the Hyde Amendment were the same and had applied to federal employees for the last thirty years, I faced strong resistance when applying those principles to the general public's purchase of private insurance on the exchange. And though the Stupak Amendment would only apply to those individuals receiving a federal subsidy to purchase health insurance on the state or federal exchange, the thought of preventing private citizens who were not federal employees from purchasing a health insurance policy that would not include elective abortions was deemed too restrictive and an expansion of the Hyde Amendment. Many of the same arguments that I had overcome in the House debate were hurled at me with even more vitriol from some of the Senators. The Senate also did not contain a large enough majority in favor of the Stupak or Hyde Amendments to generate the support necessary to overcome the legislative obstacles and survive a Senate vote removing the amendment from the health care legislation.

The RTL groups and the US Conference of Catholic Bishops had not developed strong enough support among Senators to survive a challenge to remove the Stupak Amendment.

On December 9, 2009, I was with Scott and Laurie as we were viewing the Christmas decorations throughout the first floor of the White House. The White House was wonderful and even though Laurie and I had attended the White House Christmas Party, it is difficult to see the magnificent decorations with the large crowd of more than 500 Members of Congress and their guests. We were just beginning our self-guided tour when my cell phone buzzed. It was Erika, who explained that I was going to receive a call from Senate Majority Leader Harry Reid and that the Senate was including the Stupak Amendment in its health care bill. I asked Erika to repeat what she had just told me because I did not necessarily believe the Senate would accept my amendment without a fight. Erika repeated that she had been told that Senator Reid would be calling to tell me that the Senate was accepting the Stupak Amendment without any changes. Even as Erika repeated the statement that Senator Reid was accepting my amendment, I did not believe her. Erika suggested that I find a quiet room to speak with Senator Reid when he called.

My relationship with Erika was strained. She remained my health care legislative assistant, which meant that organizations and Members of Congress still followed the congressional protocol of contacting her first instead of going directly to the Member of Congress.

After I ended my call with Erika, I told Scott and Laurie the "great news" that the Senate was accepting the Stupak Amendment and Senator Reid would be calling me shortly to discuss it. I advised Laurie and Scott that when he called I would leave them and find a quiet corner. We continued our tour and within twenty minutes I received a call from the Senator's staff asking if I could speak to him. I walked over to the front entrance of the White House that faces Pennsylvania Avenue; I was away from the touring guests and was able to speak to Senator Reid in private.

Besides "Hello," Senator Reid asked if I was alone. I told him that I was. Senator Reid then said, "Do not tell the press that we had this call. If I am asked, I will deny that I ever called or talked to you." Right then and there I knew that the Senate was not accepting the Stupak Amendment.

Senator Reid then went on to state, "We are accepting your amendment." He then explained the Capps Amendment to me, wherein people could select whether they wanted to purchase a health insurance plan on the exchange with or without abortion coverage by using private funds to pay for the abortion coverage. Senator Reid further explained that abortion would be a covered benefit under the essential health benefits.

In other words, abortion would be an essential benefit in all health insurance plans offered on the Exchange, but at least one health insurance plan would not include abortion coverage. Even though a health care plan in the Exchange did not include abortion, the insurance premium would be sufficient to pay for abortion offered in the other health care plans. The insurance premiums would be the same for health insurance plans whether abortion or was a covered in the policy or not. The Federal Government would be promoting, encouraging and paying for abortion coverage in all but one plan offered on the Exchange in violation of the Hyde and Stupak Amendments.

I responded to Senator Harry Reid, "Senator, your explanation describes the Capps Amendment. The House rejected the Capps Amendment and replaced it with the Stupak Amendment." Senator Reid said that he was accepting my amendment and the Capps Amendment and he would allow the citizens to make the decision on whether they wished to purchase a health insurance policy with abortion coverage. I responded that the Stupak and Hyde Amendments state that the federal government cannot promote or offer health insurance plans that cover abortions and that no federal money could be used to pay for any part of the health insurance policy that offers abortion coverage. Senator Reid responded that the federal government was not making the decision on whether abortion was included in the coverage; the individual citizen would make that decision. I responded that is fine if the citizen is paying one hundred percent of the cost of the health insurance policy but if one dollar was allocated for abortion coverage or to set up the Exchange with abortion coverage then, under current law, the federal government is excluded from providing, promoting or paying for any part of the policy or the benefit.

The Senate amendment as explained by Senator Reid violated the Hyde Amendment and the Stupak Amendment, which had already been passed by the House. Senator Reid explained that the Stupak Amendment would never pass the Senate. I told Senator Reid that he had to give the Senators a vote on the Stupak Amendment and if it failed, we could discuss it in conference. Senator Reid said he understood but this proposal was the best offer he could give me and I must accept it. I told the Senator that RTL, the Bishops, and I would never accept this language.

Senator Reid then asked, "Who is going to offer the Stupak Amendment in the Senate?" I replied, "I expect Senators Ben Nelson or Bob Casey would be willing to offer the Stupak Amendment." Senator Reid said that Senator Casey was working on modifying the Stupak Amendment and I responded, "I know that Senator Casey is working to find a compromise and I am willing to explore all proposals. But I cannot accept the proposal you just explained. The Stupak Amendment repealed Capps and the House will not accept the alternative that you outlined."

Senator Reid said, "Remember, we never had this conversation."
I simply agreed. I went back, found Scott and Laurie and explained
that the Senate was not accepting the Stupak Amendment. Erika was
wrong and I was back to square one with the Senate. While we all
enjoyed the White House Tour, my mind was on the Senate and how
Senator Reid had tried to wrap a bullshit gift.

I was disappointed in Senator Reid because he had voted more
than once in his career to protect the sanctity of life and Richard
Doerflinger had insisted that Senator Reid would support the Stupak
Amendment. It certainly did not sound like Harry Reid was accepting the Stupak Amendment nor did he even want anyone to know
that we had discussed it.

When we arrived back at my office from the White House, I
called Senators Ben Nelson and Bob Casey and explained my conversation with Majority Leader Harry Reid. Both Senators felt that
Majority Leader Reid would eventually allow a vote on the Stupak
Amendment, knowing full well that it would never pass the Senate.
Senator Casey advised that he was struggling to find some common
ground on which all the parties could agree. I thanked the Senators
for their efforts and asked that they keep working on the issue. I
closed the conversation by reminding them that the Senate could not
pass health care legislation without their vote and to please not give
their vote for health care unless the Stupak Amendment was inserted
in the legislation. The Senators acknowledged my request but also
indicated that they had other issues with the legislation that needed
to be resolved to the benefit of their states.

Within twenty-four hours of my conversation with Senator
Reid, I received a call from the Senate Majority Whip Dick Durbin
(D-IL) of Illinois. I served in the House with Dick and we saw each
other often on airplanes when I flew to DC through Chicago O'Hare
Airport.

Like Harry Reid, Dick started the conversation by telling me,
"This conversation never occurred and if you mention the call I will
deny it." I asked Dick, "What's the problem? I do not hold press con-
ferences after every phone call I receive from Senate leaders." Senator
Durbin explained that it was not about me but that they did not

need the women's groups coming down on them for trying to find a solution to the abortion issue. I accepted the Senator's explanation but thought that they also owed an assurance to the RTL groups and Bishops that they were at least attempting to address their concerns.

Senator Dick Durbin made the same offer that Senator Harry Reid had made. My response was the same to Durbin as it was to Senator Reid: I could not accept the proposal.

After my conversation with both Senators Reid and Durbin, I wrote a letter to Speaker Nancy Pelosi requesting that I be placed on the conference committee to advocate for the House's overwhelming support of the Stupak Amendment. Republican House Leader John Boehner (D-OH) also went to the House floor and asked Speaker Pelosi to place me on the conference committee.

Once again, the information I received from Erika Smith concerning the Stupak Amendment was filtered through her bias and not truly reflective of the facts. I do believe that Senator Reid's staff told Erika that the Senate was going to accept the Stupak Amendment. However, Erika did not have the courage to question the Senate staffer as to what the Senate meant when it claimed it was accepting the Stupak Amendment. I went to Scott and told him that Erika should be let go as she had lost her objectivity. Scott argued against letting Erika go because the Senate was in the middle of passing health care and I needed someone to stay on top of the issue. Plus, with the holidays coming up, it would not be appropriate to fire Erika. Once again, I left the personnel issues in Scott's hands and I told him that we would discuss Erika's employment status after the first of the year.

CHAPTER 48

★★★

Senate Passes Health Care
(December 23, 2009)

S enate Majority Leader Harry Reid struggled to garner the sixty votes needed to pass the Senate Health Care Legislation. Senator Reid had promised to pass health care reform well before Christmas and predicted that the final health care legislation would be on President Obama's desk by the end of the year. Senator Reid ordered the Senate to stay in session through the weekend of December 19 and 20 to work on health care. It was the weekend before Christmas.

The Senate legislation was premised on the concept that individuals and small businesses could purchase mandated health care insurance through an Insurance Exchange. Reid was having trouble securing the sixty votes needed for cloture to prevent a Republican filibuster. Cloture limits Senate debate on legislation to no more than thirty hours, thus precluding a filibuster. An immediate vote is then held on the proposed legislation. Majority Leader Reid also cut side deals with Democratic Members of the Senate to win their support for health care reform. Unfortunately, no Senate Democrat used the Stupak Amendment as a bargaining chip for their vote on health care. Instead, the Senate held a straight up vote on the Stupak

Amendment offered by Senator Ben Nelson of Nebraska. It was soundly defeated 45-54.

Following the defeat of the Stupak Amendment in the Senate, Senator Reid still needed sixty votes to invoke cloture. Senator Nelson continued to hold out. Nelson then negotiated a deal with Reid that his home state of Nebraska would receive the expanded Medicaid coverage provided for in the House and Senate health care legislation without Nebraska's having to pay its state share of the cost. In other words, Senator Ben Nelson's state of Nebraska would receive the benefit of expanding Medicaid to include more of its citizens without having to pay for it. The federal government would pick up the entire state share of the cost of Medicaid in Nebraska. This sweetheart deal was immediately labeled the "Cornhusker Deal," as the other forty-nine states were required to pay their state share (approximately 35% of the cost) of the Medicaid expansion.

With this agreement, Senator Nelson also announced that he had negotiated a compromise to the Capps Amendment, which would create a "firewall" to segregate taxpayer funds from individual private funds to pay for abortions in the Senate health care legislation. The Right-to-Life community, the Catholic Bishops, and the congressional Right-to-Life Caucus were all opposed to this accounting gimmick of the segregation of funds. The Nelson compromise also violated the Stupak Amendment because taxpayer dollars would be used to pay for basic health insurance coverage, which promoted and encouraged abortions.

On Saturday evening, December 19, Senators Ben Nelson, Bernie Sanders (IND-VT), and Sherrod Brown (D-OH) announced that they would vote for cloture to prevent a filibuster and support the proposed Senate health care reform package. The Senate could now proceed with debate and final votes on the health care legislation scheduled for December 23, 2009. As the Senators debated the Senate Health Insurance Exchange Plan, a major winter storm dumped approximately sixteen inches of snow on Washington, DC. The storm labeled "Snowpocalypse" shut down the city. The only congressional staffers who could be counted on to staff the Members of Congress were those hearty enough to wade through the snow.

During the same time that Washington, DC was being hit with Snowpocalypse, extremely cold weather hit northern Michigan. Still, Laurie and I went out for our usual morning run at Henes Park. I was confident that the Senate had now secured the sixty votes necessary to pass the health care legislation. The House and Senate health care bills were vastly different in their approaches to providing health care for all Americans and, therefore, a Conference Committee would need to be convened to work out the differences between the two bills. As I ran, my thoughts focused on how I could convince the Speaker to place me on the Conference Committee. I had already written a letter to Speaker Pelosi requesting placement on the Conference Committee, but she never responded.

Republican Minority Leader John Boehner had also requested that I be placed on the Conference Committee. Boehner's request probably hurt me more than helped me as the Speaker may have been led to believe that I may be voting with the Republicans. Chris Smith and Joe Pitts had also mentioned to Boehner that I should be placed on the Conference Committee as a Republican selection. If I went on the Conference Committee, my charge would be to advocate for the inclusion of the Stupak Amendment in the final health care bill and not to advocate for the position(s) of the Democratic Party. As I finished my morning run, I continued to hold out hope of being placed on the Conference Committee.

When Laurie and I returned home, my hopes of being placed on the Health Care Conference Committee by the Democrats were dashed when I heard the profanity-laced message on my answering machine. The President's Chief of Staff, Rahm Emmanuel, had left a profane tirade on my voicemail, cussing me out for my press statement, which declared that the US House of Representatives would never accept the Senate version of the Heath Care legislation with its permissive abortion language. Further, my statement to the press vowed that I would fight the Senate legislation with Right-to-Life and the US Conference of Catholic Bishops. I had never approved a press statement or release regarding the Senate Health Care Legislation. I instantly realized that my legislative assistant, Erika Smith, must have written something and attributed it to me.

313

Of course, Rahm believed that I had put out the press statement because he saw an email sent from my office. In his tirade Rahm stated, "The ink isn't even dried on the Senate bill, what the F--- are you doing putting out an F------ email/press release? Call me, you mother f-----!"

I did not immediately call Rahm- I called Scott. I asked him what was going on and he said that Phil Schiliro, Director of the White House Office of Legislative Affairs, had called his cell phone screaming at him saying, "What the hell is going on? You're going to kill our health care bill! What the hell are you doing?" Scott and I had never heard Phil raise his voice, much less cuss, but he was very angry. After Scott had calmed him down, Phil stated that Erika Smith had sent out an email to my Right-to-Life contacts and Members of Congress, asking, "...when are we going to hear opposition to [Senator Ben] Nelson's proposal?" Scott assured Phil that he would get to the bottom of this matter and that he would call him back with an explanation. Of course, Phil thought that I had authorized the email. Interestingly, neither Scott nor I had been copied on Erika's email message encouraging RTL to oppose the Nelson abortion agreement in the Senate health care bill.

Scott then called Erika on her cell phone. She was at her home on Capitol Hill. Scott demanded that she go into the office and immediately recall her email message. By this time, her message had already been distributed to the national media. Erika claimed that she could not get into the office because of the snow. Scott told her that she was going to go into the office and that he "would f------ come and get her if he had to" but she was going into the office and recalling her email. Scott was angry and realized that it had to be done immediately. Even though the police were urging people to stay off the roads, Scott drove in from his home in Springfield, Virginia, approximately twenty miles away, to deal with an obstinate, rogue staff person.

When Scott arrived at the office, Erika was already there. Within minutes of his arrival, his private phone line rang. It was Rahm. According to Scott, the "discussion" consisted of just three lines, "What the f--- are you doing? Why is your staff person sending out emails trying to kill our bill? F------ fix it!" Rahm slammed down his phone and Scott never had a chance to utter a word. The call was truly reflective of Rahm's best diplomacy.

After Rahm's call, Scott called me at home. I had already received my own voice message from Rahm. We agreed that if the White House had the email, the national media also had it and would report on it. We decided to put out a press release explaining what had happened and that Erika's email was sent out without my authorization.

Laurie and I prepared a press release stating that one of my staff persons had released an unauthorized email and attributed statements to me without permission. My press release also clarified the fact that I had not yet reviewed the Senate language on abortion or their health care legislation.

I wanted Erika fired. I was extremely angry with her. Once again, she had acted as if she was the Member of Congress and her actions had placed me in a very difficult position. Erika had put out an unauthorized statement on abortion without even telling anyone. At that time, abortion was the most divisive issue among the Democratic Members of Congress as we struggled to pass national health care reform.

There was no doubt in my mind that with Washington, DC shut down due to Snowpocalypse, and with the upcoming Christmas holiday, Erika believed that I would not be able to respond to her email before the media printed the statement. She also believed that her statement would be attributed to me. The longer it took me to retract Erika's statement, the more difficult it would be to explain the unauthorized statement. She was clearly attempting to undermine my authority and destroy my credibility.

The silver lining during this embarrassing fiasco was that it occurred on a weekend. Most of the reporters had already filed their reports on the Senate's ability to obtain the sixty votes needed to invoke cloture. They had gone home for the weekend and did not see Erika's statement.

Scott and I decided that we would discuss Erika's employment status after the holidays. Any chance I had of being appointed to the

Conference Committee went out the window with Erika's statement. My press release could not be explained away with a claim that "a member of my staff had sent out an unauthorized statement without my knowledge when the House offices were closed." The Speaker certainly was not going to buy it nor did she appreciate my RTL position.

I did not talk to Erika that day. As I explained to Scott, "If I talk to Erika, I will fire her even though it is Christmas." Scott indicated that Erika told him that she knew that I would not agree to the Senate language on abortion and the RTL groups wanted Congressman Stupak to make a statement against the Senate legislation, so she did it for me.

The United States Senate passed its Health Insurance Exchange health care bill on Christmas Eve, December 24, 2009, by a vote of 60-39. They left Washington, DC and Snowpocalypse behind. The final health care legislation would languish, stalled in the legislative process for another three months, as unforeseen events temporarily derailed health care.

CHAPTER 49

———— ★ ★ ★ ————

Pressure Cooker (January 2010)

E ven though the focus of the town hall meetings centered on the House and Senate health care plans, I did not limit constituents' questions to health care. My town hall meetings were not listening sessions- they were interactive and lively discussions on health care and other topics of concern. The national reporters were surprised that during my health care presentation, I only included one slide on the Stupak Amendment. It also surprised them that my constituents did not find it out of the ordinary that I would sponsor and pass the Stupak Amendment.

The town hall meetings in Ironwood and Ontonagon went fairly well. There were very few Tea Party agitators present. I did expect a problem with the Tea Party antagonists at the Houghton town hall held on the campus of Michigan Technological University on January 7, 2010. Based on experience, I knew this would be a difficult meeting because the participants there tended to be either university liberals or conservative evangelicals.

When I arrived at Tech, the maintenance crew was opening the room divider to accommodate the large overflow crowd. Before I entered the expanded room, I took a deep breath and headed into the lion's den. C-Span was broadcasting this town hall meeting live.

After a quick mic check, I said a few customary opening remarks and updated the audience on legislation passed during the previous year.

I reminded the audience of all the meaningful legislation the Democratic Congress had passed in the first year of the Obama Administration. I began with the passage of the Lilly Ledbetter Act. Ledbetter guaranteed that on federal jobs and contracts women would receive equal pay for equal work. In the US workforce, women earned twenty-two cents less than their male counterparts working the same job. Congress had also passed the Economic Recovery Package, a.k.a. the Stimulus Package. This package of bills slowed and eventually reversed the massive job losses Americans were experiencing every month. Other significant legislation signed into law over the past year included the expansion of the Children's Health Insurance Program which covered an additional ten million children, loans for General Motors and Chrysler aimed at saving the auto industry, and cash for clunkers, removing older-model vehicles from the roadways and depleting the backlog of vehicles in inventory. The economy was picking up again, and I credited the Obama Administration for the brighter economic forecast.

I also gave special praise and a thank you to the local National Guard unit, the 107th Engineering Battalion, for their distinguished service in Iraq. My salute to these service members received the loudest and longest applause of the evening.

It was time to dive into my health care presentation. With the passage of the Senate health care legislation on Christmas Eve, my slide presentation had expanded from the initial nineteen slides to thirty-nine slides. The health care presentation went well. I was confident and on top of my game; I completed my presentation and went right into questions. As the C-Span cameras panned the room, I searched for friendly faces to call on for questions.

As the questions began, the Tea Party activists started to utter comments, hurl insults, and accuse me of lying because I did not have specific slides on every health care question asked. Their crude comments were clearly an attempt to irritate me. They sat in the front row and positioned their chairs so that they could see and be seen by the crowd. I answered questions on health care, the economy, and government spending. With each answer, the comments from the Tea Party activists grew louder and interrupted my train of thought. They complained about the fact that I had not yet recognized them. Finally, about two-thirds of the way through the town hall meeting, I interrupted my answer, turned to my right and stated somewhat sarcastically, "Look, I appreciate the sound effects, but let me finish, okay?" The Tea Party member continued to complain, but I held my ground and said, "I am going to answer this gentleman's question. Please keep your comments to yourself."

I was certainly not going to recognize the Tea Party antagonists now and reward them for their efforts at interrupting me. Despite their continued snide comments over the course of the meeting, I chose to ignore them.

Like all town hall meetings, I try to relate topics of discussion back to my congressional district and constituents. As to health care, I stated that the Big Three automakers paid more for health care per employee than they did for all the steel that went into making one vehicle. At the time of the health care debate, there were two operating iron ore mines in my district, which sold most their iron ore pellets for steel to the automakers. Steel, cars, jobs, and health care were all topics that my constituents could relate to.

In responding to my constituent questions, I would often weave local citizens into my answers. At the Houghton town hall meeting, I mentioned the local hospital administrator, Jim Brogan, and the president of Michigan Tech University, Glenn Mroz. I always tried to relate legislation and issues back to my district and constituents, a valuable lesson I had learned forty-three years earlier from Senator Robert F. Kennedy.

I believed that C-Span chose to cover this town hall meeting because of my role in the passage of the controversial Stupak Amendment. During my slide presentation, I spent only a minute or two on the abortion issue and received a couple of questions from the audience regarding abortion coverage in the health care legislation. I promptly answered the questions and moved on.

An astute constituent asked how I could justify threatening to block health care if I did not get my Right-to-Life Amendment when 45,000 Americans died every year because they did not have access to basic health care. This question accurately reflected my internal tug of war. How could I justify denying health care to 45,000 Americans just because I was holding out for passage of an amendment? Another question I struggled with was, if another vote on the Stupak Amendment was defeated, could I vote for final passage of the health care legislation if it allowed public funding for abortions?

Another constituent asked if I would right then and there pledge to vote against the final health care bill if it allowed for abortions. I ducked the question by stating that I would wait to see what the final bill said, but added, "I probably would be hard pressed to vote for it. I probably would not vote for it." It was obvious to the audience that I was struggling with my moral and ethical dilemma concerning public funding of abortion and health care for all Americans.

At the conclusion of the Houghton town hall meeting, I received a nice round of applause from my constituents. I remained at Michigan Tech another sixty minutes to answer questions from individuals. I believe that the local and national media coverage of this town hall meeting accurately reflected the majority of my interactions with my constituents on health care and other issues of concern.

Throughout all my town hall meetings on health care, I made it crystal clear that I supported health care reform. It seemed that I was always being asked either/or questions: would I vote for health care with abortion rights or kill the legislation with my No vote? Or, would I still vote for health care if during the consideration of the legislation I was given a vote on the Stupak Amendment but lost? These questions were always either/or, but I wanted it both ways. I wanted to accomplish both objectives: health care reform *and* no public funding for abortion. The US House of Representatives proved that both principles could exist in harmony when it passed the Public Option Plan with the Stupak Amendment on November 7, 2009.

I would try again to have it both ways with the Stupak Amendment in the final passage of the health care legislation. The bitter polarization of the issues resulting from the vitriolic banter by both the pro-choice and pro-life zealots would not prevent me from continuing the fight. I don't know how many times I asked myself, "How can I pass health care and still protect the sanctity of life?"

When confronted with these either/or questions, I explained that as Congressman, I would do what I always did when contemplating my vote on a major piece of legislation. First, I would read the legislation; second, I would determine how the legislation affected the people of the First Congressional District of Michigan; and third, my vote would be based on what I believed to be in the best interest of the district and the United States knowing that not everyone would be pleased. The easy votes came when the legislation was clearly in the best interests of both the district and the country. The difficult votes occurred when the legislation was in the best interest of the country, but not the district. Would I put the country first or my district? What about my personal feelings and my own moral compass? Where did they come in? I found that I usually voted to put the country first and then went right home to explain the vote to those constituents most upset by it. Most times I found that the constituents who were angry just wanted to vent and let me know that they were upset by my actions. However, once I explained my position, they usually understood. They didn't agree, and they were still angry, but they were glad that I came to explain my position.

It was obvious from the constituents who attended the town hall meetings throughout the First Congressional District of Michigan that they did not trust the federal government to pass a health care plan that would be beneficial to them. I was not deterred by the skepticism, and continued to hold town hall and tele-town hall meetings on health care.

In one interesting note from the Houghton town hall meeting, a constituent stated that I was mentioned on the Rush Limbaugh Show that day. I joked that I was mentioned, "in vain, probably."

"No," the constituent stated. He said that Limbaugh had said that I was more outspoken against the health care bill than any Republican in Congress.

I was not surprised by the Limbaugh comment. I was aware of the fact that following passage of the Stupak Amendment, I became the darling of the political right wing, and the bane of the left. Following passage of the Stupak Amendment, I had conducted interviews with both right- and left-leaning radio talk shows, television programs, and print media. In each interview, I focused on what message I hoped the audience would take away from the interview and what I hoped the Democratic Leadership would hear. I was adamant in my belief that we must pass health care and also find a way clear for the Stupak Amendment. In other interviews, I threatened to take down the health care legislation if it did not contain the Stupak Amendment. Many times, the manner in which I answered the questions depended on where the negotiations stood on the Stupak Amendment.

I also realized that supporters on each side of the abortion issue would see me as political fodder for demonizing the other side. Truthfully, I was not on either side. I believed that Congress could find common ground on both abortion and health care. I never viewed abortion as a single-issue litmus test, nor did I believe that anybody who disagreed with me was the enemy. In politics, there is an old saying that if both sides of an issue are mad at you, then the legislation must be good and you had cast the correct vote.

My interviews ranged from the Mike Huckabee Show to the former LA Mayor Tom Bradley Show. Even former GOP vice-presidential candidate Sarah Palin singled me out in her speech to the Tea Party Convention in February 6, 2010, when she told the assembled audience, "When people are willing to meet halfway and stand up for common sense solutions and values, then they wanna work with them. And in that spirit, I applaud Independents and Democrats like Bart Stupak who stood up to tough partisan pressure and wanted to protect the sanctity of life and the rights of the soon-to-be-born. I applaud him for that."

As the days and weeks went by and no votes occurred on health care, many outside groups and Democratic Party supporters pressured me to drop my opposition to health care without the abortion language. Several union officials called and informed me that they would not support me in my re-election efforts if I continued my opposition to the health care legislation.

The campaign pollster with Greenberg Research who had worked with me over the past three election cycles- six years- called and told me that the firm was dropping me as a client due to the passage of the Stupak Amendment. My pollster apologized profusely but stated that one of Greenberg's largest clients, a national union, had threatened to pull all their business from the firm if they continued to keep me as a client. My campaign pollster provided me with names of other pollsters who worked for moderate to conservative Democrats. He stated that he believed one of these other polling firms would be willing to accept me as a client. I thanked him for the names and never contacted any of the other pollsters; I knew I would not be running for re-election.

As February moved into March of 2010, the multi-faceted attack from the Democratic Party was becoming unbearable. My campaign pollster dropped me. Unions and other large donors publicly threatened to withdrawal their support for my next election. Local, state and national Democrats actively recruited a primary challenger and a few local Democratic parties kicked me out.

The Members of Congress who rented a room at the C Street house became the subjects of an Ethics Complaint claiming that we were not paying a fair and reasonable rent. Six years earlier, the same complaint had been filed and we were all exonerated. Once again, we had to demonstrate that we paid rent that was considered reasonable and customary and we did not receive any excessive privileges not covered by our monthly rent payments.

Another attack came from the IRS when my 2008 campaign was audited for not paying federal employment taxes on campaign volunteers and independent contractors. The IRS ruled that these workers should be considered as campaign employees and the campaign was required to pay federal taxes on them.

It is my understanding that Stupak for Congress was the only campaign audited to determine if volunteers and independent contractors would be determined to be employees of the campaign. The IRS determined that the college students who worked for a stipend during the summer months were also considered employees of the campaign and that the campaign would be responsible for taxes on these volunteers and independent contractors. Every campaign uses volunteers and independent contractors. I repeatedly asked the auditor, "Who made the complaint or decided that I should be audited?" The auditor's response was, "you can figure it out."

What the IRS audit demonstrated was that if I sought re-election, my political opponent(s) would have been able to claim that I was under an IRS investigation and use the audit to smear my good name and integrity. The IRS would have simply claimed that I was being audited and an unidentified source would have claimed that I did not pay my taxes or that I was being audited for illegal activity. The whole audit was an attempt to destroy my credibility and defeat me in the next election.

During this time, I took solace in a short poem that I had taped to my congressional desk. It is said that President Kennedy kept a copy of the poem in his wallet. Kennedy mentioned it in a speech the day he learned of Soviet missiles in Cuba. The poem is simple but speaks volumes for those of us who are not afraid to stand up for principles, knowing that we will be condemned for our actions and that we are alone in the fight.

> "Bullfighter critics ranked in rows
> Crowd the plaza full;
> But only one is there who knows;
> And he's the man who fights the bull."

Domingo Ortega

The Senate leadership insisted that the House accept the Insurance Exchange model without the Stupak Amendment. President Obama agreed with the Senate yet sided with the House that the sweetheart deals given to Senators for their support of health care must be removed from the final health care legislation. As President Obama and the Democrats coalesced around a health care plan, it did not include the Stupak Amendment. Instead, the Administration and House leadership focused on stripping away support for the Stupak Amendment with the last few RTL Democrats who stood with me.

As it became apparent that the Democrats would actually come together to support one health care plan, the individuals, groups and organizations that had supported the Stupak Amendment became adamant that my small group of RTL Democrats and I vote against the entire health care legislation. The Stupak Amendment became the battle cry for "kill the bill." The National RTL, Family Research Council, the Tea Party, their support groups, right-wing talk radio and the Bishops were convinced that the House could not pass health care without the support of the Stupak Twelve. Therefore, it became preferable to kill the bill.

I believed that eventually Speaker Pelosi would bring the final health care legislation to the House floor when she had the necessary votes, including the ones in her pocket. The questions became when health care would come to the floor and whether my small group would continue to hold together after witnessing all the pressure being brought to bear on me for standing up for my principles and beliefs. "But only one is there who knows; and he's the man who fights the bull."

CHAPTER 50

★ ★ ★

Who Is Listening?

As I stated in Chapter 10, nothing is ever off the record; the press always get the story even if they are not in the room. I should add the caveat that you never know who is listening in on your town hall meeting.

On Monday, January 11, 2010, I left Menominee very early in the morning to fly back to DC to move from my one room at C Street SE to a two-bedroom apartment on A Street NE. The pressure from our constituents to move out of C Street just got to be too much for Mike Doyle and me. As much as we loved the C Street boarding rooms and the other C Street residents, it was better personally and politically if we moved. Mike and I promised to continue to meet with our small Fellowship group on Tuesday nights as we had for the past twelve years. I spent Monday afternoon and Tuesday morning fixing up my room in the two-bedroom apartment Mike and I had leased; Mike still did not know that I would be retiring from Congress at the end of year.

For Mike and me the A Street NE apartment was bearable. We had searched for apartments during the month of December with limited success. The A Street apartment was the best we could find for our limited resources and it was a walkable seven to eight blocks from our offices and the Capitol.

We inspected the apartment before we signed the lease. Mike and I mentioned to the landlord that we noticed quite a bit of cat hair and cat smell in the vestibule of the old house when we entered the front door. The landlord assured us that the vestibule and the narrow stairway leading up to the second-floor apartment would be free of cat hair before the first of the year. However, the vestibule was never thoroughly cleaned and there was always the smell of cat and clusters of cat hair as we walked up the narrow steps to our apartment.

The A Street apartment was very small and dingy but it contained two bedrooms. As the senior Member in the apartment, Mike gave me first choice and I chose the larger bedroom. The larger bedroom had probably functioned as a formal dining room at one time and it had two doors. One door led out into a hallway and the other door opened into the living room. To discourage anyone from mistakenly entering my bedroom, I blocked the door with my golf clubs and a small table.

There was one large window in my bedroom, which led outside to the fire escape. The fire escape was easily accessed from the bedroom by simply opening the window and stepping outside. I actually tried this when contemplating the security risks following my vote in favor of the Affordable Care Act. I realized then that the reverse was also true. It would not be difficult for an intruder to climb up the fire escape, enter my bedroom, and rob or ransack the apartment. Of course, at the time we moved in, Mike and I had few security concerns. It wasn't until after I cast my vote in favor of health care on March 21 that the death threats became serious. The threats and subsequent criminal investigation are not part of this book. However, it is important to note that after they materialized, I slept with one eye open and fixed on the fire escape. It would have been quite easy for a perpetrator to harm me and then slip back into the dark of night without ever being noticed. For me the apartment at A Street was a security nightmare.

Laurie and Susan Doyle were not part of the apartment selection committee, nor did they visit the A Street apartment prior to our move. When Laurie saw the apartment, she made it very clear that she would not spend a single night there. I understood, as A Street was clearly not the nicest apartment in Washington, DC.

Once I was settled into the A Street apartment, I walked over to my congressional office in the Rayburn Building, reviewed paperwork, and looked over the schedule for the Democratic Caucus that would be held in the new Capitol Visitor Center (CVC).

The Capitol Visitor Center is a gorgeous underground complex extending east from the Capitol to First Street SE, north to Constitution Avenue and west to Independence Avenue. Directly across the street from the CVC is the United States Supreme Court. One way to judge the actual size of the CVC is the fact that the entire US Capitol could fit inside the CVC and there would still be room left over. It is rumored that the House Chamber will someday be remodeled and the US House of Representatives will meet in the CVC's 450-seat theater to conduct legislative business.

The CVC Theater served as the location for our Democratic Caucus as the Majority Party on January 14, 2010. The Democratic Leadership stressed that it was extremely important for all Democratic House Members to attend the Caucus meetings, billed as the *Democratic Issues Conference and Job Summit.* In addition to jobs and the economy, health care and the two competing plans- Public Option versus Insurance Exchanges- would be discussed.

The first half-day of the Caucus was taken up by leadership laying out the legislative plan for 2010, with the promise of immediately moving health care legislation in early February following the special election to fill Senator Edward Kennedy's seat. The Democratic House Caucus did not appear to be in any hurry to begin work on health care, even though it was our number one issue. Speaker Pelosi had not yet appointed House Members to the Health Care Conference Committee.

President Obama wrapped up the first day of meetings and focused on health care in his remarks. Surprisingly, the President received some pushback from Members regarding provisions in the health care legislation where policy disagreements existed. For instance, Congresswoman Anna Eshoo (D-CA), who sat next to me on the Energy and Commerce Committee, challenged the President on the appropriate length of time allowed for biological patents in health care. The Energy and Commerce Committee had already passed Congresswoman Eshoo's version of twelve years of patent protection, but President Obama and Chairman Waxman demanded a six-year patent protection for the pharmaceutical companies. Congresswoman Eshoo and President Obama conducted a lively exchange of words over the issue. In the final bill, biological patents received a twelve-year period of protection.

The next morning, President Bill Clinton was scheduled to close out our conference. The massive theater was full and, as usual, I sat in the back. President Clinton began to address the group and persuasively argued that $300 billion in health care was wasted each year on paperwork and administrative costs. He claimed that those costs could be eliminated if we required all health care providers and insurance companies to accept a one page, double-sided, medical insurance claim form. President Clinton also discussed the Children's Health Initiative Program that Congress had passed a year earlier, and stated that it must be included in the final health care legislation. President Clinton also mentioned that he understood that health care reform was difficult and that the Congress was struggling with two plans, one from the House and one from the Senate. He pleaded with us not to give up, and to find a way forward.

Then President Clinton said, "I heard the best explanation of health care ever one day recently when I was sitting in my office in Harlem. Like you, I am a political junkie and I had C-Span on and I heard this voice that I was familiar with. I stopped and watched this town hall meeting on health care in the Upper Peninsula of Michigan. Now, C-Span was not there because Congressman Bart Stupak was an authority on health care. They were there because they wanted to see what would happen when he brought up the abortion issue. Well, Bart, is he here? I saw him earlier today."

From the back of the theater I raised my hand and the President continued, explaining how I defined the health care problem the country was facing, that I described the House and Senate health care plans and how they differed, what I thought about each plan and that I wanted to see health care passed. President Clinton told my colleagues my Power Point presentation was the best explanation on health care he had seen.

President Clinton reminded my colleagues that C-Span and all the media were covering the town hall meeting because they wanted to see how I handled the abortion issue. As President Clinton said, I had spent maybe a minute or two on the abortion issue and had gone right back to health care. In summation, the President said, "It was great, I sat and watched the whole thing. I tell you, get a copy of his health care slide presentation, it is great."

I was bursting with pride as President Clinton praised my presentation on health care. With the President's praise of my command of the facts on this critical issue, at least my House Democratic colleagues would view me as knowledgeable about the legislation and not as a single-issue Neanderthal. The lesson here was that you never know who may be listening when you give a live presentation covered by C-Span. I expected at some Members to call my office asking for my Power Point presentation, but very few ever did. The Members who did call were advised to modify my presentation by inserting their own demographics and statistics describing the status of health care in their states and congressional districts.

I was disappointed with the lack of response from my Democratic colleagues. If they were experiencing a tough time selling health care in their districts, President Clinton had endorsed a presentation that walked them through the highlights of the greatest social issue they would probably ever vote on. Their lack of response may have come from the fact that many Members were no longer holding town hall meetings on health care. I took the opposite approach to addressing health care issues; I continued to hold both town hall meetings and tele-town hall meetings because I wanted to afford every constituent an opportunity to learn about health care directly from their Congressman and not through social media.

By the end of January 2010, I was looking forward to a few days in Menominee during the Republican Legislative Retreat. I returned home on Thursday, January 28, the day after President Obama's State of the Union address. I knew I had to drive to Iron Mountain on Friday to attend the funeral of former State Representative Jack

Gingrass. Jack and I had remained close friends and political allies for many years and I was moved when the Gingrass family called to personally inform me of Jack's passing.

I put on my suit, walked outside into the cold, and slid behind the steering wheel of my black Oldsmobile Aurora. Then, I just froze. I could not turn the ignition to start the engine. I knew I had to start the car to drive the sixty-five miles to Iron Mountain, but I just sat there behind the wheel, not moving. After a few minutes, I slid out of my car and walked back into the house. A stunned Laurie asked me what was wrong. I told her I could no longer drive my car. Laurie simply asked me to give her a minute to change her clothes and she would drive me to Iron Mountain. I did not protest, saying simply, "That would be great." On the way to Iron Mountain, Laurie asked me if I was okay. I told her, "I am okay, but I just can't drive around the congressional district anymore. I no longer want to come home for only twelve hours and then jump in my car and drive to the ends of the earth. I just cannot do it anymore."

At that time, Laure and I had been married thirty-six years. I had spent thirty-one years of our marriage driving around Michigan-eleven years in the Michigan State Police, and twenty years in politics. I looked forward to retiring; I wanted to stop the madness of coming back to Michigan every week but never really staying home. I wanted the health care debate to be over and I wanted to come home and stay home. No longer could I continue to drive like a madman to some chicken dinner hundreds of miles away and spend the night in a cold motel room.

With reapportionment on the horizon and the drawing of new congressional district boundaries, my district was expected to become even larger. It was time for me to retire. I was the longest-serving Congressman from the First Congressional District and I was burned out. The good Lord had reminded me, once again, that I could no longer continue my hectic pace. The Gingrass funeral that Friday re-affirmed my decision to retire at the end of the year and I couldn't wait.

I continued my demanding public appearance schedule during February and March, never giving anyone any indication that I would not be seeking re-election. No one gave it a second thought when I stopped fundraising in 2010. I didn't hold my annual fundraiser on my un-birthday, February 28. I was born on Leap Day, February 29, so once every four years I held a real birthday fundraiser. For three of the four years when February 29 never came, I held my un-birthday fundraiser. In February of 2010, it was an un-birthday year and nobody missed my event.

I also continued with my live town hall meetings on health care through March 8, 2010. My last live town hall meeting was held in Tawas, 380 miles from my home. To accommodate the expected crowd, the meeting took place in the high school auditorium. Over 200 people were in attendance and the meeting lasted over three hours. Tea Party activists waved signs in opposition to the healthcare legislation and asked several questions. However, probably due to the heavy police presence, no altercations took place. I flew back to Washington the following day; the House of Representatives was scheduled to remain in session through March 26, 2010, with the votes on health care scheduled for the weekend of March 20-21.

CHAPTER 51

★ ★ ★

Frantic Friday (March 19, 2010)

M ost of the events of this unbelievably hectic day are not recorded on my original calendar. Although my schedule was laced with interviews, meetings and votes, the most significant discussions and events could never have been anticipated.

As the day's events began to unfold, I realized once again that I would need to fly solo. Pressure from my Washington staff and a rapidly eroding lack of trust in my health care legislative assistant put me at a disadvantage. There were very few people I could still trust.

My day began with an ABC News interview with George Stephanopoulos at 6:45 a.m. The interview went well; George was supportive and optimistic. Not a bad start to what would become another brutal day, which ultimately would make or break health care. None of the players in the drama realized that Friday, March 19, 2010, would become D-Day for the passage or failure of the Affordable Care Act.

At 9:00 a.m., the leadership scheduled another Democratic caucus on health care in the Cannon Caucus Room. At least one caucus had been called every day over the past couple of weeks. Therefore, I did not feel bad when I arrived late, as I had been engaged in a phone interview on health care with Todd Spangler of the *Detroit Free Press*. When I joined the caucus, I sat in the back, surveyed the Democratic

Members, and asked myself: did the Democratic Members of Congress possess the courage necessary to pass such sweeping legislation? More importantly, did we trust and believe in each other enough to take the final steps to pass health care reform? Would we capture or squander the moment? Did we have the strength to carry on when others walked away? Could we actually pass health care? How could we succeed when so many had already failed? What did we possess that others did not? What faith or fate brought us together at this critical time in our Nation's history? As usual, nothing happened at the caucus that would have convinced Democratic Members to change their votes on health care.

I was exhausted and convinced that it was incumbent upon the Obama Administration to make the next move. All day long, I had been stating that there were no current discussions or meetings scheduled between President Obama and Pro-Life Democrats on resolving the impasse. With each interview, I was determined to keep on message. I wanted to pass health care reform, but I could not vote for legislation that included taxpayer-funded abortions.

Scott urged me to accept the Senate language and attempted to convince me that the Senate language was essentially the same as the Stupak-Pitts Amendment. I was not buying it. Scott was getting desperate for an agreement- any agreement. He was under tremendous pressure from friends, constituents, and our own district and DC staff. Like most of my staff members, Scott is Pro-Choice. He believed that I had carried my opposition too far and my name was becoming mud in Democratic circles. He warned me that I would probably be getting a Pro-Choice primary opponent. My response was the same as always: bring 'em on.

The bells rang to call Members to the floor for votes, and the Capitol Police were outside my door, trying to keep the hallway clear so staff, members of the public, and Members of Congress could walk down the corridor. Activists from the Tea Party and Religious Right zealots were camped out in front of my office. They were holding prayer vigils and demanding that I meet with them. They were rude and obnoxious. My staff and I tried to reason with them and informed them that although we appreciated their concerns, no votes had been scheduled and I was still working on ways to protect Life. In the meantime, they needed to stop blocking access to my office and holding prayer sessions in the foyer and the hallway. They also needed to stop the constant calls to my office from their cell phones.

Our request fell on deaf ears as these so-called good Christians continued to block the hallway and doorway to my office. When the Capitol Police arrived to clear the hall, they claimed to be holding a prayer vigil. They accused the Capitol Police of infringing upon their "freedom of religion" when they attempted to clear the hallway and my office foyer and maintain some semblance of order on the second floor. After the police cleared a path so that business could still be conducted, the activists continued to call my office from the hallway, jam the phone lines and carry on with all types of disruptive behavior.

By Friday afternoon my staff was totally frustrated and asked if we could lock the office door. We could no longer conduct business. I called the Capitol Police and advised them that we were shutting down the office and locking the front door. They assured me that police officers were patrolling the halls, trying to keep traffic moving.

After we locked the front door, the demonstrators opened the mail slot and sent messages through. They held it open, prayed out loud, and preached to my staff. It was hard to discern their prayers other than an occasional Our Father; the demonstrators' arguments mostly consisted of unintelligible ad lib invocations and chanting. We were eventually forced to tape the mail slot shut from both sides, and staff members felt compelled to leave the office through a door in my inner office. When my staff stepped into the hallway, they were bombarded with questions from demonstrators wanting to know where I was and reminding them to be sure to tell me that they were continuing to pray for me and that I had to kill the health care bill. We could no longer freely move in and out of the office without being harassed, and no one could call into the office because the phone lines were jammed. The fax machine was constantly running out of paper. Fortunately, we had a couple of private phone lines and a private fax machine that we could rely upon to conduct business.

The staff took thirty-minute shifts answering the non-stop phone calls. The chaos that swirled around us caused everyone to be on edge.

My Chief of Staff Scott Schloegel, my Executive Assistant Rachel Stevenson, and my front desk person Loren Aho were constantly dealing with the Christians holding prayer vigils through our front door mail slot. When they needed a break from the chaos outside my office and the constant ringing of the phones, they would step out of the office through an unmarked door. One time these three loyal staffers left through the unmarked door, and were asked by the prayer group in front of my office if they worked for Congressman Bart Stupak. Immediately, Scott said, "No." As they continued down the hallway, Scott was again asked if he worked for me and again Scott said, "No." By the time they walked the twenty yards to the elevator, Scott was again asked if he worked for me. Again, Scott said, "No." Scott, Rachel and Loren entered the elevator and broke up in laughter as Scott had denied me three times. It was during the Lenten season and two weeks before Easter; the irony was not lost on them. This is just one of the many funny stories that circulated amongst staff members and the occasional humor helped break the tension within the office.

Serious congressional work was also conducted in my "hideaway" and it became a staff refuge. The hideaway is an extra room that House leadership provided some senior House Members. Mine was on the same second floor as my congressional office but on the opposite end of the Rayburn building. My staff and I held constituent meetings in the hideaway when we had no room to seat people in my office suite. During the last few weeks of the health care debate, Scott and I encouraged our staff to use the hideaway to escape the mayhem of my office. Staff were warned not to allow anyone to follow them to the hideaway and that no friends were allowed access to it. Everyone honored the rules except Erika. She tried very hard to turn the hideaway into her own work station; on more than one occasion, Scott and I were obliged to remind Erika that she could not set up shop there.

Since Thursday, March 18, 2010, the Capitol Police had become a constant presence in our hallway, ensuring access to offices and protecting Members of Congress and our staffs. The Capitol Police would tag along as I walked over for votes, walking alongside me as we proceeded through the tunnel that led from the Rayburn Office Building to the Capitol Building. The entry point of the Rayburn tunnel was a police checkpoint and from there we could move quickly to the Capitol building to record my votes.

As the security concerns and threats multiplied, I was ordered by the Capitol Police not to leave my office without a police escort. I could no longer walk outside when votes were called. Sgt. Dwight Sturdivant of the Capitol Police was constantly by my side once I moved outside my office. Sgt. Sturdivant and the other officers wasted no time in moving me through the Capitol complex for meetings and never allowed me to become engulfed in the hysteria surrounding my office.

With each passing hour on Friday, March 19, 2010, tension and security concerns increased considerably. The President and the Speaker did not have the necessary votes to pass health care. While I was aware that the "Stupak Twelve" was diminishing in number, the media continued to report that the Speaker could not move the legislation without us. While leadership had pretty much figured out the last Stupak holdouts, each Member knew and was thankful that I never made public the names of my remaining holds.

CHAPTER 52

★ ★ ★

Divide and Conquer and Defection

Dwight and I walked over to the House floor. Votes had been called and I joined my colleagues in my usual location in the Pennsylvania corner. Suddenly, Congressman Steve Driehaus of Ohio came running over to me asking, "Where were you? Where were you?" All I could say was, "What the hell are you talking about?" Joe Donnelly of Indiana quickly joined us.

Both Steve and Joe were solidly with me on Pro-Life issues and we often discussed how to explain our positions and votes to our constituents back home. Steve and Joe were not looking for justification on their Pro-Life votes, they just felt that I had been dealing with Pro-Life issues politically longer than they had and I had a knack of explaining complex legislation in the simplest of terms. I was always looking to compare notes on legislation and learn what the folks were saying back home in Michigan, Ohio, and Indiana. Joe represented the University of Notre Dame and was in contact with Father Hesburgh, who was very understanding and encouraged us to find a way to provide health care coverage *and* protect the unborn. One of my more enjoyable evenings in Congress was attending a Notre Dame reception with Congressman Joe Donnelly honoring former Notre Dame President Father Theodore Hesburgh. It was a memorable evening cut short by votes back at the Capitol.

Steve Driehaus explained that he met with the President yesterday afternoon and the President asked if he would agree to an executive order enforcing the Hyde language in the health care legislation. Steve said he did not agree but would be willing to look at it. Steve explained that there had been a meeting about the executive order in one of the Speaker's offices and he wanted to know why wasn't I there? Now the White House was offering an executive order to the Affordable Care Act. In return, the Pro-Life Members present were required to vote for the health care legislation.

As Steve Driehaus explained the meetings, Congressman Mike Doyle was listening in. Steve said, "I asked the White House attorneys where Stupak was and they said they did not know. The bastards never told us you weren't invited." Steve continued, "Then, they read us all these flowery, great-sounding 'wherefores' and 'therefores' and we just looked at each other and said we wouldn't agree to anything without Stupak and that we didn't know if it was even legal. The executive order didn't sound too bad, but we don't know the law like you do, so we told them, we won't agree to an executive order without Stupak's okay." I was pleased to hear that my core team was holding together and I imagined they were under tremendous pressure to accept the executive order and accept it now, as the health care vote was to be called within the next twenty-four to forty-eight hours. Time was running short and the 218 votes necessary to bring the legislation to the floor were proving elusive for the Speaker.

Both Congressmen asked if I was aware of the executive order and I said no, but that Rahm had offered me one last fall when I was working on the Stupak Amendment. I had said no- that I wanted a clean vote on my amendment. Donnelly and Driehaus said, "Well, it's clear to us that the White House is trying to divide us from you, work around you, and isolate you."

With Congressmen Oberstar and Kildee both agreeing to support the Senate language on abortion, the White House could pick off just enough Pro-Life Members to pass health care over the weekend. I reassured both of them that we still had six or seven Members hanging with us on the abortion language and that leadership could not pass the Rule without us.

I said, "If we stick together we will be fine. It is not over yet. Now the fun begins- who is going to blink?" These staunch Pro-Life Midwestern Democrats assured me they would not vote for anything without my approval. I knew I could count on them and I thanked them for their courage and commitment to the RTL cause.

I then told them that I saw Congressman Dale Kildee on the floor and I was going to talk with him. They just said, "Good luck."

Congressman Dale Kildee of Michigan was a solid Pro-Life vote over his thirty-three years in the US House of Representatives. He had put out a press release that Wednesday stating that he was voting for the health care legislation and that the Senate language on abortion was acceptable to him. In his press release Kildee mentioned that he had attended the seminary, consulted with his priest and carefully studied the Senate language on federal funding of abortion. He was comfortable that no taxpayer dollars would be used to cover abortions under the Affordable Care Act.

Dale Kildee was sitting in the second row, right of center from the Speaker's rostrum alongside Congressman Jim Oberstar, another staunch Right-to-Life Democrat. Congressman Oberstar had also put out a press release stating that he was Pro-Life and that he was comfortable with the Senate language on abortion and he was voting for the health care legislation.

These two gentlemen were stalwarts in the Democratic Pro-Life circles. It was Jim Oberstar who had encouraged me to take over the chairmanship of the Pro-Life Democrats. Jim had also relinquished his co-chairmanship of the Congressional Right-to-Life Caucus and recommended me for that position. I often consulted with Jim Oberstar on Right-to-Life issues. We would discuss Chris Smith and the Republicans and their extreme views on some of their Pro-Life amendments. I could always count on Oberstar to provide me a detailed, thoughtful opinion and analysis on my inquiry.

Jim Oberstar had worked on Capitol Hill for more than fifty years, starting as a staff person for Congressman John Blatnik in 1963. Jim succeeded Blatnik upon his retirement in 1974 and represented the "arrowhead" of northeastern Minnesota. Jim's district was adjacent to mine and very similar; our two districts contained the last three working iron ore mines in the United States. Jim served as Chairman of the Transportation Committee and I relied on him to help pass my legislation to protect the Great Lakes, expand the Soo Locks, and construct the Coast Guard buoy tenders and the new ice breaker, *Mackinaw*. Jim was a great friend and great legislator and had helped me many times throughout my career.

But now I needed to confront two of my friends and two stalwarts of the Democratic Pro-Life Caucus. Dale Kildee and Jim Oberstar had just abandoned us and it would not be a pleasant conversation.

I decided to try a little humor on my senior colleagues and as I approached them, I repeatedly said, "Tell me it ain't so Joe. Tell me it ain't so."[1] Congressman Dale Kildee immediately became defensive and told me that I was wrong and he knew more about being Pro-Life than I did. I rebutted Kildee and said that I thought he took a cheap shot at me in his press release. I also told him that he could have at least warned me before jumping ship and putting out his press release. Dale just fired back that he did not have to explain anything to me and he had made his decision. It was obvious that he was agitated and uncomfortable with me confronting him on the issue. I told him how disappointed I was in his decision and that I and the other Pro-Life Members deserved the courtesy of a phone call and that we felt blindsided by his defection. Now, the Obama Administration was using his announcement to further divide the remaining Pro-Life Democrats. Dale simply got up and walked away. I sat down next to Congressman Jim Oberstar.

Jim simply said that he had no choice. As the Chairman of the Transportation Committee, leadership had demanded his vote. I will never forget the pain on Jim Oberstar's face. He then said, "Keep up your fight, you will figure this out and do what is right. I have faith in you." I squeezed his hand, looked him in the eye and said, "thanks." Congressman Jim Oberstar died unexpectedly in the fall of 2014. I lost a great friend and he is truly missed.

---

1   The famous quote of a young boy to Shoeless Joe Jackson as the Chicago Black Sox were accused of throwing the 1939 World Series for money.

I got up and went back to the Pennsylvania corner, realizing that my little group of twelve was now down to about six. The Stupak dozen that the press kept referring to was shrinking fast; I was not sure how much longer I could continue to hold onto the last few remaining Democratic Pro-Life votes. The fight may very well have been over; the President and Speaker Pelosi were doing a masterful job of peeling my group apart.

It was obvious in my brief discussion with Congressman Oberstar that his Chairmanship was in peril if he continued to stand with me. I could not compete with the inducements and threats put forth by the Administration and the Speaker. All I had to offer was the personal satisfaction of standing up for the principle of protecting the sanctity of life *and* providing all Americans with access to quality, affordable healthcare. Each of us was committed to these principles, which were now colliding with each other. How long could I hold the group together with leadership splitting us apart? How much longer before it was Bart Stupak and his group of none? How much longer could I hold enough votes to force leadership to negotiate?

The White House had attempted to negotiate with the last remaining holdouts and had intentionally excluded me. It was clear to me that the last remaining remnants of the Stupak dozen were squarely within the crosshairs of President Barack Obama and Speaker Nancy Pelosi.

I had just returned to the Pennsylvania corner when Congresswoman Marcy Kaptur (D-OH) approached me and said that she had just announced that she would be voting for health care but would still support me on the Life position. I was dumbfounded by Marcy's statement. I asked her, "How can you support health care and the Stupak Amendment when the Stupak Amendment needed to be resolved BEFORE the vote on health care?" I really did not know what to say. Marcy always voted with us on Pro-Life issues and I knew she took constant grief from the Democratic women Members of Congress. Marcy had always voted with me and I counted on her to stand with me until the Life issue was resolved. Marcy had no answer; she would just say, "When you need my vote, I will be there."

It looked like the fight was over. I believed that the White House and the Speaker had enough votes to pass health care and the Rule; it appeared that the fix was in. For fifteen months, RTL Democrats had warned, pleaded, and demonstrated our ability to stop legislation that had not contained our traditional Pro-Life Riders. Last November, the US House of Representatives overwhelmingly supported the Stupak amendment, which reflected the wishes of the majority that taxpayer funds not be used to pay for abortions. Now, after all this time and courageous effort, I believed the Speaker had the votes necessary to pass the Affordable Care Act, which would include coverage for elective abortions.

More votes were scheduled for later in the afternoon. I was convinced that by the end of the day, at least one additional member of the Stupak dozen would defect and declare support for the Affordable Care Act. I feared that the noble fight to protect the sanctity of life was over. The political bulls would prevail; I could not compete with promises from the White House and threats from the Speaker.

Maybe Scott and Mike were correct. Maybe it was time to throw in the towel. I knew that I would not be seeking re-election to Congress. I had fought a noble fight and held true to my beliefs.

As I lingered in the Pennsylvania corner, I counted over and over, again and again the remaining Members of my coalition. I had Donnelly, Driehuas, Rahall, Mollohan, Dahlkemper, and me. Six votes. Was that enough to block health care from coming to the floor?

As I mentioned previously, the Speaker always carried votes in her pocket, like John Tanner, Jim Cooper, possibly Lincoln Davis, Bobby Bright or maybe Charlie Melanchon. The Speaker's "pocket votes" were those votes held by Members who did not want to vote for the legislation but at the same time would not allow the legislation to fail by one or two votes. Therefore, based on a prior agreement with the Speaker, the Member agreed not to allow the legislation to fail. So I asked myself, how many votes did the Speaker still have in her pocket?

From my perspective, everything was spinning out of control. I could no longer hold my coalition together and force the hand of the President and the Speaker. But I had one more chance. A few days earlier, I had drafted a Technical Correction Bill that required cooperation from Republican Senators and my good friend, Senator Tom Coburn. Coburn was my Senate lead on this legislation. It was time to check back with him.

A Technical Correction Bill is legislation to correct or address an obvious oversight, clerical error, or mistake made in previously passed legislation. A technical correction bill must be approved by both the House and Senate and presented to the President for his signature before the legislation that the Technical Correction Bill corrects is signed by the president. Under the Affordable Care Act, the Senate had to pass the Technical Correction Bill first and then send it over to the House for final consideration. My Technical Correction Bill would have inserted the Stupak Amendment in the Senate version of the Affordable Care Act. Since the House overwhelmingly passed the Stupak Amendment and the Senate had not, the Technical Amendment would have to begin in the Senate. The Technical Correction Bill would not be possible without the overwhelming support of the Senate Republicans. Thus, I had to rely on my friend and C Street colleague Senator Tom Coburn to convince the Senate Republican leadership to support my Technical Correction legislation.

I immediately called Senator Tom Coburn's private number from the Democratic cloakroom and caught him in his office. Senator Coburn said he had spoken with Minority Leader Mitch McConnell within the last twenty-four hours and McConnell was not willing to allow the Senate Republicans to vote for my Technical Correction Bill. Tom explained that he was disappointed, but that Senate Republicans would not support my Technical Correction Bill if it was sent over from the House. I asked Tom to double check with his leadership on supporting the Technical Correction Bill. I also informed him that the White House had proposed an executive order promising continuation of the Hyde Amendment in the health care legislation. Tom quickly added that an executive order would not cover federal community health centers and I agreed with him. Still, my only chance of protecting life now was my Technical Correction Bill, which needed the support of all the Senate Republicans and a handful of Senate Democrats. Neither option would be as strong as the Stupak Amendment, but these were the only options I had left if we wanted to pass health care.

I told Tom that Kildee and Oberstar were now going to vote for health care and that the Administration and Speaker were really pressuring Members to vote for the health care package. Tom asked me how many votes I had left and I told him that I could count on six or seven. He quickly responded, "Then they don't have enough votes." I said don't forget that the Speaker always carries a few in her pocket and that Marcy Kaptur was now voting for health care. I explained that Marcy was willing to support any action I took to force a vote on a Technical Correction Bill or the Stupak Amendment, but I was running out of options and I felt that the health care vote was imminent.

I asked Tom to go back to McConnell one more time. He said he would go back to both McConnell and John Kyl (R-AZ), but that the Senate had already adjourned for the weekend. I told him I needed a promise from the Senate Republicans to support the Technical Correction Bill and that I had already faxed the bill over to Senator Ben Nelson.

Senator Ben Nelson and Democratic Pro-Life Senators supported the idea of a Technical Correction Bill because the bill could pass with a simple majority. I had completed the research. I needed Republican Senators to support the Technical Correction Bill just as I had previously discussed with Senator Coburn. I assured Tom that I had faxed the bill to him earlier and that it was bipartisan legislation. I had to have the Senate Republicans support it.

Tom asked me to fax him the Technical Correction Bill with the bipartisan cosponsors listed so he could show his leadership. I told Tom that I had introduced the bill earlier in the day and that it would be printed in the Congressional Record. He said he would go back to McConnell and Kyl and give it one last try; it was our last legislative opportunity to insert the Stupak Amendment into the health care legislation. It was very late in the legislative process, but Tom and I had discussed the Technical Correction Bill more than once. He was familiar with the process and had encouraged me to amend the Senate version of health care. It was late in the game on Friday afternoon, March 19, 2010.

I was very forceful but respectful with Tom as I stressed that if he and the Senate Republicans were truly committed to protecting the sanctity of Life, now was the time to act. I needed a commitment to keep the remaining members of the Stupak Dozen united to stall the weekend vote on health care until the Senate would come back next week. Once again, I was holding onto a long shot, but it was still a shot.

With the Tea Party activists demonstrating outside, the atmosphere surrounding the Capitol was becoming more and more intense. The Tea Party was making its presence known with their impromptu rallies against health care. As the day wore on, more and more Tea Party activists and evangelicals were congregating around the Capitol and outside my Rayburn office door. The reception area in my congressional office remained the site of prayer vigils and demonstrations. Citizens from around the country were descending on my office and demanding to see me. None of the participants in the prayer vigils who insisted on meeting with me were from the First Congressional District of Michigan. According to the evangelicals camped out in my reception area, they had traveled to Washington, DC to save me and the country from enacting a socialist health care program forced on us by the atheist President Barack Obama. As ridiculous as these claims were, there was no reasoning with the Tea Party activists or the "good Christians" parked in front of my office.

After the afternoon votes were completed, many Members remained on the House floor discussing health care, the disruptive antics of the Tea Party, the constant demonstrations outside, and the intense scrutiny by the media. Members of the US House of Representatives had been advised that we would not be returning home to our congressional districts over the weekend and that at some point, probably Sunday, we would be voting on health care. However, no one knew when the votes would occur as everyone understood that Speaker Pelosi still had not secured enough votes for passage. Members were actually handicapping as to when the votes would occur and how many votes the Speaker still needed to pass the health care legislation. I could see the strain on the faces of the Members of Congress who were lingering on the House floor after the votes. Each Member understood that history would be made one way or the other: either health care passed against the wishes of the Tea Party protestors or the Democratically controlled Congress would fail to pass health care.

I remained on the floor to discuss strategy with some of the Democratic Right-to-Life Members. We huddled in the Pennsylvania corner and discussed a possible executive order; I told the group that I was still not ready to go down that road.

Once again, Rahm was floating the idea of an executive order to address the concerns of the Right-of-Life Democrats. During the past year, Speaker Pelosi had overplayed her hand in denying the traditional Pro-Life Riders on the appropriations bills. I had proven my point with the passage of the Stupak Amendment. Sixty-four Democrats had stood with me in affirming Hyde language in the health care bill. I was not ready to give up on a statutory solution and I was still pushing the Technical Correction Bill through Senator Coburn.

As Members slowly drifted off the House floor. I noticed my friend, Congressman Mike Doyle, hanging back. He was quietly sitting in the top row of the Pennsylvania corner. Mike quickly asked me, "If you could write an executive order, what would you put in it?" I answered, "The executive order would need to include the Hyde language, conscience clause, language concerning federal funding for abortions in community health centers, and the Weldon language." Then Mike said, "Why don't you write up what you need in an executive order and I will get it over to the White House." I told Mike, "Thanks, but I have never written an executive order." He said, "Just write down your ideas on what you need and get it to me." I said, "Okay. I will call you later."

Slowly, I walked back to my Rayburn office thinking about an executive order and wondering if Senator Coburn was making any progress with the Republican Senate leadership. When I was back in my office, I called Tom. The conversation was very short. Tom said he checked back with Senators McConnell, Kyl and Hatch and the answer was a final, definite NO. The Republicans in the Senate would not support my Technical Correction Bill. Tom was emphatic, "it is no longer about Life. We are not going to give Obama a victory."

The Republicans preferred to kill the health care bill and start over; I told Tom that was not going to happen. I said that Senator Orrin Hatch (R-UT) had offered to work with me on a new bill last fall but I had rejected the idea then and I rejected it now. I truly believed in health care for all Americans and we were closer now than we had ever been. As we ended our conversation, I told Tom I was not going to kill the health care bill.

Senator Tom Coburn said, "Well, then you are on your own. The Senate has already left for home and we are done for the week." For nearly a hundred years, presidents had been calling on Congress to pass national health care. This was the closest Congress had ever come to passing national health care and I was not going to be the person responsible for killing it now.

It occurred to me that by standing my ground and insisting that the Stupak Amendment be made in order last fall resulted in the passage of the Rule for the health care legislation. Once on the floor, the health care legislation passed in a bipartisan fashion because of the Stupak Amendment. Now, it was obvious that a determined Republican Party was not going to give President Obama a victory and would use the Stupak Amendment to kill the health care legislation. The Stupak Amendment went from ensuring bipartisan support of health care to a bipartisan vote to kill health care. I was not about to allow my amendment to be turned upside down and become the death of health care. By killing the Stupak Amendment, the Republicans were willing to allow 45,000 living, breathing Americans to die needlessly because they did not have access to basic health care. They would let 45,000 Americans die rather than give President Obama a legislative victory. I would not be part of a heartless scheme to kill health care; I became more determined to find a way forward. In my dogged determination, I was still convinced that Congress could pass national health care and protect the sanctity of life.

My next phone call was to my most trusted adviser, Laurie. Not unlike most political couples, I always turned to my wife when I needed truly honest input about something. I trusted her judgment implicitly and valued her sound practical advice. Laurie had served as Mayor of Menominee and guided our city through a very difficult transition from a traditional mayoral form of government to a city manager-led administration. Still, as Mayor, Laurie was considered the highest elected official of our city of approximately 10,000 citizens.

Laurie and I discussed the day's events. I told her about the abandonment of the Technical Correction Bill by Senate Republicans, my conversations with Senator Coburn, Congressman Driehaus asking why I wasn't at the secret meeting with White House Counsel on the executive order in the Speaker's office, and now Doyle asking me to draft an executive order. Laurie's comments were concise and thoughtful.

> "For the executive order, put in everything that you need to be able to vote for health care," she said. "Make sure you can vote for the health care legislation after you negotiate the executive order. Make sure you get everything you want and realize that you will never be able to please the Bishops. Bart, you ran for Congress to pass health care. You can do this. This is the closest we have been to passing national health care. It is now or never. You have worked too long and too hard to watch it all fall apart now."

As usual, Laurie was right. She gave me the confidence I needed to begin drafting an outline of an executive order that my small group of Right-to-Life Democrats could support. Each Member of Congress who stood with me had a stake in this executive order; these Democrats had to have faith in the President to uphold the order and that it would withstand judicial review.

Earlier in the day these Members of Congress had soundly rejected a proposed executive order put forth by the President's legal team and informed the White House Counsel that they would not support an agreement without me. Congressmen Donnelly and Driehaus were not impressed with the executive order presented earlier in the day; why would they be impressed with mine? The answer lay in the question. They trusted me and followed my lead on Right-to-Life issues. After eighteen years of fighting with Democrats, Republicans, and presidents on abortion issues, I had a firm grasp of both the law and the politics surrounding the abortion issue.

I called Scott into my office and we discussed the proposed executive order. He offered to conduct the necessary research and pull together some recent executive orders for reference. I asked him to pull up President George W. Bush's order on stem cell research. It was agreed that I would take the first cut on an outline of issues that needed to be addressed. Then Scott, Nick Choate, my legislative director, and I would go over the draft before I sent it to Doyle.

Scott asked about Erika and I told him that I did not want her involved. I made it very clear that she would not be included in the negotiations on the executive order. The Bishops wouldn't agree to one and I did not need Erika undermining my efforts. She would only sound the alarm to National Right-to-Life and the US Conference of Catholic Bishops; I knew that I could not trust her to keep my work on an executive order confidential. I should have fired Erika by this point but I just did not have time to deal with her; I was focused on health care and would address the problem after the legislation passed. I also did not need all the interest groups that opposed health care but supported the Stupak Amendment to be gathering in front of my office. Even as we spoke, the evangelicals were praying outside my office door and attempting to send notes and prayers through the mail slot.

Scott and I discussed whether Doyle actually had permission from the White House to ask me to draft an executive order. Scott knew that there were only three people I truly trusted on this issue; him, Mike Doyle and Laurie. Scott also knew that Mike was my closest friend in Congress. We both understood that he was our go-between with the Speaker and now the White House on the health care legislation. We also believed that if Mike told me the Speaker did not have the votes to pass health care, the Speaker did not have the votes. Mike Doyle was present last fall when I negotiated with Nancy Pelosi on a compromise to the Stupak Amendment; he would not mislead me now.

Scott and I wondered whether Rahm Emmanuel and our White House Congressional Liaison, Dan Turton, were involved in this executive order strategy. I knew that I did not trust Rahm; I respected him and his abilities, but I could not believe a word he said.

I liked Dan Turton and had known him from my early days in Congress as a member of Majority Leader Dick Gephardt's (D-MO) staff. Dan was Director of Floor Operations, US House of Representatives. Even after Democrats lost the majority in the 1994 elections, Dan stayed on as Director of Floor Operations and also covered Rules Committee for Leader Gephardt. When President Obama was elected, Dan was part of the White House Legislative Affairs Team.

I realized that Laurie and Mike were right. The last opportunity to pass health care was an executive order. The Senate Republicans had moved from protecting Life to politicizing it to defeat health care and the Obama Administration. Anyone who walked by and listened to the prayer vigils in front of my office understood that the purpose of the prayers was to defeat health care by insisting on the inclusion of the Stupak Amendment.

CHAPTER 53

★ ★ ★

The Executive Order

There was a knock on my office door and in came a smiling Erika with Jayd Hendricks of the US Conference of Catholic Bishops. Erika and Jayd claimed that they were just checking in to see how things were going.

After Erika sent out the email blasting the Senate health care bill without my permission, she had lost my trust and confidence. She could no longer be trusted to keep my thoughts and ideas on health care private. She was too close to the issue, too close to the Bishops, and too close to the Republicans. Erika's role in health care was greatly diminished and she resented it.

I summarized my conversation with my Democratic RTL Members; Jayd stated that the Bishops knew about the proposed executive order and that they had rejected that idea a long time ago. He said that he knew that the executive order was circulating but was unaware that it had been presented to some of the Members.

I pressed Jayd on what he would put in an executive order if he could write one. He just kept insisting that the Bishops would not accept it. The Bishops viewed the Stupak Amendment as their one and only opportunity to codify the Hyde Amendment. If the health care legislation did not contain the Stupak Amendment, then they would just as soon kill the health care bill. I raised the issue of social justice and how health care was the number one priority listed on the Bishops' website. We were so close to passing health care, their number one issue- yet they would not consider accepting an executive order abiding by the Hyde Amendment.

It was obvious as I pushed Jayd regarding what he would include in an executive order that he was uncomfortable with the discussion. I believe that he sympathized with me on this issue but that his superiors would not allow him to contribute or discuss an executive order. Jayd just kept repeating the company line: no executive order and no health care without the Stupak Amendment.

The afternoon was quickly drawing to a close, as was our conversation. Unfortunately, I have neither seen nor spoken with Jayd since that Friday afternoon in my office. I always felt that he could be reasonable and practical on social justice issues but that he was restrained by Richard Doerflinger.

I dismissed everyone from my office so I could concentrate on drafting the proposed executive order. I quickly realized that it was ludicrous for me to attempt to write one, so I began to outline the principles I needed to include in the order. I quickly pulled up the Stupak Amendment on my computer, along with past statements supporting the Weldon and Church Amendments on the conscience clause. I reviewed some of the legal analyses provided over the past couple of years by National Right-to-Life and the US Conference of Catholic Bishops. The more I wrote, the more I cut from my original draft outline. I then included the Hyde language that the House and Senate had previously accepted and noted the amendment's history. I also included the most recent appropriations bills that contained the traditional RTL riders protecting the sanctity of life. I completed my outline and understood the legislative history and logic behind each point. I then shared my outline with Scott and Nick, but not Erika.

Then, I emailed my most trusted advisor. Laurie said it looked good. She did not understand all the legal provisions but each point was succinctly stated. She asked what would happen next and I told her that I really did not know, other than I was going to send the document to Mike Doyle. She wished me luck.

I then emailed my outline to Mike on his private congressional email account. The ball was now in his court. A short time later, he called and asked, "Where are we going to eat? We have one more series of votes and then let's have dinner." I told Mike, "Let's head down to the Club immediately after votes; I will drive." Then I added, "Let's go over early, just the two of us, before any other Members join us." He said it sounded good and to bring the van up to the Capitol.

Mike and I drove over to the Democratic Club. A small group of us, Pascrell, Capuano, Doyle, Holden (D-PA), John Larson (D-CT), Carolyn McCarthy (D-NY), and me, frequented the Club during session days. We felt that since we had to eat when we were in DC, we might as well spend our dollars at the Democratic Club as opposed to any of the other high-priced DC restaurants.

The Democratic Club is located at 30 Ivy Street SE in Washington, DC. It encompasses the first floor of the three-story building owned by the National Democratic Committee. The Club, however, is a separate, private entity from the DNC.

Patrons of the Democratic Club enter from Ivy Street S.E. and walk down a short corridor with a coatroom and a small office on the left. At the maître d' post, Michelle greets guests in her thick French accent. Since our small group of US Representatives frequents the club for dinner at least once a week, Michelle has permanently reserved our favorite table, the only large booth in the dining room. The east wall of the club is lined with booths built to accommodate two people. In the middle of the row of booths is the large booth, which comfortably seats eight to ten. From our booth, we can survey the entire dining room and bar area.

Our booth is the most popular table in the club and is constantly visited by the other patrons and Members of Congress. If a Member of Congress appears at the club alone, he or she is invited to join us at our booth. It is not unusual to see a minimum of six to twelve Members of Congress sitting at our reserved table on a Tuesday, Wednesday or Thursday evening. Mirrors extend from the top of the booth to the ceiling. Our booth in the center is graced by the large NDC emblem etched into the mirror.

As stated earlier, Members of Congress are creatures of habit and gravitate to their usual table at the club. For instance, Members of the Black Caucus pull together two tables and sit right behind the maître'd post. The women Members of Congress prefer to sit at the tables in the center of the dining room, which seat four. If a Member of Congress held a fundraiser earlier in the evening, tables were pulled together so their staff and guests could enjoy dinner afterwards. The union lobbyists, if not in the bar area, occupy the three booths that back up against the south wall that separates the bar from the dining room.

The club's dinner menu consists of a variety of entrées, including the favorite dishes of various Members of Congress, which are periodically rotated. My menu dish was a tenderloin steak and mushrooms with a side of asparagus.

For the twenty-four years that I have been a member of the club, Joseph the Bartender has manned the bar. With a thick middle-eastern accent, Joseph from Lebanon runs a tight ship and serves his patrons in the dimly lit bar. Each day at 5:00 p.m., many lobbyists, union leaders and local card-carrying Democrats stop to see Joe for their favorite beverage before heading home or venturing out on the fundraising circuit.

There are two medium-sized televisions at each end of the bar and two larger televisions in the dining room. The televisions are always tuned to a sporting event or the evening news. When the House is in session, at least one television in the club is tuned to C-Span live coverage of the House floor. When votes are called, Joseph, Michelle and the wait staff immediately advise Members of the pending votes. Interestingly, Members of the Democratic leadership and Members of the Senate seldom come to the Democratic Club for lunch or dinner.

It is considered rude to "lobby" Members of Congress while they are enjoying lunch or dinner at the club. Members of Congress sincerely appreciate the club's "No Lobbying Zone," as they know that they will not be hassled or interrupted while enjoying a meal.

Mike and I did not take our usual table but sat at the bar to have a beer. It was well after 5:00 p.m. and since the regular patrons had already left the club we were alone. The conversation quickly turned to health care and Mike asked, "How many votes do you believe you can deliver if we can work out an executive order?" I told Mike that I could deliver six to eight votes and he seemed surprised. Mike repeated the question, and my answer was the same. Mike then said, "If you just deliver six votes we have enough votes to pass health care." I told Mike, "I am well aware of that, but then you never know how many votes the Speaker has in her pocket." Mike assured me, "She does not have enough to pass health care without your votes. Some people who she thinks will vote for health care will not. If you can deliver those votes, you will get whatever you want in the executive order." He went on to explain that the White House had my documents and they were working on a draft executive order based on my outline.

Mike's Blackberry buzzed and he stepped away to take the call. He came back and said that the White House Counsel wanted to meet later that night. I asked when and where and he said that we would have to find a place that the media did not have staked out. The White House was therefore off limits and so were Mike's and my offices. I added that the Speaker's office was also off limits and we both just laughed.

Mike said, "We will use my hideaway on the fifth floor of the Cannon Building and no one will bother us there." We went on to discuss how the White House Counsel could drive right into the Cannon garage and take an elevator up to the fifth-floor storage room area and avoid the media. Mike placed a call and said, "The meeting is set for 11:00 p.m. in my hideaway." He said that he would have his staff set up a table and some chairs for us to work on. We agreed that there would be no personal or committee staff members included in the meeting; only the Members of Congress who we invited would be allowed.

Mike asked whether I knew White House Counsel, Bob Bauer. I replied that Bauer's former law firm worked on a couple of Election Commission issues for me and that I had a favorable opinion of him. Mike said, "I do not know the guy." I said, "Well, I guess you will get to meet him tonight in your hideaway." We both laughed.

I then advised Mike that I needed to call the six remaining Members of my group; I did not want them to think that I was holding this meeting without them. Also, we all had to agree to the executive order. Our little group stuck together despite tremendous pressure and I was not proceeding without them. He agreed and I excused myself and started to make phone calls from the Club to Donnelly, Driehaus, Dahlkemper, Ellsworth, Rahall, Mollohan, and Costello. I asked each Member to keep the meeting in strictest confidence and invited them to join us at 11:00 p.m. The Members' initial reaction was that 11:00 p.m. was awfully late to start a meeting but they would try to make it.

CHAPTER 54

★ ★ ★

Eye to Eye

We arrived at Mike's hideaway on the fifth floor of the Cannon Building shortly before 11:00 p.m. with our paper cups filled with hot coffee. It was obvious that Mike's staff had straightened out the room. There were file boxes in varying heights stacked against the back wall. There was one beat up old desk with an equally battered desk chair accompanying it. The desk had a phone on it, which Mike claimed actually worked. There were more file boxes stacked in front of the desk. Mike's staff had cleared away the center of the room and placed a folding table with six chairs around it. The lighting was poor, dust covered some of the file boxes that had not been moved in a while, and staff obviously had not had time to sweep the floor before setting up the folding table and chairs. Given the short notice and the limited staff available around after 8:00 p.m. on a Friday night, I was pleased with the setting. The press would never dream that Members of Congress and the President's Legal Counsel would be in a musty old hideaway off a little-used hallway in the Cannon Building negotiating the executive order that would make or break health care. Bob Bauer and a young attorney, Danielle Gray, were already seated on one side of the table. Mike Doyle and Dan Turton were sitting behind the White House attorneys. We made our introductions and with me were Donnelly,

Driehaus, Mollohan, and Dahlkemper. Donnelly and Driehaus pulled up chairs next to Mollohan and me and Dahlkemper sat on file boxes off to the right of us. With an uneasy "we don't trust you" tension filling the air, Bob Bauer began the discussion.

Bob Bauer did not mention the earlier meeting and instead handed me a three-page draft of an executive order. He mentioned that that he had tried to incorporate the language that I had drafted. Bauer asked us to review the proposed order and then we could discuss it. To our surprise, the executive order encompassed all the points I had outlined. When I finished reading the draft, Bauer asked me to explain my rationale behind the language. I told him that the draft was a good first step but there were certain areas that needed clarification and expansion. The tension lessened a bit.

Methodically, I went through the executive order paragraph by paragraph explaining the legal, legislative and political basis for each point that was important to us as Right-to-Life Democrats. I explained that we needed the Hyde Amendment, the conscience clause and a prohibition on abortions from being performed at community health centers all addressed in the executive order. After my twenty-minute explanation on how the federal government had been banned from promoting, advocating, supporting, or paying for abortions over the past thirty-three years, Bob Bauer stated that he thought the draft executive order adequately covered the points I raised. I did not necessarily disagree with Bob, but I spent a little more time explaining not just to him but also for the benefit of our little group, including my good friend Mike Doyle, that each paragraph had a purpose, a legislative history, and a moral conviction that should not be lost on anyone in that musty hideaway. I specifically pointed out how we would need stronger language to prevent taxpayer funding of abortions in community health centers, the high-risk pool, and under federal grants awarded under the Affordable Care Act. Under the Stupak Amendment, federal grant money could not be used for encouraging, promoting or performing abortions.

While the draft executive order was well written, I still needed the language clarified. For example, I added the words "federally qualified health care clinics" in a couple of places in the draft. Federally qualified health care clinics were the same as community health centers, but the executive order had to clarify this fact.

White House Legislative Affairs Director, Dan Turton, asked us, "If the changes I asked for were placed in the executive order, would we all vote for health care?" I told Dan, "The language, while close, is not enough to win over our votes, so we would need to see the final language. Also, I need to conduct a colloquy with Chairman Waxman on the House floor so there will be a record of the congressional intent and purpose behind the executive order." Dan responded that the order would speak for itself. I said, "No, I need the colloquy so there will be no question as to the purpose and function of the executive order." Bob Bauer then chimed in, "The colloquy on the House floor is a reasonable request and I will recommend it to the President and Chairman Waxman."

Once again, my small group and I were pressed on whether we would vote for the Affordable Care Act. Once again, I told Dan Turton and Bob Bauer that we would reserve judgment until the executive order was finalized and accepted by the President. Bob Bauer then claimed that he believed that the President would sign it; his more immediate concern was whether the women Democratic Members of Congress would accept the executive order. I asked if the Pro-Choice Caucus knew about this meeting and Bauer stated that they did not.

Bauer further explained that the women's groups knew that an executive order had been drafted and presented earlier in the day, but that it had been rejected by the Members present in the Speaker's office meeting. I asked, "Why I was not invited to the meeting?" Bauer answered that he had not created the invitation list and that I should have been included in the meeting." Turton did not say a word about the previous meeting in the Speaker's office. The other Members spoke up and stated that there would be no more meetings or proposed executive orders without Bart Stupak's approval. Bauer and Dan Turton assured us that they would only work with us and try to finalize our suggested edits by tomorrow after they checked with the President on our proposed changes.

We then agreed to meet the next day and that Congressman Doyle would notify us of the meeting time and location. Before our initial meeting broke up around 1:00 a.m. Saturday morning, all the copies of the proposed executive order were collected and given back to Bob Bauer with the understanding that no one would have anything that the media could obtain. Further, we agreed that no one would mention the meeting or the executive order to the media; we would only share this information with our most trusted staff and they too must agree to the media blackout.

I caucused briefly out in the hallway with my small group. We were generally pleased with the executive order and the proposed changes we had suggested. Mollohan wanted to know about the Bishops and if I could get their support. I told Alan and the group that the Bishops were adamantly opposed to an executive order, as they would only settle for statutory language. The Members with me objected to this line of thinking and stated that the Bishops were being unreasonable because the Senate would never pass the Stupak Amendment. The consensus was that the Bishops never really wanted health care to pass. I cautioned the group that we should keep our powder dry and work on improving the executive order; at this point, it was the only vehicle still available that protected the sanctity of life.

Congressman Alan Mollohan then said that he had served in Congress for twenty-five years and had attended countless meetings, yet had never seen as commanding a display of knowledge and persuasive argument as I made to Bob Bauer on the language in the executive order. Alan added that he had never seen me in action before and that I had to be a "hell of a prosecutor." He went on to say that he did not know about the rest of the group but that he would not agree to anything unless I agreed. He was proud to stand with me. The other Members agreed with Alan's sentiments and after a few slaps on the back, we walked down the empty halls of the Cannon building wondering what tomorrow, or rather later today, would bring. As we left the Cannon Building we were hopeful that maybe we could find a way to protect the sanctity of life and provide access to health care for all Americans.

Around 1:30 a.m., we stepped into the dark night and not into the glare of television camera lights; we were pleased that the media had not learned of our secret meeting. As we left the Cannon

Building, I believe it was Joe Donnelly who joked, "Hell, are we the only fools still up at this time of night?" We all laughed and walked into the early morning hours. It had been another exhausting day. Mike Doyle and I drove my Explorer back to our apartment over on A Street without saying a word.

The executive order was a start and our first meeting went well. Our little group suggested some changes and I had asked for a colloquy to be conducted on the House floor. The executive order was far from a done deal, as the only person who had to agree and could actually sign it had not been in the room. Plus, I felt the colloquy might be too much of a stretch for the Speaker and Chairman Waxman. But if the Speaker truly needed our votes, then our request for a colloquy on the House floor was not an unreasonable request.

I needed to check with the House Parliamentarian on the rules governing a colloquy referencing an executive order. I would check with the Parliamentarian or my Jefferson Manual the following day. At that moment, it appeared my best opportunity for protecting the sanctity of life and providing all Americans with health care would be to cut a deal on the executive order. The Technical Correction Bill was still a possibility and I would introduce it tomorrow.

As my brain swirled with my "to do" list for the next day, I wondered if health care would ever pass.

CHAPTER 55

★ ★ ★

Saturday, March 20, 2010

As I climbed into bed close to 2:00 a.m., I knew it was going to be another sleepless night. Physically I was exhausted but my mind kept whirling, replaying the day's events. When the day started, I had hopes of inserting the Stupak Amendment into the final health care legislation. I had ten Members of Congress standing with me and we could block the Rule and health care from coming to the floor if Speaker Pelosi did not allow the Stupak Amendment. Six hours later, I was hanging onto six Members and that number may be optimistic.

I never dreamed I would be sitting across from the President's legal counsel, arguing over the nuisances of a proposed executive order, which was possibly my last and only option.

I ticked off the legislative options that had looked promising at the beginning of the day. Now, that moment seemed like a long, long time ago. I had no options left. The principle of protecting the sanctity of life was no longer important to the Bishops or National RTL. Now, the failure to codify the Hyde language in the health care legislation meant these organizations now demanded that I use the Stupak Amendment to defeat health care. I worked so long and so hard to get these groups to embrace health care reform by doggedly fighting for the Stupak Amendment. Now I had to fight these same groups to give health care legislation a chance at life.

When President George W. Bush signed the executive order limiting stem cell research, the Bishops and National RTL fell all over themselves praising the President and the strength of the order. Now, these same groups were adamantly opposed to an executive order in principle and would not even assist in drafting the strongest possible language to protect the sanctity of life.

For over thirty years, there had been a truce between the Pro-Life and Pro-Choice Caucuses stipulating that neither side would expand or codify the Hyde Language. With the Stupak Amendment, the Hyde language moved the closest it had ever been to being codified. The truce had now been called off and both sides were at war with each other. Did these groups lose focus and common sense, or did I? The opposing groups' inability to agree on the abortion language in the health care legislation was not a reason to kill the bill. I kept asking myself whether it was right to destroy the whole bill if my amendment was not attached to it. When did ideology trump moral and social justice?

The maximum number of votes that the Stupak Amendment could garner in the Senate was forty-five- not the sixty needed to pass the amendment. I repeatedly warned the Bishops' lobbyists that the Stupak Amendment would never be accepted in the Senate. Why couldn't they understand this reality? Why and when did the Stupak Amendment become the "means to the end" for health care legislation? How could these organizations, which constantly lectured Americans on social justice, turn their backs on health care because they did not receive their one amendment? If we could not help everyone, shouldn't we at least try to help some?

Every year 45,000 Americans died because they did not have access to basic health care. Why couldn't the Bishops join me and explore ways to provide health insurance coverage under the Affordable Care Act? Based on the meeting this evening with the White House Counsel, I believed we could protect the sanctity of life through an executive order *and* provide health care. Why wouldn't the Bishops even try to develop a strong executive order that addressed their concerns?

What was I missing? The US Senate never came close to passing the Stupak Amendment when it was offered by Senator Ben Nelson. The Senate had departed Washington, DC and left the legislative decisions on health care in the hands of the House of Representatives. The Senate Republicans who had encouraged the Technical Correction Bill bailed on the idea at the eleventh hour. Senate Republicans said that it was no longer about protecting life but about denying Obama a political victory. The evangelicals and zealots were outside my office door, praying that the Stupak Amendment would defeat the health care legislation. The Bishops were adamantly opposed to an executive order. Where and when did this issue become our way or the highway?

Yes, it was going to be another sleepless night and I did not have visions of executive orders dancing in my head- I had the bitter seeds of betrayal by the US Conference of Catholic Bishops stuck in my throat. It was not a good feeling.

I rehashed the day's events and tried to figure out how I could do better the next day. I rehashed every word I uttered, every press interview I gave and every conversation I had with Members of Congress. As my eyes grew heavy, I looked forward to my early morning workout, which had become my quiet sanctuary.

After hitting the gym in the morning, I went up to my office to catch up on paperwork before my staff came in. Since it was the weekend and the office buildings were technically closed, Scott would only have a skeleton crew working to keep the office running and thankfully, there should not be any prayer vigils outside my office door. The staff needed a break from the upheaval of the past few weeks. It had been brutal on everyone's time, patience and commitment to public service.

I was way behind in reviewing and signing the constituent mail. I had put off reviewing the letters, as I was under tremendous pressure to either pass the Stupak Amendment or defeat the health care legislation. I wanted to accomplish both goals, but my friends and allies were at war with each other and I was the man in the middle, trying to find a solution to please both sides. I looked forward to burying my head in paperwork, which I hoped would take my mind off the internal and external struggles swirling about me. The pressure of health care must have gotten to me because no one in his right mind looks forward to doing paperwork. I saw it as an escape.

A few years ago, I had allowed my staff to directly answer constituent mail without my review. The experiment only lasted six months and was a complete failure. Answers to constituent mail were sent based on speed rather than the quality of the response. Plus, I felt that I had lost contact with the issues my constituents were concerned about. When staff answered a constituent inquiry within ten days but never actually responded to the concern, the inept correspondence was a negative reflection on both my office and me personally. Seldom do constituents send letters to their congressman but when they do, they deserve a thoughtful answer to their concerns. I was a stickler on mail and it helped me to stay connected with my constituents throughout my vast rural congressional district. I also took pride in jotting personal notes on letters so that my constituents knew that I personally read their communications.

The US House went into session at 9:00 a.m. and recessed until 10:30 a.m. Great- more time to do my paperwork. When the House resumed session, a number of suspension bills were debated and then called for votes. Voting on the suspension bills lasted for about an hour and then Congressman Sandy Levin (D-MI) called up the Tricare Affirmation Act, which stated that Tricare health insurance met the minimal essential standards of coverage under the proposed Affordable Care Act. The proposed legislation also clarified that coverage for our military men and women and veterans would not come under the Affordable Care Act. Members of the military and veterans received their health insurance coverage and health care system through Champus and the Veterans Administration, respectively.

When I heard the title of the bill my ears perked up, as it sounded like the Democrats were moving to amend the Affordable Care Act under a suspension of the Rules and pass the Tricare Affirmation Act. I thought the Speaker had made it very clear there would not be any amendments to the Affordable Care Act.

I started to question the Democratic leadership floor staff. The staff claimed no knowledge of the legislation being debated on the floor. I did not believe them and they knew that I would not accept

"I don't know" as a valid answer. I started to look for the Speaker. If the Speaker allowed this Tricare Amendment, would she allow my Technical Correction Bill or the Stupak Amendment? Suddenly, my two pending pieces of legislation had found renewed legislative life. I had to find Speaker Nancy Pelosi.

As I listened to the debate on the House floor, I learned that the Tricare Amendment to the Budget Reconciliation Package had been introduced shortly before midnight and came immediately to the floor as a suspension bill. The Democrats were constantly told that there would be no amendments to the three bills sent to us from the Senate.

It was this Budget Reconciliation Package that House Members would amend to strip the Second Louisiana Purchase, the Cornhusker Deal, the Florida payoff, and the many other payoffs that the Senators had placed in the health care legislation in exchange for their support. So why was Congressman Levin offering an amendment to the Budget Reconciliation Package when there were to be no amendments?

I then noticed Armed Services Chairman Ike Skeleton (D-MO) speaking in support of the Tricare Affirmation Act. Ike was publicly opposed to the health care legislation, but was now speaking in favor of an amendment to the legislation. My Democratic Pro-Life friend, Ike Skelton, was on the floor debating an amendment to the Reconciliation Package. I intended to find out why Ike was allowed an amendment and I was not.

I knew that my only chance to talk with the Speaker would be on the House floor, if she showed up for votes. It is customary for Speakers not to vote on legislation even if they are on the floor when votes are occurring. However, Speakers will often come to floor to discuss issues and other legislative matters with Members.

I was confident that Speaker Pelosi would show up on the floor for a vote on the Tricare Amendment, as she was still strong-arming Democratic Members to vote for the Budget Reconciliation Package.

By attaching the Affordable Care Act to the Budget Reconciliation Package, the Package would only require a simple majority of fifty-one votes in the Senate for passage. This parliamentary scheme had been concocted by President Obama, Senate

Majority Leader Reid, and Speaker Pelosi after Scott Brown's victory for Ted Kennedy's Senate seat. With Republican Scott Brown's Senate victory in the heavily Democratic state of Massachusetts, the Democrats had been dealt a severe blow to passing national health care. The Democrats no longer had their filibuster-proof sixty votes as they had prior to the election of Scott Brown.

Democratic leaders had already declared that House Members would be required to cast votes on three separate pieces of legislation to pass national health care. The Rule to allow the debate on health care also allowed votes on the three Senate bills: the Senate health care bill, now referred to as H.R. 3590, the Patient Protection and Affordable Care Act, the Budget Reconciliation Act, and H.R. 4872 The Health Care & Education Reconciliation Act, which stripped the outrageous Senate inducements from the legislation. All three of these pieces of legislation needed to pass the House without any changes.

The Senate had adjourned for the weekend, which signaled that the Senate would not be accepting any amendments to these three pieces of legislation. The fate of health care rested with the Members of the US House of Representatives. The Speaker had made it crystal clear that there would be no amendments to this carefully choreographed trio of bills.

Why then was Congressman Ike Skelton offering an amendment to the Reconciliation Package? Ike was arguing that there had been an oversight in the Reconciliation legislation and he wanted to make it clear that veterans and members of the Armed Services would not be included in the health care legislation. It had already been stated repeatedly that members of the Armed Services would continue to receive health care benefits through the Department of Defense and veterans through the Veterans Administration. Apparently, there was still confusion as to whether this held true under the Reconciliation legislation. Congressman Ike Skeleton was therefore on the floor Saturday afternoon to amend the proposed health care legislation through the Budget Reconciliation Package to calm the fears of our military personnel and veterans.

I was livid! I spoke with leadership staff, which informed me that Mr. Skelton was only correcting an oversight and that the health care legislation would not pass without his amendment. I asked about my amendment and I was curtly told that the Senate did not agree with my amendment. I would not be allowed to offer it today or ever. The Stupak-Pitts Amendment had passed the House last November with a 240-194 vote and now the wishes of most of the Members of the US House of Representatives were not being honored.

I saw Speaker Pelosi along the back rail approaching the Pennsylvania corner and I seized the opportunity to press my case for my amendment. It was around 2:00 p.m. on Saturday, March 20, 2010.

I asked the Speaker why I could not offer my amendment and she simply responded, "No amendments are allowed." I asked her, "What was Ike doing offering an amendment?" The Speaker said that she did not know what the amendment was all about and she saw it as a "technical amendment" and it really "was not an amendment." I was now irate.

I told her that I found it hard to believe that the Speaker of the House on such an important issue was either unaware or had not given Ike permission to offer his amendment. The Speaker just said that we had to do this one amendment. I countered that I had drafted and introduced a Technical Correction Bill to correct the mistake of allowing taxpayer funds to pay for elective abortions. My Technical Correction Bill would correct the Senate language on abortion and the health care legislation would reflect exactly what the House had passed with the Stupak Amendment. The Speaker said that there was no way the Senate would go along with my Technical Correction Bill. I countered, "If the majority of Senators would pass my Technical Correction Bill, would you allow a vote in the House?"

"No, you cannot have your bill or your amendment," she said. I took her "No" as a "maybe," for I had been down this road before.

The discussion turned sour when I confronted her about excluding me from the meeting in her office with the White House Counsel and Right-to-Life Democrats. She claimed that she had no knowledge of the meeting; I told her that I did not believe her and asked why I was not included. She said she had no idea what I was talking about. I told her that was bullshit and if she or the White

House thought that they could separate the RTL Democrats and roll them on some nice-sounding executive order, it wasn't going to happen. If she wanted health care, she had to deal with the abortion issue and not ignore it.

Out of the corner of my eye, I could see Members clearing the area as our discussion was becoming more and more intense. I also saw the press corps watching from its perch above the Speaker's rostrum; other reporters had their noses pressed against the glass doors separating the House floor from the Speaker's lobby. It was not going to be a pretty picture if the reporters wrote about the confrontation between the Speaker and me on the House floor with the debate on health care expected to begin soon.

I suggested to the Speaker that we step into the red copy room just off the Pennsylvania corner to finish our discussion; she understood why I was suggesting that we leave the floor and move out of the glare of the press. As we walked into the copy room, she reiterated that she knew nothing of the meeting in her office with White House Counsel and the RTL Democrats. I told her that I found that hard to believe but I still wanted my amendment and reminded her that the remaining RTL Democrats were not going to agree to an executive order without me. The Speaker said that without an agreement with the Senate, I would not be allowed to offer the Stupak Amendment or the Technical Correction Bill. I pushed the Speaker on the Technical Correction Bill and she said that she did not understand the nuances of a Technical Correction Bill and would not agree to it.

The Speaker left and I waited a few minutes to figure out my next step. It was getting too late in the legislative process to execute any changes. As I left the red copy room the hecklers from the Pennsylvania corner started in on me. "Did you and the Speaker have a good time? Did you kiss and make up?" As the chuckles rose from the corner, I responded with "screw you" and kept walking to the cloakroom.

Maybe the Technical Correction Bill strategy was still a possibility. First, I needed to go back to the House Parliamentarian to gain a clearer understanding of the complex legislative maneuver that I wished to undertake.

CHAPTER 56

--- ★★★ ---

Obama Pep Rally

M aybe my Technical Correction Bill strategy still had a chance. First, I would need to set up a meeting with the House Parliamentarian so that I could understand the complex parliamentary procedure necessary to implement my Technical Correction Bill. The Parliamentarian said that the House was in recess and to come right over.

I immediately remembered that there was a Democratic Caucus scheduled with a "special guest." The special guest was President Obama.

I told the Parliamentarian that I needed to attend the Caucus first and I would come by immediately afterward. The Parliamentarian was gracious and said that he would be in his office all day to answer any questions I may have on the parliamentary procedures on Technical Correction legislation.

The House chamber was empty, so I headed through the tunnel from the Capitol Building to the Cannon Building. I walked up the back stairwell to the back door of the Cannon Caucus Room. The back door was secured by the President's security detail, but they recognized me and allowed me to enter through the back of the room just as the President was addressing my Democratic colleagues.

As usual, President Barack Obama was extremely eloquent. He recited the one hundred-year history of former presidents requesting and Congress failing to pass national health care legislation. Now was the time to act. The President admitted that a few more details needed to be worked out, but these issues would be resolved and the House would cast its historic vote for health care tomorrow, Sunday, March 21.

The President acknowledged the tremendous pressure that Democrats were facing from opposition forces vowing to defeat the health care legislation. He argued that we could not turn our backs on the American people. If we did not pass health care now, it would be twenty-five years before any meaningful efforts would be undertaken again by Congress.

I stood in the back of the Caucus Room and listened and snapped a photo of the President speaking to the Democratic Caucus. I wanted the photo to preserve the moment, to preserve history, and to remind me of my personal struggle.

I left the Caucus as soon as the President finished speaking. I was pleased that President Obama did not mention the negotiations underway concerning the proposed executive order.

I still did not know if there would be another meeting on the proposed order or whether the Speaker had obtained the last few votes needed to pass the Rule. I left the Caucus wondering what would happen next on health care. I knew I had to talk to the Parliamentarian, Chris Smith, and Joe Pitts. I had just about run the course on protecting the sanctity of life in the health care legislation.

CHAPTER 57

★ ★ ★

Damn the Sixty-Vote Rule

I did not need Speaker Pelosi's permission or the approval of the Rules Committee to offer the Technical Correction Bill if I defeated the Rule. With the Rule defeated, I would immediately seek recognition by the Speaker Pro Tempore. The Jefferson Manual on House procedures states that upon defeat of a Rule the Speaker Pro Tempore should recognize the leader of the opposition to the Rule. The leader of the opposition to the Rule would be me. It was a long shot but I had to try.

If I could hold my six Democratic RTL votes and if the Speaker did not carry votes in her pocket (though I figured she had to have at least a couple), then I could defeat the Rule providing consideration of the Senate health care bill, HR-3590. Immediately upon defeating the Rule, I had to be the first Member of the House recognized by the Speaker Pro Tempore. If I defeated the Rule, the Speaker Pro Tempore would look first to Democratic leadership and not to the person who engineered the defeat of the Rule. I had to be recognized first and then offer my Technical Correction Bill to the Senate Health Care Bill *and* the Budget Reconciliation Package, HR-4872.

Therefore, the Rule for health care would be amended by the Technical Correction Bill and the Senate health care bill HR 3590 would then be deemed to pass the House only when and if the Senate accepted and passed the Technical Correction Bill. In other words, my Technical Correction Bill would become the poison pill to the health care legislation because the Senate had to muster sixty votes to pass it. Unfortunately, the Senate had to accept the Technical Correction Bill by sixty votes and not the simple majority of fifty-one, as I had mistakenly believed.

Upon acceptance of the Technical Correction Bill in the House Rule, both it and the Reconciliation Bill would be sent back to the Senate. Again, upon receipt of these two pieces of legislation, the Senate would first vote on the Technical Correction Bill, which must receive sixty votes. If it did, then to pass health care the Senate would have to vote on the Reconciliation Bill, which needed a simple majority of fifty-one votes to pass.

There were forty-one Republicans in the Senate. I believed that a vote in the Senate on the Technical Correction Bill would closely resemble the vote on the Stupak Amendment offered by Senator Ben Nelson (NE). Therefore, I believed that Democratic Senators Bayh (D-IN), Casey (D-PA), Conrad (D-ND), Dorgan (D-ND), Kaufman (D-MA), Nelson (NE), and Pryor (D-AR) would vote for the Technical Correction Bill for a total of forty-eight votes, well short of the sixty votes needed.

I spent some time going over the parliamentary procedures on defeating the Rule and inserting my Technical Correction Bill with the House Parliamentarian. No matter how I attacked and probed ways of getting around a sixty-vote requirement in the Senate, I could not.

Unfortunately, I had faxed the President's Chief of Staff, Rahm Emanuel, my Technical Correction Bill, along with correspondence to Speaker Pelosi asking that it be included in the Rule. In hindsight, faxing Rahm the Technical Correction Bill may not have been the smartest thing to do, but the Speaker received daily reports of legislation drafted by House Legislative Counsel, which affected the health care legislation being considered. Instead of hiding my efforts, I believed it was better to put all the cards on the table as we played heath care poker.

Late Saturday afternoon, I contacted Chris Smith and ran my strategy of defeating the Rule and then inserting the Technical

Correction Bill into the Rule and passing the health care legislation back to the Senate. Chris liked the idea, but he believed that if the Rule was to be defeated, he should be immediately recognized so he could insist on sending the legislation back to the Energy and Commerce Committee and substitute the Republican health care bill containing the Stupak Amendment. No matter how hard Chris tried to convince me that his strategy was the correct way to proceed, I knew the Democratic Speaker Pro Tempore would never recognize a Republican Member of Congress to insert the Republican provisions into the Rule on health care. Upon defeat of the Rule, I had a better chance of being recognized by the Speaker Pro Tempore than Republican Chris Smith. While Chris was excited about the possibilities and the mischief we could make on the floor with the Rule, I knew that neither he nor I would be recognized if we defeated it.

As I witnessed throughout my career, if it appeared that a Rule or a piece of legislation offered by the Majority was headed for defeat, a Member of the Majority immediately moved to adjourn before the vote was finalized. If the House adjourned, then the vote on passage was never recorded and the Rule or the legislation was not defeated but could be brought up at a later time. A Member may move at any time during debate to adjourn the House. Asking for an adjournment is a time-honored practice used by both parties to slow down floor proceedings or to save a Rule or legislation from defeat.

After my discussion with Chris, I realized that I really had no practical legislative options left. Reluctantly, I was down to an executive order and I had not heard back from Congressman Doyle or the White House Legal Counsel. Maybe the President had rejected the changes we had offered? Maybe my demand for a colloquy with Chairman Waxman was asking too much? Maybe we were back to blocking the Rule? Did we even have enough votes to block the Rule? Maybe I would hear from Doyle or Bob Bauer requesting another meeting. I just did not know what was going to happen next. I knew that we had few options left.

CHAPTER 58

★ ★ ★

Round Two on the Executive Order

The secret negotiations between the "Stupak Twelve" on the executive order were no longer a secret in the media, the RTL Groups, or the bishops. Still, the media could not figure out when or where our little negotiating group was meeting. Early in my career when I spoke at the White House without the press present, they still managed to get the story. Not this time. Doyle's fifth-floor hideaway in the Cannon Building was the perfect refuge for our secret negotiations away from the constant badgering and probing by a demanding press corps.

By 1:00 p.m. on Saturday, March 20, my office was flooded with emails and faxes from National RTL, US Conference of Catholic Bishops, Susan B. Anthony Organization, Family Research Council, and every conservative RTL group claiming that an executive order would not supersede statutory language. My response to these groups was basically, "no shit, but explain to me how we get to sixty votes in the Senate?" The Senate could only garner forty-five of the needed sixty votes to pass the Stupak Amendment, and Senate Republicans had abandoned me on the Technical Correction Bill. In my exchange with Speaker Pelosi, I raised the Technical Correction Bill but I had not formally met with House Leadership regarding the proposed legislation. I had to ask for my Technical Correction Bill.

Each Member of the Stupak Twelve realized that we were now much less than a dozen votes against the Rule. Our diminishing number only served to commit and bind us to each other and vote as a block rather than as individuals. I had no idea how many votes for the Rule the Speaker carried in her pocket after Kildee and Oberstar caved, and I was no longer confident we could even defeat the Rule. As individuals, we were easy marks for the President or the Speaker to persuade us to vote for the Rule and the health care legislation. As a block, we could deflect the political pressure by leaning and hiding behind each other or behind me.

Early Saturday afternoon, I received a call from Kristen Day, Director of the Democrats for Life, who was outside my office but could not gain access due to the rowdy, fervent Christian crowd praying and blocking access. The crowd was deep in prayer, demanding that I kill the health care legislation. If I listened closely and long enough I may have heard an occasional Our Father or Hail Mary, but most of the prayers were whatever one or more of the group thought was appropriate to say out loud. Many of the impromptu prayers were imploring Jesus to kill the health care bill. Kristen was outside my office and wanted to encourage me to vote for health care.

Finally, Kristen called me on my cell phone and Scott went out and escorted her and her young daughter, Kate, through the back door to my inner office. Kristen could not believe the madness outside but once inside and away from the noise, my inner office was peaceful. Kristen laughed at how the staff and I were at ease with the crowd. My staff offered Kate some cookies, crayons and paper to draw on; she sat down at the coffee table, ate cookies, colored and was at peace. Kristen and I discussed the executive order and she encouraged the Right to Life Democrats to negotiate strong language and pass health care. I appreciated Kristen's sentiment, though the Democrats for Life were not a political force in the congressional districts and would not sway a Member of Congress to vote for or against health care legislation. Kristen was sincere in her support and it was appreciated. Her daughter Kate did not want to leave my office because it was peaceful and quiet and removed from the chaos outside. Plus, we served cookies!

The homemade cookies that Kate enjoyed were provided by a Republican staffer who had brought them to the office earlier that day. The kind staff person knew it would be a long day and believed that my staff would enjoy a thoughtful snack. The Republican offices and staffs assumed that I would vote against health care and were being very kind to me. It was no longer important to them that I protect the sanctity of life, only that I controlled the votes to defeat heath care legislation. The staff person never said that cookies were in trade for a "No" vote on the health care legislation; it was just assumed by the Republican staffer that I would do the "right" thing and kill the health care bill.

The next day, Sunday, when it was reported in the media that I had reached an agreement with the President on the executive order and would vote for the health care legislation, the same Republican staff person who delivered the cookies on the previous day actually came back to my office to demand that we return them. Unfortunately, my team appreciated the thoughtful gesture of the Republican staffer so much that by Sunday morning, a little RTL Democrat and my un-apologetic cookie-filled staff had already eaten every one.

After the President left Capitol Hill, the House reconvened the legislative session. Members of Congress made their way over to the House floor, listened to the proceedings, and waited for the expected vote on a House Resolution "Urging a Moment of Silence for Military Personnel." The Resolution recognized March 26, 2010, as "National Support Our Troops Day." The debate was expected to be cordial and the Resolution in support of our troops would pass unanimously. Unfortunately, the debate on the Resolution quickly turned ugly and epitomized the tension between the parties; the raw emotions over health care spilled into the debate on supporting the troops.

Throughout the day, the Tea Party held demonstrations and leveled threats of political reprisal against any Democratic Member who dared to vote for the health care legislation. The Tea Party only further poisoned the atmosphere around Capitol Hill with their antics. Some Republican Members of Congress stepped out onto the House balcony located just off the Speaker's lobby and actually encouraged the unruly behavior of the Tea Party activists. This only further infuriated the Democrats.

The debate on the Resolution honoring our military personnel should have been met with praise and passed without a dissenting voice. Instead, it was more about health care than the sacrifices of our veterans. The arguments were not addressing the Resolution but instead concerned the health care legislation; the minority was using the sacrifices of veterans as a reason not to pass health care. While I could not listen to all the debate, it was not one of the US House of Representatives better moments.

Congressman Mike Doyle called early in the evening and asked if we would meet again in his Cannon hideaway at 9:00 p.m. to go over the changes the White House had made in the executive order. I agreed and told Mike that I would invite the same Members who attended the previous night's meeting. I added that I would meet him there, as I was in discussions with Democratic Congressman Dan Lipinski and Republican Congressman Joe Cao. I hoped to convince both of these strong RTL Members to vote for the health care legislation if I could obtain an executive order enforcing the Hyde language. Mike simply wished me luck with these two Members of Congress who were listed as "No" votes on everyone's tally sheet.

The meeting on the revised executive order took place at 9:00 p.m. Congressmen Donnelly, Driehaus, Mollohan and Ellsworth came along with Congresswomen Kaptur and Dahlkemper. Bob Bauer presented the changes and pointed out a few other areas that he and his legal team thought were appropriate to add or delete language.

We again discussed the colloquy and it was understood that Chairman Waxman and I would both take part. Bob Bauer, Dan Turton and I briefly discussed the colloquy and the rationale behind it; neither Bauer nor Turton would suggest any language other than to encourage me to work it out with Chairman Waxman. It was my understanding that Chairman Waxman was made aware of the colloquy and had no objection to it.

After reviewing the negotiated changes made by the White House Counsel, RTL Democrats were generally pleased with the executive order. I made a few minor suggestions concerning the community health centers and clarification of the conscience clause.

When we finished our discussions, Dan Turton again asked, "If the suggested changes are made to the executive order, will each of you vote for the Rule and the health care legislation?" I quickly said that I would like to see the final order prior to confirming, but "Yes, I would vote for the Rule, though I have some doubts on the legislation, which I am still reviewing."

I asked Bob Bauer, "Has the executive order been run by the congressional Pro-Choice women's groups?" Bob Bauer responded, "They [women] are aware that the possibility of an executive order has been discussed, but they have not seen it nor are they aware of the meetings taking place in this room." Bob further explained, "If you do not agree with the executive order, there is no reason to alarm the women's and Pro-Choice groups."

Bob Bauer said that he would contact the Pro-Choice Democratic women Members of Congress since we agreed that the executive order was close to being finalized. Further, he said that we should meet the following morning to go over the final wording. We all agreed, shook hands, left the storage room, and stepped into an empty hallway. Once again, we had evaded the media and barrage of staff. This executive order was truly a sincere negotiation between White House Legal Counsel and a handful of Democratic Members of Congress.

As we stepped into the hallway, the RTL Democrats asked me again about the Bishops and if they were aware of the executive order. I explained that Richard Doerflinger had made it very clear that the Bishops would not accept an executive order and they would not even review a proposed draft of one. I believed that if the Stupak Amendment was not in the final health care legislation, the Bishops would demand that we kill the bill. Further, I explained that despite my comments in the meeting, I would vote for health care legislation because I believed we needed to pass it for the benefit of all Americans. I was not going to tell Turton that I would vote for health care until we had everything we needed to protect the unborn child and a clearly defined conscience clause in the executive order.

I invited the group down to the Democratic Club, as I had plans to meet Dan Lipinski there. They declined the offer and Mike and I drove down to the Club. We found Dan sitting at a table just off the bar area. We said hello to Joseph and ordered a beer. Dan indicated that he did not want anything to drink.

Dan asked, "What was the meeting about?" I explained, "We [RTL Democrats] have come a long way and we plan to meet again tomorrow morning with White House Counsel to finalize the executive order, which includes the Hyde Amendment." I had been pushing Dan to support the health care legislation that would be reinforced by the executive order. Dan suddenly became very silent and seemed to have problems focusing his eyes. I asked him if he was okay; he responded by stating that he was having a diabetic reaction and needed to get some sugar immediately.

Dan sank to the floor; I knelt by him and got him a Coke. Dan said he would be fine; it had been a long day and he had not eaten very much. The sugary drink seemed to stabilize him and he said that he was doing better. I offered him a ride back to his apartment, which he said he would welcome but he just wanted to sit there on the floor for a bit and finish his Coke.

I could not help but wonder what would happen if Dan was not a Member of Congress and not tuned in to his body. Would he have the financial means to treat his diabetes and pay for his insulin? Even if he had the means to pay for his medication, what were the costs? How many Americans suffered from diabetes and could not afford medical treatment? Unlike most of the American public, Dan had immediate access to health care through the House physician at the Capitol at little or no cost to him.

Dan does not drink alcohol and usually went to the House gym in the morning to exercise. He is tall and thin and did not carry excess weight, which could exacerbate his diabetes. Still, here he was, having a diabetic episode while discussing national health care with other Members of Congress. However, he still could not see the ethical, moral, or social value in providing health care for all Americans so that they, too, could overcome their illnesses and suffering. I wanted to scream at Dan, "What don't you understand? There are Americans who suffer from diabetes like you and they are not Members of Congress or employees of large corporations. They cannot access the best health care in the world. We cannot save everyone, but 45,000 Americans die every year; one American dies every twelve seconds because he or she do not have access to basic health care."

When and where did we leave our moral compass? Even the US Conference of Catholic Bishops website listed health care for all Americans as the number one priority, yet they want me to kill health care because the Senate would not accept the Stupak Amendment. If the Bishops did not get the language they wanted, then no one would have health care. The Bishops would not even review or suggest language that would help protect the sanctity of life in the proposed executive order. I thought the Bishops might oppose or criticize the language as inadequate, but to not even consider the executive order was wrong.

It had become clear to me that the Bishops would rather stick their heads in the sand and pretend health care legislation never existed. Even the unborn child needs health care to be delivered into this world. Because the Bishops were unable to pass the Hyde Amendment in the Senate, they turned a blind eye to the unborn child and turned their backs on the American people.

After Dan had his Coke and regained his strength, Mike and I drove him home safe and secure with his "No" vote for health care for all Americans. I nonetheless invited him to the Sunday morning meeting on the executive order with the White House Counsel. I had not given up on Dan or Joe Cao.

So ended Saturday, March 20, 2010. My day had run the gamut from the innocence of a child drawing pictures and eating cookies in my office while her mother encouraged RTL Democrats to provide health care for all Americans to Congressman Dan Lipinski's ability to access the best health care in the world while denying other Americans access because of political fear and intimidation.

It was late before Mike and I returned to our apartment on A Street. We were both physically and mentally spent and longing for a deep and restful sleep. Only one of us would achieve his goal, and it would not be me.

Back home in Menominee, Laurie was forced to remove the phone from its cradle so it would not be ringing all night. For the past week, the phone had been disconnected to avoid the late-night, bar-closing obscene phone calls. The caller would berate me for my Right-to-Life views or claim I was not doing enough to protect life and to kill the health care bill. Laurie had learned from her experience last November when the Stupak Amendment was pending in the House: whether people were for or against the amendment, they would call at all hours of the day or night to vent their frustrations.

One of the more humorous calls received one Saturday after-noon was from California. Laurie realized that the call was not our son calling from the West coast so she let the answering machine pick it up. The caller left this succinct message, "Tell your husband not to listen to that schmuck from Sherman Oaks!" The schmuck from Sherman Oaks the caller was referring to was Chairman Henry Waxman.

Another message came from a caller in Florida, who implored me to vote against and defeat the heath care legislation. The caller insisted that if I killed health care they would make me a hero like they did for Marco Rubio. Laurie asked me, "Who is Marco Rubio?" I explained that he was the Tea Party candidate in Florida who would probably be elected to the US Senate. Laurie just told me, "Don't even think of voting with the Tea Party, you are better than that." All I could say was "Amen."

Many of the phone calls that got through to Laurie were obscene or threatened my life or my political demise if I did not do what the caller demanded. Laurie heard some of the worst in humanity. She received no calls in support of my efforts to protect the sanctity of life. She always reminds me that a person "gets more with honey than vinegar," but that sound advice, along with civility, has sadly disap-peared in politics today.

Even though my home phone was off the hook most of the time during the last couple of months leading up to the final vote on health care, these two calls are a small sample of the intrusions that constantly flooded my home. Laurie was not inclined to put up with phone calls at all hours of the day and night from individuals who did not even live in Michigan or the First Congressional District.

CHAPTER 59

★ ★ ★

Upon A Prayer

A fter another sleepless night, I woke up on Sunday morning and quietly drove over to St. Peter's Catholic Church on the Hill, a block down from the Cannon Office Building. It was too early for Mass and the Church doors were locked.

I just wanted to pray and think about the dawning of a new day, which would give birth to national health care. But more importantly, I wanted to ask Jesus if I was doing the right thing. Was I upholding the sanctity of life by negotiating an executive order in which President Obama promised to protect the sanctity of life? How could I be sure that the President would keep his word? Jesus, am I doing your work here on earth?

If health care for all Americans was the number one priority of the US Conference of Catholic Bishops, why then wouldn't they help me with the executive order to produce the strongest possible language protecting the most vulnerable among us? What was I missing?

There are those Americans who did not trust President Obama when it concerned abortion, as he is known to be the most Pro-Choice president in history. I had to trust the President; what other option did I have left? Speaker Pelosi had not allowed one traditional

RTL amendment and if I killed health care, she would *never* allow one.

If I did nothing, I would get rolled. If I voted against health care, then all the work that I has done throughout my twenty years in elected office would be for naught. Even if I voted against health care without an executive order or the Stupak Amendment, the Speaker might still prevail depending on the number of votes in her pocket.

It was too early for St. Peter's on the Hill to hear my thoughts and prayers, and it was too late to turn back. I had no choice but to move the country forward and pass national health care with the only legislative vehicle I had left to protect the sanctity of life: the presidential executive order. I had to trust President Obama with his promise to protect the sanctity of life and the conscience clause.

I know in my heart and in my mind that Father Patrick Wisneske would have agreed with my decision to accept an executive order, as did my parish priest Father Ron Sufka and many more members of the Catholic faithful. I am sure that my father, who had instilled a deep social conscience and passion for public service in me, would have encouraged me to negotiate the best possible executive order and pass health care legislation.

I know that Laurie and Ken wanted me to pass health care for all Americans. I had done what Laurie encouraged me to do- to get what I needed in the executive order so I could vote for health care. I could no longer sit helplessly by while 45,000 Americans died every year because they lacked access to basic health care.

I was not seeking re-election; I did not have to worry about political fallout. I did not ask the President or the Speaker for any-thing in return for my support of health care. I remained true to my belief that an individual should base his or her vote on the legislation itself and not what he or she can negotiate in return for a vote. Legislation should rise or fall on the quality of the bill and not on a quid pro quo.

I headed over to the House gym to get a workout in as it looked like it would be another long day. I was finally comfortable with my decision to support the executive order and health care for all Americans.

I arrived at the House gym before it was technically open. It was difficult to push the weights as my mind was swimming with thoughts of health care and the executive order. I was not focusing on my workout, so I gave up, shaved, showered and headed to 2268 Rayburn, my congressional office.

As I arrived at my front door a young female reporter who had been covering health care asked in a cheerful voice, "I hear you and the President are close to an agreement. When will the executive order be finalized?" With an angry scowl I replied, "If you would leave me alone, I could get it done." I slammed the office door and locked it behind me.

I went to my desk and started to read the constituent mail. I had asked my staff to pull the letters from constituents I knew personally who had recently written on health care. As always, I wanted to know what people were saying back home. After five minutes, I got up from my desk and stepped into the hallway to apologize to the reporter for acting like an ass. She was nowhere to be found. To this day, I feel bad about the way I reacted to her question. She was only doing her job and I was not professional in my response.

Soon Scott came into the office and we discussed the previous night's events with the executive order and Congressman Lipinski's diabetic episode in the Democratic Club. I told Scott to have a statement and press release prepared, as I would agree to the executive order and vote for the Patient Protection and Affordable Care Act.

Scott was pleased and peppered me with questions, from what time the next meeting with White House Counsel would be to when and where I wanted to hold a news conference, who would be invited, and whether had I spoken to the Bishops. As always, Scott was thorough in his questions and I knew he would have staff prepare a press statement and set up the news conference in the Members' Press Room in the Capitol. I told him that I only wanted to invite the half dozen Members who had negotiated the executive order to the press conference.

Scott said we would shoot for a 1:00 p.m. press conference, as I expected to hold the final meeting with Bob Bauer at around 11:00

a.m. The conference would be two hours after my meeting with Bauer and before the start of the Michigan State Men's Basketball Team versus Maryland in the NCAA basketball tournament in the "Elite Eight" flight.

I was so absorbed with the legislative maneuvering that I had completely missed the Michigan State Spartans' three-point victory over New Mexico State on Friday. The victory advanced the Spartans to the second round against Maryland.

With the support of the remaining half-dozen Stupak holdouts, history would be made with the passage of health care coverage for all Americans nearly a hundred years after President Teddy Roosevelt called on Congress to pass such a law.

After the final meeting on the executive order with White House Counsel Bob Bauer, I could relax and watch the Spartan game. I needed the distraction from the health care debate and the upcoming vote.

As word drifted out that an impending agreement with President Obama by the remaining Stupak holdouts would ensure passage of the health care legislation, my office phones, fax, and email were sent into a frenzy. Fortunately, the Rayburn Building was closed to the public and there was limited access to the building.

Sgt. Dwight Sturdivant of the Capitol Police came to my office to check on my safety and make sure I had free passage throughout the Capitol Complex. Dwight was adamant that I not walk outside, as the demonstrations had become ugly. I advised Dwight that I would be heading over to the Cannon Building through the tunnels and then back to my office. Further, I would be holding a press conference over in the Capitol later in the afternoon. Dwight said that he would walk me over to my Cannon Building meeting, wait for me to finish, and then escort me back to the Rayburn Building. He advised me that throughout the day and evening Capitol officers would always be close as I went about my business and traveled through the Capitol Complex.

The only condition placed on me was not to go outside. My appearance outside would further incite the already angry Tea Party demonstrators and there were not enough police officers to hold back a rushing crowd. I had become radioactive and there was concern for my safety. By now the outside demonstrators understood that I had reached a deal with the President. Even though the demonstrators had no idea what the agreement with the President consisted of, it angered them to know that the health care legislation would be voted on and passed later in the day. As word circulated of the agreement, law enforcement became more concerned for my personal safety.

I received a call from Bill Livingood, Director of the Sergeant at Arms and Capitol Security. Bill and I had become fast friends as he was former Secret Service Agent and I was a former Michigan State Police trooper. We understood each other's concerns and the challenges facing law enforcement with crowd control and the personal safety of Members of Congress. Director Livingood advised me not to go outside and stated that I would remain under the watchful eye of the Capitol Police. I thanked Bill for his concern and promised that I would not take any risks that might jeopardize my safety or that of my staff.

I understood what Bill and Dwight were telling me. They would give me the space I needed to do my job, attend meetings, and hold my press conference, but I needed to conduct business within the confines of the Capitol so they could control the space around me. I did not want to cause them further concerns for my safety or their own.

CHAPTER 60

★ ★ ★

Final Negotiations

A s agreed upon, we met in Mike's hideaway one last time and gave the executive order a final review. The meeting began around 11:00 a.m. and I invited Congressmen Dan Lipinski and Joe Cao to join my small group. Dan and Joe leaned against the door during the meeting and acted as though they wanted to escape. The regular Stupak holdouts were present: Congressmen Joe Donnelly, Steve Driehaus, Alan Mollohan and Nick Rahall, along with Congresswoman Kathy Dahlkemper. Members took their usual positions; Driehaus sat to my left, Donnelly and Mollohan to my right. Nick and Kathy were sitting on the file boxes. Marcy Kaptur also joined us and stood behind Donnelly and me. With Dan and Joe present the musty hideaway was very crowded.

By now we were comfortable with White House Counsel Bob Bauer, Danielle Gray, and Dan Turton. As always, Mike Doyle sat at the cluttered desk in his battered office chair. Dan Turton sat on the file boxes in front of the desk.

Bob Bauer stated that the President was in complete agreement with the executive order; the White House legal team had finalized the changes we had requested and asked us to review it one last time.

The entire team was given a copy of the final draft of the executive order. I went right to the order and reviewed the changes against the suggestions we had made only twelve hours prior. The executive order accurately reflected our changes and we were good to go. I asked to add one word for clarification and Bauer said the change would be made.

I then looked to my team, all busy carefully reading the executive order. After all the Members finished reading, I stated that I was fine with the order and if the President would sign it, we had an agreement. I looked at each member present and they all nodded in agreement and said they were okay with the executive order.

I asked Bob Bauer whether the Democratic Pro-Choice Caucus had approved the order and Bob said, "No, we are going there next to explain it to them." I was quite surprised and asked again whether they had seen the order and Bauer said, "No." I asked what would happen if the Democratic women Members of Congress did not agree with it. Bauer said if that was the case then we would have no agreement. Bob could see the disappointment in my eyes and he said that it would not have been fair to present the executive order to the women until we, the Members present, had reached an agreement with the President. If we did not agree, then there was no reason to put the order before the Pro-Choice Caucus. Bob once again clarified that the Democratic women were aware of the negotiations but were not aware of the substance or the location of the discussions on the executive order.

Dan Turton chimed in and explained that House Leadership was aware that the negotiations would be finalized this morning and they were calling a meeting of the Democratic women Members of Congress. Dan turned and looked at Kaptur and Dahlkemper and said, "You are invited." Kathy quickly replied, "No, thank you. I would not be welcomed." Marcy Kaptur quickly added that Kathy was right and there was no need for them to attend the meeting.

Turton next asked whether we would all vote for the health care legislation if the President agreed to sign the executive order. Dan was asking the question again because Rahall, Lipinski, and Cao were present for the first time. Rahall said he would but Lipinski said that he would not vote for the health care legislation without statutory language on the Stupak Amendment. I turned to Lipinski and said it was impossible to include the Stupak Amendment because it had only received forty-five votes in the Senate and the Senate had also rejected the Technical Correction Bill. Dan just said that he was not in favor of the health care legislation and would not vote for it without the amendment. He said the only way he could justify a "Yes" vote was if the legislation specifically included the Stupak Amendment.

Joe Cao simply said that he would not vote for the legislation. I reminded him that the issue was popular in his district and if he had any chance of winning re-election he should vote for the health care legislation. Joe said that he had announced the other night on the House floor that he would not vote for the health care legislation. I asked him why he had made that statement when he knew we were trying to work things out with the President and the Catholic Bishops; Joe said that he was getting tremendous pressure from the Republicans not to vote for final passage as he had voted for the House version of health care back in November. Joe said the Republican Party was not about to let him vote again for health care and make it a bipartisan bill. Plus, Joe said that without the statutory language of the Stupak Amendment and the support of the Bishops he could not support health care. In response, I stated that the Bishops were opposed to the executive order and wanted the Stupak Amendment included or no bill at all.

Joe Cao and Dan Lipinski excused themselves from the meeting. As soon as they left the room my last statement set off a course of protests from Steve Driehaus, Donnelly and Alan Mollohan. They again asked, "Are the Bishops really against the executive order?" I assured them, "The Bishops will not even look at it."

Alan Mollohan insisted that I call Richard Doerflinger right then and there as he did not believe that the Bishops would not even review the executive order and provide us with their input. Alan insisted that we had all been through so much as a group and had withstood so much by sticking together; he could not believe the Bishops would abandon us now.

I said, "All right, I will call Richard right now and you can hear it for yourselves. The Bishops will not accept the executive order and they want us to oppose the health care legislation."

As I stood up to go over to the phone that was in Mike's hide-away, Bob Bauer said that he would leave the call to us and that he had to meet with the women's group. He then said, "Wish me luck."

We all shook hands with Bob and his team and wished them luck as they left for their meeting with the Democratic women Members of Congress. He told us that the President would be briefed later in the afternoon and that they would recommend that he sign the executive order. Dan Turton said that the tentative plan was to pass health care today and then two or three days later sign the order.

I asked Dan if the President would invite our group, whichhad negotiated the executive order, to the White House for a signing ceremony. Dan said that my request was reasonable and he would make the recommendation.

The President's legal team left to meet with the Democratic women Members of Congress, minus RTL Members Kathy Dahlkemper and Marcy Kaptur.

As soon as Dan Turton, Bob Bauer and the White House legal team left the secret storage room, the Stupak team jumped me and asked why I had invited Lipinski and Cao to the meeting. No matter how hard I tried to convince my colleagues that it was worth inviting them to try to convince them to vote for the health care legislation, they were not buying it. Dan and Joe had not built the relationships that I had built with the Members of Congress present and it was hard for them to accept Members into our little group who had not been present for the earlier negotiation meetings on the executive order.

I apologized to the Members and said that I was trying to make the vote on health care bipartisan and pointed out that Cao had voted with us back in November. I did not know that on the previous night he had announced on the House floor that he would not vote for health care.

As always, I attempted to win more votes for health care and to take the pressure off the "Stupak Dozen."

CHAPTER 61

★ ★ ★

Seeds of Betrayal, Bitter Fruit

My colleagues quickly turned their attention to the US Conference of Catholic Bishops. Congressman Mollohan and Driehaus were insisting that I call Richard Doerflinger at home and ask him to review the final copy of the executive order that Bauer had left with us. I explained, "It will not do any good but if you want me to call Richard, I will."

I picked up the phone and dialed the number. I joked that he was probably at Mass but that I would leave a message. Richard answered his home phone. I explained that I was concluding discussions with the White House Counsel on the executive order. Further, that I was with Congressmen Mollohan, Rahall, Driehaus, Donnelly, and Congresswomen Dahlkemper and Kaptur. I said that we would like him to review the order before it was finalized and asked whether I could fax or email it to him. Richard simply said, "No." I asked him why he would not review it. Richard said, "The Bishops will not support the executive order and will not support the health care legislation without the Stupak Amendment." I repeated back Richard's answers for everyone in the room to hear.

I countered by stating that the Senate would never accept the Stupak Amendment and that we were twenty votes short of passing it in the Senate. Furthermore, the best that we could negotiate to

394

protect the sanctity of life in health care legislation was the executive order. I asked, "Even though the Bishops will not accept the order, would you please review it and help us improve upon it? We want to make sure that it prevents elective abortion in health care."

Richard just stated that he would not even look at the executive order. I pleaded with him that we needed his input; he simply said that he could not help us.

I told Richard that I would conduct a colloquy with Chairman Waxman during the debate on the health care legislation to establish the intent and purpose of the executive order. Richard finally responded positively and said that the colloquy would be critical to any legal challenges as to the President's authority to issue the executive order. I agreed and I thought for a moment that Richard wanted to help us but could not because his employer, the US Conference of Catholic Bishops, opposed our position on the executive order. In my notes of the meeting with Bauer I wrote down Richard's comments on the planned colloquy. I again asked him to review the executive order to make sure that we did not miss anything. He again said that he could not.

Next, I tried to persuade Richard to help us by pointing out that health care legislation was listed on the Bishops' website as their number-one issue. We were close to passing their number one social justice issue- health care for all Americans. Wouldn't they help us achieve their stated top priority? Richard said, "I am sorry but I cannot help you nor will I review the executive order." We were on our own.

I thanked Richard for answering the call and told him that we were disappointed with the position of the Bishops. I assured him that my small group of RTL Democrats would accept the President's executive order and that we would pass health care later tonight. Richard said he understood but his hands were tied.

As I hung up the phone, it occurred to me that the US Conference of Catholic Bishops were acting just like our Bishop of Marquette had forty years earlier, when Parochial Aid was defeated in Michigan. Back then, the Bishop had not gotten his way and subsequently declared that all Catholic high schools in the diocese would close at the end of the school year. History does have a tendency of repeating itself.

In hindsight, I feel that Richard fundamentally agreed with me, the executive order, and with the passage of health care, but his hands were truly tied by the US Conference of Catholic Bishops. I have not spoken to Richard since that phone call. I hope to someday sit down and talk with him, as I am sure he was also experiencing his own health care hell.

After the call, my colleagues expressed their bitter disappointment with the Bishops and Richard Doerflinger. Some claimed that the Bishops were nothing but a front for the Republicans, just like National Right-to-Life. The Members present felt that for all the years we carried water on RTL issues, when the chips were down, they abandoned us.

It is worth noting that no RTL legislation had ever passed during my eighteen years in Congress without the critical support of RTL Democrats. The Members of Congress gathered in Mike Doyle's hideaway never wavered in their support of Right-to-Life legislation. These brave Members of Congress defied the President and the Democratic leadership and stood on their principles despite threats to their political careers. They stood up for social justice and equal-opportunity access to health care coverage. They stood up to protect the sanctity of life when the legislative hurdles became too great for others. They persisted in their efforts to find a way for their principles to coexist in providing health care for all Americans *and* protecting the sanctity of life. When other Members of Congress gave up, they insisted on finding a way forward. They made history, knowing that their political careers within the Democratic Party and in the United States Congress were in jeopardy. Still, without hesitation they stood up for what they believed in. They have my utmost respect. The true heroes of health care for all Americans were Joe Donnelly, Steve Driehaus, Brad Ellsworth, Alan Mollohan, Nick Rahall, Kathy Dahlkemper, Jerry Costello, Marcy Kaptur, and, especially, my friend Mike Doyle.

CHAPTER 62

——— ★ ★ ★ ———

Do You Trust the President?

I instructed my staff to set the Stupak Press Conference for 1:00 p.m. on Sunday, March 21, 2010, in the House Press Conference Room on the third floor of the Capitol. The purpose was to announce the agreement with President Obama on the executive order and that the remaining seven Members of the Stupak Dozen had pledged our support in favor of the Rule and the Patient Protection and Affordable Care Act. It was my understanding that Speaker Pelosi was three or four votes short of the needed 218 votes to pass the Affordable Care Act. The seven RTL Democrats who pledged to support the health care legislation were invited to appear with me to announce the agreement with the President.

At around 12:30 p.m. Scott advised me that the President had not yet signed the executive order and that our press conference may be premature. Scott cautioned me about getting out ahead of the President; plus, we did not yet know whether the women's groups had agreed to the executive order.

I argued with Scott that if my colleagues and I were ready to make the announcement of the agreement on the executive order, then the pressure shifted to the women Members of Congress and the President to accept the compromise if they wanted to pass health care. There was no more room for further compromise: either the women Members of Congress and the President accepted the executive order as written, or the agreement would be off. The seven Stupak votes would not be cast for a Rule to bring forth the Affordable Care Act for a final vote. The ball was in their court and we would follow through with our No votes on the Rule if they betrayed us on this compromise. I had unfortunately witnessed this scenario the previous fall, when Speaker Pelosi reneged on our agreement, which could have ended all this drama.

Scott said he understood but he recommended against the press conference until we heard that the President had accepted the final draft of the executive order. Reluctantly, I agreed and postponed the press conference until later in the afternoon. When the press release went out announcing the time change, it immediately sent the media into a frenzy of speculation that the agreement with the President had fallen apart.

My press secretary started to field calls from the media inquiring what had happened to the agreement. Michelle Begnoche and Nick Choate simply stated that we were waiting for the President to sign off.

Chris Smith called and wanted to know if he could discuss the executive order with me. I advised him that we had an agreement and I would not reverse my decision. The RTL Democratic Members who had negotiated the executive order with me were firm in their position as well. We had done the best we could to protect the sanctity of life and we all supported the Affordable Care Act. Chris asked if we had seen the position papers of National Right-to-Life and the US Conference of Catholic Bishops written by attorneys on the illegality of the executive order. I replied that I had seen them and did not agree with their conclusions. Chris argued that these folks were the real experts on the legality of executive orders and that I should follow their legal advice.

I responded that if I followed their legal argument, the executive order on stem cell research signed by President George W. Bush was also illegal. These same groups had heaped praise on President Bush's stem cell executive order; now they were claiming that President Obama's executive order was not worth the paper it was written on from a legal perspective. I explained to Chris that he could not have it both ways. These groups were claiming the President's executive order was illegal, yet had never even seen the final document.

To further thwart some of the opponents' legal arguments, I had negotiated a colloquy on the executive order to be conducted during the debate on health care. Therefore, the opponents could not claim that President Obama had exceeded his authority by issuing an executive order that is "incompatible with the express or implied will of Congress."

Finally, the legal arguments presented by Chris and the RTL groups fell short because every president of the United States had issued hundreds of executive orders and only two or three had ever been declared unconstitutional by the Courts.

I agreed with Chris that the best way to protect the sanctity of life was through the Stupak Amendment, but added that there was no way the Senate would accept the Stupak language. I asked Chris, "How do we get to sixty votes or even to a simple majority of fifty-one votes on the Stupak Amendment in the Senate?" Chris admitted that we could not get to fifty-one, let alone sixty, votes in the Senate. I told Chris that the executive order was the only means we had left to protect the sanctity of life. He asked if I trusted the President to enforce the executive order and I said, "Yes."

Chris pleaded with me not to vote for the health care legislation. I told Chris that the Stupak holdouts and I would vote for health care and that I believed the legislation would pass. Chris and I ended the call on civil terms.

At about this time I received a message from Laurie. I called her and she told me that the Archbishop of Detroit had called our home phone and wanted to speak with me about health care. When Laurie explained that I was in Washington, the Archbishop asked Laurie to relay the message that he wished to speak with me and that I should not vote for health care.

I did not return the call. It was the first and probably the last time I will ever receive a call from an Archbishop. It was now after 1:00 p.m. and we still had no word from the President. I was starting to get that sinking feeling, wondering if President Obama was going to agree to the executive order. I turned on the Michigan State Basketball game to distract me from my troubled thoughts.

Scott stepped into my office and said President Obama would be calling me around 4:00 p.m. I told Scott to set the press conference for 4:30 p.m. He said he would get it done and ducked back into his office. I turned my attention back to March Madness and my Michigan State Spartans.

CHAPTER 63

★ ★ ★

President Obama's Call

At approximately 4:00 p.m. the President called and thanked me for my leadership on health care and for working to reach an agreement with him. The President said, "You win, I will sign the executive order." I wanted to shout with joy, we won! But I knew it was time to be humble and gracious, for everyone had given something up to get to this point. Plus, I never felt that my position was against President Obama. No, I did not feel like bragging nor did I feel like I had forced the President to do what he said he would do all along when he said, "I'm Pro-Choice, but I think we also have the tradition in this town, historically, of not financing abortions as part of government-funded health care. My main focus is making sure that people have options of high quality care at the lowest possible price."

I responded, "It is the American people who won and now thirty-two million more Americans will now have access to quality, affordable health care."

The President went on to say he considered the executive order an "iron-clad commitment" that there would be no public funding of abortions in health care. He was instructing his administration to honor the executive order. I thanked the President for his commitment and then mentioned that the conscience clause was also in the order.

The President commented on the history of the conscience clause and was surprised to learn that the original author was Senator Frank Church, a Democrat from Idaho. I simply said that I knew about Senator Church's involvement because I had been working these issues over the past twenty years and that I appreciated his willingness to include the conscience clause. I also expressed my appreciation to the President for his willingness to work with us RTL Democrats so that health care legislation could be passed.

I asked the President if he would schedule a signing ceremony on the executive order with the RTL Democrats. He promised to do so and that his staff would set it up. The President then explained that he would sign the health care legislation immediately, probably the next day, and then would sign the executive order a day or two later. The President indicated that the health care legislation had to become law first with his signature before the executive order could be implemented.

I agreed and assured the President that I understood the timing. I also discussed the upcoming colloquy on the executive order with Chairman Waxman, which would take place during the debate on health care. President Obama indicated that he knew about the colloquy and thought it was a good idea.

I thanked the President for the call and stated that I was now going to meet with the press. I said that I would mention his call, that we have an agreement on the executive order, and that we, RTL Democrats, would vote for the health care legislation. The President thanked me for my leadership and wished me luck with the media.

As I spoke on the phone with the President, I stood with my knee bent, the bottom of my right foot resting on the windowsill. I wanted to hold onto the moment forever. The sun was setting, the Capitol Dome was ablaze in lights, and it felt surreal. I was so proud of the Right-to-Life Democratic Members who stood with me, who had kept their word. We would now pass health care. My last promise to the voters when I first ran for Congress almost twenty years earlier- providing health care for all Americans- would become a reality. The setting sun reminded me of my fading congressional career, yet the blazing Capitol Dome told me that there was an even brighter future beyond my office window. I was proud to have played a part in providing health care for all Americans. Now, it was time to go home.

CHAPTER 64

★ ★ ★

Final Press Conference

Immediately after my call with the President, my staff and I called the RTL Democratic Members who helped to negotiate the executive order and invited them to join me at the press conference announcing our agreement with the President. We agreed to convene at 4:30 p.m. on March 21 in the House Press Conference Room. Word of the compromise agreement concerning the executive order had been reported in the media, with a couple of the Democratic women already condemning the agreement in the press. The press corps was calling my office requesting confirmation of the agreement. My staff simply invited the callers to the 4:30 p.m. press conference.

The convening of our press conference proved even more challenging than anticipated, as the women's groups had already put out their press releases condemning the executive order as a meaningless, worthless piece of paper. Their sentiments were echoed by both National Right-to-Life and the US Conference of Catholic Bishops. The delay of our press conference until after my call from the President resulted in complications due to the senseless actions of NARAL (the National Abortion Rights Action League) and the rest of the Pro-Choice groups, which made it more difficult to explain our compromise. Instead of graciously accepting a compromise in an effort to pass health care, the women's groups chose to poison the well.

For the remaining seven RTL Democrats, NARAL and the other Pro-Choice groups were no better- probably worse than- the Right-to-Life groups in condemning us. NARAL and the Pro-Choice groups just could not accept the fact that the executive order was proper and the only vehicle that allowed us to reach consensus on a divisive issue. Instead of embracing the executive order as a compromise to move the health care legislation forward, they condemned the messenger and the message. I personally caught the brunt of their ire.

As I called Members to come to the press conference, more than one RTL Democratic Member expressed an interest in calling off the agreement with the President. I certainly understood their sentiments but then we would be no better than the women's groups that were spreading falsehoods concerning the legality of the executive order. The order had been negotiated by their Pro-Choice president through his White House Counsel and the President had personally called and committed his support of the agreement. Like the RTL groups they condemned, the Pro-Choice groups were even worse and did not respect anyone's view but their own. It is groups like NARAL and Right-to-Life with their small-mindedness that foster the hate and contempt of any person or group that does not adhere to their position one hundred percent of the time. We knew the press conference would be rough, but we had given our word and we had found a path forward. A path that we were proud of, regardless of what single-minded organizations thought. Unlike our critics, we left our opponents with their dignity. We did not try to tear them down or discredit them as they did to us.

The press conference went without a hitch and I was joined by Nick Rahall, Alan Mollohan, Kathy Dahlkemper, Marcy Kaptur, Steve Driehaus, and Joe Donnelly. I purposely kept my comments short. I was excited and happy but very, very tired as I started the press conference.

I thanked my colleagues for their courage in standing with me and negotiating the executive order with the President of the United

States. We had kept the faith and held true to our beliefs and the beliefs of the majority of Americans that federal funds should not be used to finance abortions. Now, thirty-two million Americans would have access to health care in this Pro-Life legislation.

Next, I thanked Chairmen Waxman and Dingell, President Obama, Speaker Pelosi, and Leader Hoyer. I also thanked my congressional staff, both in Washington, DC and back home in Michigan. But most importantly, I thanked my wife, Laurie, and my dear friend and colleague, Mike Doyle, and regretted the hell that I had put them through. It was Laurie's love and support and Mike's commitment and friendship that had sustained me during the difficult times as we fought to protect the sanctity of life and provide health care for all Americans.

After the appropriate "thank yous," I explained that with the help of the courageous Members of Congress standing behind me, we had reached an agreement with the President that there would be no public funding of abortion under the Affordable Care Act. The agreement would be enforced through an executive order, which included the Hyde language, the conscience clause, and would prevent community health centers from performing or funding abortions in the Affordable Care Act. With this executive order, the Members standing with me pledged to vote for and thereby ensure passage of the Affordable Care Act.

As a group, we were pleased that our principle of maintaining current law that no public funds would be used to pay for abortion would be enforced and honored under the Affordable Care Act. The real victory was not for us Members of Congress but for the American people.

As I introduced each Member of Congress to give remarks, I reminded the reporters that throughout this long ordeal, each Member had repeatedly expressed support for the health care legislation but insisted that there should be no public funding of abortions. We had withheld our support of health care only because public funding of abortions would occur under the health care legislation voted on in the US House. Therefore, we had passed the Stupak Amendment. Also, we believed that public funding of abortions would occur under the Affordable Care Act. Thus, we negotiated the executive order with the President's legal team to guarantee that no public funding would be used to pay for abortions in health care.

In response to reporters' questions, we highlighted the positive aspects of the Affordable Care Act, including the Patient's Bill of Rights, the provision for children staying on their parents' insurance until age twenty-six, no lifetime caps on health care costs, ending discrimination for pre-existing conditions and injuries, and making it very difficult for insurance companies to rescind health insurance policies without legal due process.

After the press conference, Wolf Blitzer of *CNN News* asked for and was granted a one-on-one interview. After the reporters and my colleagues left the press conference, Wolf interviewed me in the House Press Room. The interview began with Wolf stating that he knew I was a big Michigan State Spartans fan and he was aware that I had not had an opportunity to watch the end of the MSU game.

Wolf had a monitor set up and played the last thirty seconds of the Michigan State vs. Maryland basketball game for me. With time expiring, Michigan State's guard Korie Lucious hit a three-pointer at the buzzer as MSU won 85-83 and advanced to the next round of "March Madness." I thanked Wolf for the taped replay.

When I told Laurie about seeing the last shot of the MSU game on Wolf's monitor, she said that she had been running between two televisions that she had on at home. The small television in the kitchen was tuned to *CNN* with our press conference and the larger television in the living room had the Spartan game on. She was wise to have the larger television tuned to the Spartan game.

I told Wolf that like Michigan State's win, so will the American people win with the passage of the Affordable Care Act later that night. Wolf and I then went into the details on how the executive order came about and he asked what I expected with the votes tonight on final passage of the health care legislation. He asked all good questions and I responded that I expected a close vote on the passage of HR-3590, the Affordable Care Act.

After leaving the pressroom, I went back to the office to see if there had been any progress with Chairman Waxman's staff on the colloquy. My staff informed me that Chairman Waxman was insisting that I limit the colloquy, as my original submission was way too long. After a few drafts back and forth between our staffs, Chairman Waxman and I finally signed off on it. Chairman Waxman was on the House Floor managing HR-3590. I tucked the latest copy into my brown accordion health care folder and went to the House floor to engage Waxman in a colloquy.

By definition, a colloquy is a formal discussion or a written dialogue. Judges often use a colloquy during formal court proceedings to make sure the defendant understands what is occurring and understands his/her rights. In the United States Congress, colloquies are common when a Member of Congress wishes to clarify or highlight a point of interest to the Member's congressional district. I have engaged in colloquies with the Chairmen of Appropriations to advocate for financial support of a project or clarify the intent of a legislative provision urging a federal agency to take an action beneficial to my congressional district.

It is unusual to use a colloquy to express the intent of the whole Congress on a major piece of legislation. Here, in the Affordable Care Act, it was very important to state the legislative intent and understanding of the Congress that under the executive order, the traditional Hyde Amendment and the conscience clause would be enforced and prevent public funding for abortion. The colloquy stated the intent of Congress and how the Administration would administer the law. The colloquy served as a legal defense to prevent a legal challenge to the validity of the executive order.

In the over 200-year history of executive orders, more than 13,000 have been issued by presidents since 1789. The US Supreme Court has only struck down two executive orders. On these two occasions, the Court struck down the orders because the president had overstepped his legal authority by requiring action that the Congress of the United States had neither considered nor rejected. The first executive order overturned by the Supreme Court was President Truman's 1952 order taking control of the nation's steel mills to continue production during the Korean War. In striking down the executive order, the Supreme Court ruled that President Truman was making law and not executing an existing law.

President Clinton's 1995 executive order was ruled illegal by the Supreme Court when he ordered that companies that hired permanent replacements for striking workers would not be entitled to bid for or carry out federal contracts. Clinton's executive order was contrary to a 1935 law that Congress had passed stating that employers could replace striking workers with permanent replacements.

The constitutional authority reserved for Congress cannot be usurped by the Executive Branch. In other words, executive orders are valid only if they are consistent with the laws already enacted or considered by Congress. Executive orders are used to inform the American people and Congress how a president will "faithfully execute the laws of the United States."

CHAPTER 65

★ ★ ★

Rule Vote, Colloquy and Obey's Porch

The first crucial vote on health care occurred on the Rule that would allow the House to debate and vote on the three pieces of legislation that the Democratic leadership had "tie barred" together to secure passage of health care in the Senate with only fifty-one votes. Therefore, at approximately 6:00 p.m. on March 21, 2010, the House of Representatives called the question on the Rule that allowed for consideration of H.R. 3590, Service Members Home Ownership Act of 2009, and provided for the consideration of H.R. 4872, Health Care and Education Reconciliation Act of 2010.

RTL Democrats believed that if they voted en bloc they could defeat the Rule and prevent the health care legislation from coming to the floor. On the evening of March 21, 2010, only seven RTL Democrats remained committed to voting against the Rule if their concerns on public funding for abortion were not addressed.

These seven remaining RTL Democrats who had committed to voting against the Rule were the same Democrats who had helped negotiate the executive order. With their concerns on public funding of abortions, abortions conducted in community health centers, and the conscience clause all specifically addressed in the

1

executive order, these seven Democrats now promised to vote for the Rule.

The vote on the Rule was called at approximately 6:05 p.m. on Sunday, March 21, 2010. The Rule passed on a party line vote of 228-212. Even if the seven RTL Democratic Members had voted "No" on the Rule, it still would have passed 221-219. Since the Speaker had enough votes to pass the Rule without the seven RTL Democrats, the agreement on the executive order became even more crucial in assuring final passage of the Affordable Care Act.

It was important for me to locate Chairman Waxman to make sure that the colloquy establishing congressional intent and acknowledging the executive order was clearly stated and preserved in the Congressional Record.

In between the vote on the Rule and the debate on HR-3590, I was able to discuss the colloquy with Chairman Waxman, Energy and Commerce Committee Staff Director Phil Barnett, and Karen Nelson. Together, we made a few changes to the colloquy script.

I remained on the floor as Chairman Waxman and Ranking Member Joe Barton (R-TX) were granting a minute of time to Members of the Energy and Commerce Committee for unanimous consent to address the House and to revise and extend their remarks for insertion in the Congressional Record. It was agreed that this was an appropriate time to conduct the colloquy.

When Chairman Waxman recognized me for one minute, I asked "…to engage the chairman in a colloquy, if I may:

> Mr. STUPAK. "Throughout the debate in the House, Members on both sides of the abortion issue have maintained that current law should apply. Current law with respect to abortion services includes the Hyde Amendment. The Hyde Amendment and other similar statutes to it have been the law of the land on Federal funding of abortion since 1977 and apply to all other health care programs—including SCHIP, Medicare, Medicaid, Indian Health Service, Veterans

Health Care, military health care programs, and the Federal Employees Health Benefits Program.

The intent behind both this legislation and the executive order the President will sign is to ensure that, as is provided for in the Hyde amendment, health care reform will maintain a ban on the use of Federal funds for abortion services except in the instances of rape, incest, and endangerment of the life of the mother."

Mr. WAXMAN. "If the gentleman will yield to me that is correct. I agree with the gentleman from Michigan that the intent behind both the legislation and the executive order is to maintain a ban on federal funds being used for abortion services, as is provided in the Hyde amendment."

The SPEAKER pro tempore. The time of the gentleman has expired.

Mr. WAXMAN. "I yield the gentleman thirty additional seconds."

Mr. STUPAK. "I thank the chairman. I'm seeking the chairman's commitment that our conversations on this issue, the abortion issue, will continue."

Mr. WAXMAN. "I know this is an issue of great concern to the gentleman from Michigan and many other members of the Energy and Commerce Committee. You have my commitment to work with you and other Members in the future."

[Congressional Record – House, H-1859-1860, March 21, 2010]

Immediately following the colloquy, Joe Barton recognized Ranking Member of the Judiciary Committee, Jim Sensenbrenner (R-WI) to refute the colloquy. Sensenbrenner's response to the colloquy is also found in the Congressional Record. Sensenbrenner stated that Chairman Waxman and I misstated the law and that an executive order cannot overrule statutory law, that the executive order states that it cannot be enforced in a court of law, and even that Congresswoman Wasserman Schultz (D-FL) had appeared on *Fox News* earlier in the day stating that the executive order would not change the law.

Again, the purpose of the colloquy was not to claim that the executive order would change statutory law- it could not. The executive order reflected the manner in which the President and his Administration would implement the Hyde language with its ban of using federal funds to pay for abortions in the health care legislation. It was necessary to conduct the colloquy to state unequivocally both the President's and Congress's intent on how the law would be applied. The executive order was entitled, "Ensuring Enforcement and Implementation of Abortion Restrictions in the Patient Protection and Affordable Care Act."

Opponents to President Obama's executive order claimed that it was useless because an individual would not have a legal right to enforce the order and that the language prevented an individual from bringing a claim in court. The language in question stated that the executive order did not automatically entitle a person to bring a cause of action in our courts because he/she did not agree with the order. The civil lawsuit language found in the Obama executive order was the same language found verbatim in President Bush's June 20, 2007 Executive Order #13435 on stem cells three years earlier. It is ironic that these same groups, National Right-to-Life and the US Conference of Catholic Bishops, had enthusiastically praised President George W. Bush's executive order but condemned President Obama's, which contained identical language concerning the enforceability of civil lawsuits.

The comment of Congresswoman Wasserman Schultz that the executive order could not change statutory law was correct. But what

Sensenbrenner and Wasserman Schultz would not admit was that executive orders, when based on proper authority, carried the "full force and effect of law." The "full force and effect of law" legal principle was not lost on me and that was why I had asked for the colloquy to clearly demonstrate the intent of the President and Congress as stated in the executive order's title of "Ensuring Enforcement and Implementation of Abortion Restrictions in the Patient Protection and Affordable Care Act."

After listening to Sensenbrenner, I left the House floor and cursed the Pro-Choice women for not accepting the intent and purpose of the executive order. What did they not understand? Their false criticism of the executive order in principle gave fodder to the opponents of the health care legislation. Why didn't they understand the importance and the weight of the executive order?

They must not have realized that the most famous executive order still in existence today is the Emancipation Proclamation, issued as Executive Order #95 in 1863, which freed the slaves in the states rebelling against the United States.

In 1976, Jimmy Carter issued Executive Order #11095 outlawing the use of political assassination.

President John Kennedy issued a series of executive orders in 1962 and 1963 to impose trade and travel restrictions against Cuba. It wasn't until 1992 that Congress codified the embargo against Cuba; however, Kennedy's executive orders held with "full force and effect of law" for thirty years until they were superseded by statutory law.

President Truman used an executive order to desegregate the Armed Forces and President Franklin D. Roosevelt implemented much of the New Deal through Executive Order #7034 in 1935.

By the time I walked back to my office through the tunnels, I had already received two inquiries from RTL Democrats as to the validity of the executive order to be signed by President Obama. After a brief conversation with these Members explaining the fallacy of Sensenbrenner's argument, they accepted my explanation and stated that they would still vote in favor of the health care legislation.

I expected that I had an hour or so before the series of votes on health care would be called, so I decided to get away and go to dinner. It would not be until the next day that a law school or two would weigh in, stating that the executive order to be signed by President Obama was legal, proper and binding on the Administration.

As the night and the debate on health care wore on, tempers once again began to flare on the House floor. Members were advised that votes were expected shortly after 10:00 p.m. Members of Congress began to gather in their usual areas of congregation, which of course meant that I was standing in the Pennsylvania Corner. At approximately 10:15 p.m., the first votes on the question of whether the House would concur with the Senate amendments to HR-3590 were called.

As I walked over to the Pennsylvania corner, I was immediately approached by Congressmen Chris Smith and Joe Pitts. The Congressmen implored me not to vote for health care and not to accept the President's executive order promising to apply the Hyde language with its abortion restrictions. Chris asked me if I believed President Obama and I said "YES." Chris shook his head and kept saying that President Obama was the most Pro-Choice president ever and could not be trusted on this issue.

I countered Chris and Joe's argument by responding that health care was going to pass anyway without any restrictions on abortion. I turned the argument back on them and asked, "What would *you* rather do? Allow health care to pass with no restrictions on federal funding of abortions, or accept an executive order in which the President promised to enforce Hyde language?"

Chris said the Speaker could not pass health care without my vote and the handful of RTL Democrats who had stood with me. I told Chris that he could not be sure of that fact as the Speaker always carries votes in her pocket and neither one of us could be sure of how many she had.

Finally, Chris asked me to vote No on health care and start all over with a new bill. I explained that that was not going to happen. The Democrats had passed the health care bill through the House and the Senate and now the final version would be voted on tonight. It was too late to start over.

I told Chris and Joe that I would be voting for health care with the promise of the executive order. I agreed with Chris and Joe that we would need to make sure President Obama kept his word. However, I was not going to defeat health care and I was not going to take the chance of allowing the opportunity of providing health care for all Americans to pass us by. We were so close; I could not allow this legislation to fail.

It was obvious that Chris and Joe did not trust President Obama to apply the Hyde language to the health care legislation. Chris, Joe and I had been through many legislative battles together; now, the greatest fight was before us and we had to split ways.

The Speaker pro tempore gaveled to gain Members' attention and inform them that there were only a few minutes to vote on the Motion to Concur with the Senate amendments to HR-3590.

As I voted on the Motion to Concur, I was pleased with the day's events. Finally, I was about to achieve the last promise I had made to my constituents almost eighteen years ago: the passage of national health care legislation.

The Motion to Concur in the Senate amendments passed 219-212 on a party line vote.

The next crucial legislative hurdle to overcome was the Republican Motion to Recommit. When the Republicans provided a copy of their Motion to Recommit, I asked for a copy to make sure that immigration was not one of the wedge issues they were inserting in the Motion. I had promised my Hispanic friends that the RTL Democrats would not vote for the Motion to Recommit if it contained language offensive to them.

I reviewed the Motion and did not see any language on immigration so I knew the Hispanic Caucus would vote for the health care legislation. I breathed a sigh of relief. Suddenly, Majority Leader Steny Hoyer yelled, "Hey, Stupak- I need you to speak in opposition to this Motion." I replied, "No, someone else can speak." Hoyer quickly countered that his reading of the Motion to Recommit indicated that it did two things: took away the taxes in support of the Affordable Care Act and incorporated the Stupak Amendment. "It is your Amendment that they are trying to peel off votes with and I am going to yield you time to oppose the Motion. Get ready," Hoyer yelled as he walked to the well of the House chamber.

As always, I had my brown accordion RTL file and pulled out a tablet of paper to scribble down some notes. I thought about Kathy Dahlkemper and how she always argued that the health care bill was a Pro-Life piece of legislation. I thought about how the US Conference of Catholic Bishops and National Right-to-Life had changed the Stupak Amendment from a positive Pro-Life message to a "poison pill" to kill the Affordable Care Act. The Stupak Amendment became the means to an end. The Republicans had turned the table on the Stupak Amendment in an effort to defeat health care for all Americans. These Pro-Life Groups were politicizing the life issue. I knew what I was going to say; I jotted down a few phrases and walked down to the front of the Chamber.

Steny was finishing up his remarks in opposition to the Motion to Recommit and stated, "This motion is inconsistent with reconciliation, a process that seventy-two percent of the time was pursued by the other party. They know that this motion would not have support in the Senate, so they are indirectly trying to kill this bill. However, as well, I think they well misstate the facts.

I yield to the gentleman from Michigan."

As the Speaker pro tempore gaveled for order in the House Chamber, I asked Steny to yield his podium and he pointed for me to take the podium at the Majority table. I laid my tablet with my notes down and began my argument in opposition to the Republican Motion to Recommit.

Mr. Stupak. "I thank the gentleman for yielding." Suddenly the podium started to move forward and I realized that in the heat of the debate, someone had broken the podium and it would not stand up. The base was splintered and the tabletop of the podium was falling forward along with my notes. I quickly grabbed my papers with one hand and the podium with the other. I continued with my comments.

> "The motion to recommit purports to be a Right-to-Life motion, in the spirit of the Stupak Amendment. But as the author of the Stupak Amendment, this motion is nothing more than

an opportunity to deny thirty-two million
Americans health care. This motion is really a
last-ditch effort of ninety-eight years denying
Americans health care.

The motion to recommit does not promote Life.
It is Democrats who have stood up for the principle of [No] public funding for abortions. It is
Democrats, through the President's executive
order, that ensure the sanctity of life is protected
because all life is precious and all life should be
honored."

At about this point in my remarks, one of the Republican
Members of the Congress shouted out "baby killer!" The insult sent a
murmur through the House floor and the Speaker pro tempore gaveled me to stop my comments. The Speaker pro tempore suspended
proceedings until the Chamber settled down after the inappropriate
crude remark. The Speaker pro tempore advised me that I should
resume my remarks.
I continued:

"For the unborn child, his or her mother will
finally have pre- and post-natal care under our
bill. If the child is born with mental [medical]
problems, we provide medical care without bankrupting the family.

For the Republicans to now claim that we send
the bill back to committee under the guise of
protecting Life is disingenuous. This motion is
really to politicize Life, not prioritize Life. We
stand up for the American people. We stand up
for Life. Vote "no" on this motion to recommit."

The Democratic Members of Congress erupted out of their
seats and gave me a tremendous standing ovation. I gently laid the

broken podium on its side. I went down the aisle toward the Speaker's rostrum and turned to my left and walked back to the Pennsylvania corner as Members shook my hand and pounded me on the back as I passed by.

Congressman Jim Clyburn was the Democratic Whip and his job was to make sure that Democrats had enough votes to pass the Affordable Health Care Act. Jim loves to tell audiences that after I laid the broken podium down, I walked directly toward him. He congratulated me on what he describes as one of the "greatest, dramatic speeches" that he ever witnessed. I responded by pulling him closer and whispering in his ear, "Now, don't f--- this up!"

Steny Hoyer then spoke for less than thirty seconds and the Democrats yielded back their time. All time had expired and the Speaker pro tempore called the question and ordered a roll call vote on the previous question, the Motion to Recommit. A recorded vote was taken and on a party line vote the Republican Motion to Recommit was defeated 232-199.

Of all the procedural and substantive votes cast on the Affordable Care Act, the Motion to Recommit generated the greatest number of Democratic votes. Many of my colleagues attributed my comments against the Motion to Recommit as saving the Affordable Care Act from certain defeat as the Right-to-Life Democrats followed my lead and voted No on the Motion. I am constantly reminded by my colleagues that my comments against the Motion to Recommit were some of the most compelling statements throughout the health care debate.

It was now approaching 11:30 p.m., and my good friend and mentor Congressman John Dingell of Michigan rose as the congressional debate on health care wrapped up. Like his father before him, John Dingell had advocated for over fifty years for national health care. Dingell demanded a recorded vote on the passage of the Affordable Care Act.

The time had finally arrived to vote on health care. After eighteen years in Congress I finally had an opportunity to vote on the final promise I had made to my constituents. I finally could fulfill and vote on my belief, as stated in my very first congressional campaign brochure, that health care was a right, and not just for the privileged.

I voted to keep my promise. I voted for what I believed. I voted to protect the sanctity of life. I voted for all those Americans who did not have a lobbyist or an advocacy group. I voted for those struggling to provide health insurance for their employees in their small business. I voted for the families that are forced into bankruptcy by unforeseen medical expenses. I voted for the Americans who had appeared before my Oversight and Investigations committee, who had been devastated by an illness and had their health insurance policy rescinded by their health insurance companies. I voted for the person on the street who had no voice but still believed in the goodness and righteousness of their government. I voted for my father's admonishment that the "bum on the street, would someday be my boss." Most of all, I voted for someone I will never know.

As Members of Congress inserted their voting cards into the little brown box located on the back of the seats in the House Chamber, the green lights of the "YEA" votes quickly raced to 175 affirmative votes. The Republican red lights signifying their "NAY" votes raced to catch up. Every Member of Congress, every reporter, every citizen in the gallery stared at the House of Representatives' electronic voting board covering four sections of the wall above the Speaker's rostrum and above the reporter's gallery. Americans watching C-Span were glued to their televisions as the votes were recorded and the electronic scoreboard kept tally. Many Americans were straining to see the magic number of 218 votes, which would signify passage. At the same time, many Americans were praying that they would *not* see 218 votes for passage, which would signal the defeat of the Affordable Care Act.

As the time for the vote counted down, the votes for passage continued to climb past 218, then 220 and finally, 222 votes in favor of health care for all Americans. As the vote on the Affordable Care Act was called and gaveled into history, the Act became the law of the land with a final recorded vote total of 222-211.

As the cheers and high fives were being raised from the Democratic side of the House Chamber, I stared at the numbers and did the math. The President and Speaker Pelosi needed all seven of the RTL Democrats who had stood with me a few hours earlier and promised to vote "Yes" on final passage based on the promise to apply the Stupak/Hyde Amendment to the Affordable Care Act through the executive order. My small and courageous group of seven Democrats had delivered the necessary votes for passage of the Affordable Care Act. Without our votes, the tally would have been 215-218 and the legislation would have been defeated. I was so proud of the profound courage of our little group. I looked at the electronic voting board and I believed the lights behind the names of Costello, Dahlkemper, Driehaus, Donnelly, Mollohan, Rahall and Stupak shined a little more brightly than all the other names.

The Speaker gaveled the vote closed and announced that the unfinished business of the House was a vote on a resolution recognizing the sixty-fifth anniversary of the battle of Iwo Jima. The House unanimously passed the resolution. Voting was completed for the day, Sunday, March 21, 2010.

In comments following the vote, Congressman Nathan Deal (R-GA) announced his resignation from the House of Representatives. He decided to return to Georgia to run for Governor. Nathan had entered Congress with me in 1992 as a Democrat and then switched parties. I chose to remain a Democrat despite numerous requests from the GOP to join their ranks as well.

As the last vote on this historic day was cast, I remained in the Pennsylvania corner with my closest friends. Congressman John Larson (D-CT) came over and said, "thank you, thank you, without you, health care never would have passed."

Mr. Dingell came over and said, "Thank you, Pan Stupak." I smiled and told him, "I would not have let you down." John Dingell just smiled and said, "I know it and I love you for it. You played a hell of a poker hand and you were a team player under very difficult circumstances."

My close friend and Chairman of the Appropriations Committee David Obey asked, "Would you please join me on my balcony for a celebratory toast?" I told Dave that I would be honored to join him.

The Speaker's staff also asked if I would join the leadership team at a press conference. I respectfully declined.

I wanted to call Laurie and then join David Obey. I knew that for David Obey the passage of health care was very personal.

As Chairman of the powerful Appropriations Committee, David worked throughout his forty-one years in Congress to expand access to health care through his committee. David promised his dying sister that he would pass health care for the benefit of all Americans so they would not have to go through the physical and financial pain that her family went through during her courageous battle with cancer. When David asked me to join him for a toast, I was honored. I was proud to have helped him keep his promise to his sister.

After a quick conversation with Laurie ending in "I love you." Mike Doyle and I joined David Obey for a solemn drink on his balcony. As Chairman of Appropriations, David's office was located on the second floor of the Capitol overlooking the National Mall, the Lincoln Memorial and the Washington Monument.

David, Mike and I sat quietly sipping our glass of scotch and gazed at the historic monuments aligning the National Mall. David thanked me for my courage and my moving speech on the Motion to Recommit. I thanked David and told him, "I know that your vote was for your sister." He simply nodded as a tear came to his eye. I knew right then and there that David Obey would not be seeking re-election. I wanted to tell him that I would not be seeking re-election either, but now was not the time.

Every Member of Congress knew that David Obey was passionate about providing health care coverage for all Americans but they did not know about the last time David visited his sister in a Wisconsin hospital. As David tells the story, his sister said to him, "I hope I die by Friday." David responded to her, "That's a hell of a thing to say." His sister then explained, "My health insurance ends on Friday and I do not want to leave Jack and the kids with a bunch of medical bills." David Obey's sister died on Thursday.

As I looked at the Lincoln Memorial, I quietly hummed the *Battle Hymn of the Republic*. It was the first time I could even bring myself to think of the hymn in the ten years since B.J.'s funeral. I recalled our Holy Spirit congregation, friends, relatives, and Members of Congress singing along as we ushered B.J.'s casket down the aisle, out of church and to his gravesite. As we each quietly reflected on the day's events, we knew that the road ahead toward the implementation of Obamacare would be a bumpy one, with twists and turns and many obstacles along the way. However, we accomplished what presidents and Congresses had promised the American people throughout the past century but until now could never deliver: health care for all Americans.

Mike and I could have gone to any number of celebrations that night; we were suddenly the toast of the Democrats. We walked outside into the cool darkness. It was late and we were both exhausted. Neither one of us had enjoyed a restful night of sleep in weeks.

I had kept my promises to my constituents. My last promise, to pass national health care, was complete. I had fought the bull and now it was time to go home.

ABOUT THE AUTHOR

★ ★ ★

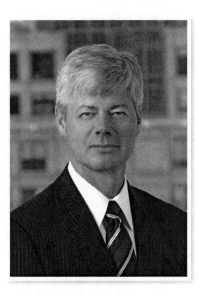

Congressman Bart Stupak served 18 years in the US House of Representatives from 1993 to 2011. During his time in Congress, Stupak engineered the passage of the Food Safety Modernization Act, Cash for Clunkers, Drug Take Back Bill and legislation governing the Protection and Preservation of the Great Lakes. Stupak's most significant legislative accomplishment was providing the critical votes necessary for passage of the Affordable Care Act.

Stupak's life-long experiences as a middle child in a large Catholic family molded his strong belief in social justice. As a law enforcement officer, Bart Stupak was injured in the line of duty and is medically retired from the Michigan State Police. As a citizen with a pre-existing injury he was denied medical coverage following knee surgery.

In his first run for Congress in 1992, Congressman Stupak pledged to fight for quality, affordable health care, *For All Americans.* While serving in the US House of Representatives, Stupak vowed not to accept Congressional Health Insurance benefits until all Americans were provided health care coverage.

Upon his retirement from Congress, Stupak was awarded a Fellowship at the John F. Kennedy School of Government, Harvard University. Stupak conducted a weekly seminar at the Kennedy School entitled "Investigate or Irritate" based on his Chairmanship of the Oversight and Investigations subcommittee.

Stupak works as an attorney in the Legislative and Government Affairs group at the Venable Law Firm in Washington, DC. He resides in Michigan and Maryland with his wife Laurie. *For All Americans* is his first book.

CPSIA information can be obtained
at www.ICGtesting.com
Printed in the USA
FFOW03n1525131017
40954FF